HYGIENE AND HEALTH EDUCATION

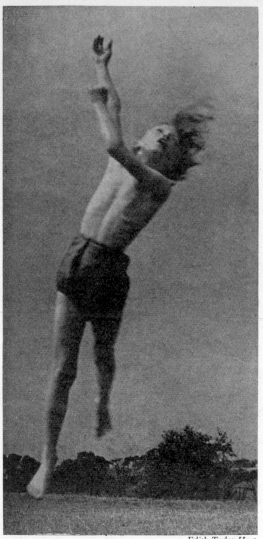

Edith Tudor Hart

A Primary School child taking part in movement training. The activity takes place out of doors on grass and with a minimum of clothing and is obviously enjoyed. The child is expressing herself in movement, and her skin gets the benefit of ultra violet rays from the sun. Note that the feet are natural in shape. There is no sign of deformity from ill-fitting shoes. The photograph suggests not just freedom from ailments but vigorous positive health.

HYGIENE AND
HEALTH EDUCATION

For Training Colleges

M. B. DAVIES, B.Sc.

*Lecturer in Health Education at S. Katharine's
Training College, Liverpool
Author of "Physical Training, Games and Athletics in Schools"*

FIFTH EDITION

With Illustrations

LONGMANS, GREEN AND CO
LONDON • NEW YORK • TORONTO

LONGMANS, GREEN AND CO LTD
6 & 7 CLIFFORD ST LONDON W 1

ALSO AT MELBOURNE AND CAPE TOWN

LONGMANS, GREEN AND CO INC
55 FIFTH AVENUE NEW YORK 3

LONGMANS, GREEN AND CO
215 VICTORIA STREET TORONTO 1

ORIENT LONGMANS LTD
BOMBAY CALCUTTA MADRAS

First Edition . . . Oct. 1932
New Impressions . Oct. 1933, Nov. 1933
Aug. 1934, Aug. 1935
Second Edition . . . Sept. 1937
New Impression . . . Oct. 1939
Third Edition . . . Oct. 1940
New Impressions . Sept. 1941, March 1942
March 1943, Aug. 1944
July 1946, July 1947
Fourth Edition . . . March 1948
New Impression . . . June 1948
Fifth Edition . . . 1951
New Impression . . . 1952
(With minor corrections)

Printed in Great Britain
SPOTTISWOODE, BALLANTYNE & CO. LTD.
London and Colchester

TO

PROFESSOR WINIFRED CULLIS
C.B.E., M.A., D.Sc., LL.D.

PREFACE TO THE FIFTH EDITION

IN this edition the opportunity has been taken to add material relating to the newer views on eye-strain, as well as on cerebral palsy, asthma clinics, anæmia and acquired heart conditions in children.

M. B. DAVIES.

October, 1950.

PREFACE TO THE FOURTH EDITION

THIS book is designed to cover the course in Health Education for Teachers in training. In this edition, the two approaches to Health Education, the social and the biological, have been kept in mind.

On the biological side, new material has been incorporated on endocrine glands, allergy, food and vitamins, the effects of sunlight, improved treatment of skin diseases, the prevention of dental decay, and the treatment of squint.

On the social side, the wide implications of the 1944 Education Act on the health of the community has been considered and a fresh section on the work of the Public Health Department of Local Authorities has been added. In addition new material has been introduced on the stages of the child's development in the practice of health, the classification of deaf children for education, the differentiation of dull, backward and retarded children and on play therapy and child and vocational guidance.

It is hoped that the book will serve students not merely to pass examinations, but will help them to lead their children, by example no less than by precept, to value and to seek a healthy way of life.

I would like to thank Miss Mabel Parry, B.A., for her help in reading the proofs.

M. B. DAVIES.

March, 1948.

CONTENTS

CHAPTER		PAGE
	Preface	vii
I.	Personal And Social Aspects of Health Education	1
II.	Bones and Joints	14
III.	Muscles	31
IV.	Blood and Circulation	48
V.	The Lungs and Breathing	62
VI.	Ventilation—Sunlight and Smoke	74
VII.	Digestion of Food	88
VIII.	Foodstuffs and Choice of Foods	100
IX.	Milk and other Beverages	118
X.	Diets and School Feeding	127
XI.	Teeth and Dental Hygiene	136
XII.	The Skin and Kidneys	148
XIII.	Clothing	162
XIV.	The Practice of Health	171
XV.	Endocrine or Ductless Glands	181
XVI.	The Brain and Nervous System	190
XVII.	Economy of Work—Fatigue—Rest and Sleep	208
XVIII.	Attitude to Health—Hysteria—Tic—Stammerers	219
XIX.	Intelligence Tests and Vocational Guidance	233
XX.	Dull, Backward and Retarded Children. Epileptics	245
XXI.	The Senses—Taste, Smell and Sight	256
XXII.	Eye Defects—Special Education for the Blind	266
XXIII.	Hearing—Special Education for the Deaf	284
XXIV.	Sex Physiology and Teaching	295
XXV.	Mendelism and Heredity—Eugenics	303
XXVI.	Alcohol in Relation to Social Problems	325
XXVII.	Infectious Diseases—General Considerations and some Special Infections	332

(ix) 1*

CHAPTER		PAGE
XXVIII.	Further Infectious Diseases	349
XXIX.	Tuberculosis	357
XXX.	Rheumatism	367
XXXI.	Maternity Welfare and the Pre-school Child	374
XXXII.	Public Health—the School Medical Service—Special Schools	385
XXXIII.	The School Building	400
XXXIV.	School Emergencies and Accidents	413
	Bibliography	428
	Index	431

CHAPTER I

PERSONAL AND SOCIAL ASPECTS OF HEALTH EDUCATION

THERE are two clear-cut yet not unrelated lines of approach to Health Education. There is the Health Education necessary for the individual as an individual and the Health Education equally necessary for every individual as a member of the community. In other words the study must be viewed from both the *personal* and the *social* angle.

Personal Aspect of Health Education

Looking at the personal aspect first, the question arises what is implied by the word person. Any attenpt to answer the question must be based on the realization that human beings have evolved both physically and mentally from simpler life forms.

In order then to understand how to ensure health for an individual, by which is meant his successful mental and bodily functioning, it is necessary to consider briefly this process of organic evolution. This is the concept, now generally accepted, that all living things, plants and animals, are related to one another and that they must have been derived from one or more common ancestors.

The reader will learn about the bodily functions of individuals, how we move, breathe, take in food, reproduce our kind, and about the mental functions how we think and feel and seek our goals. Further there will be the need to pay attention to such activity as seeing and hearing and interpreting what we see and hear. In doing this we shall find ourselves continually reminded that the way we do these things is conditioned by the way our earlier animal ancestors reacted to situations and environments, often more exacting.

1

A study of this process of the evolution of organism reveals that the physical basis of life is *protoplasm*, in the unit of the single microscopic cell, and all things that are alive are made up of from one to myriads of such cells. Protoplasm is a clear jelly-like slimy substance, which has the power of taking in food, of growing, of responding to external stimuli and of reproducing itself in like form.

No inorganic material can do all these things. A mechanism like a motor car cannot be used while it is being made. It needs to be fuelled and kept clean during use by an external agent. It cannot produce another machine of itself. The same is true of all mechanisms such as engines, wireless, aeroplanes, microscopes, gramophones.

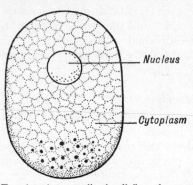

FIG. 1.—A generalized cell (based on an illustration in *Knowles' " Man and other Living Things "—Harrap*).

How life originated is not known, but it certainly branched early along two lines of development, (i) protoplasm with green colouring matter, which could make use of inorganic food substances, from which modern plants have evolved and (ii) protoplasm lacking this green chlorophyll, and needing organic food, from which *animal* forms developed. *The proofs that evolution has taken place*, and is still taking place not just in man but in all living things, are based on cumulative evidence, from a number of sources, from (i) geology, (ii) embryology, (iii) vestigial structures in the body, (iv) classification of living types.

(i) Evidence from Geology

The *geological evidence* comes from the fossil remains of animal and plant life found preserved in rocks of known relative age. To the geologist the word " rock " is a general term, including everything from granite to mud, from coal to beach sand. Roughly speaking, rocks are of two kinds, igneous and sedimentary. Igneous rocks have their origin in the white hot interior of the earth whence they are forced to the surface in a molten condition, and so there can be no fossils in them.

Sedimentary rocks, on the other hand, are formed by the wearing down or weathering of igneous or older sedimentary

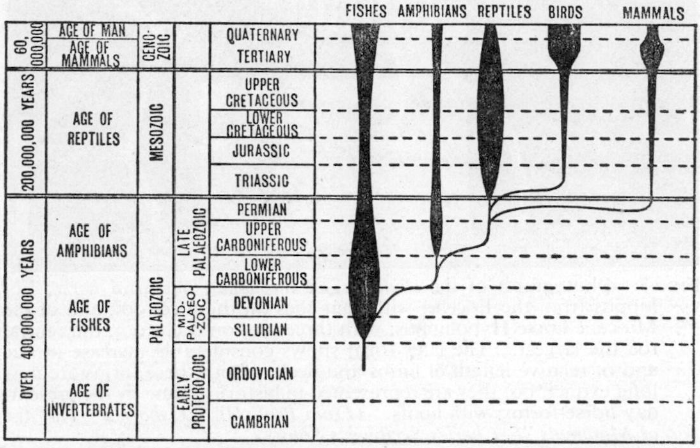

FIG. 2.—*Diagram to show the succession of the five main vertebrate classes in geological time.* The approximate length in years (deduced from radio-active minerals) of the three main epochs is given on the left. The thickness of the black columns for each class represents roughly its abundance and dominance. (Probably those for Fish and Amphibians should not contract in the Mesozoic to less than their final thickness ; and that for Reptiles should contract much more intensely at the close of the Mesozoic.) (*After Prof. H. F. Osborn's " Origin and Evolution of Life "—Charles Scribner's Sons.*)

rocks. The small particles thus produced are transported by water or other agents and laid down so as to form, according to size of the particles, muds, sands, gravels or other rocks. These deposits accumulate slowly and cover over or envelop animals and plants and it is in them that fossils are found.

The earliest known sedimentary rocks contain no unequivocal evidence of the presence of living creatures, but this is probably due to the absence of any hard parts in the organisms then living, rather than to the absence of life. However, from

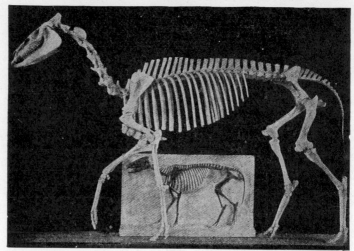

FIG. 3.—Photograph of the *skeletons of the small, ancestral horse,* Eohippus from the Eocene, with four toes on the fore-foot, and of the Miocene horse Hypohippus, with three toes on each foot, the central toe the largest. The later form shows considerable increase in size and of relative length of limbs and neck. Both these forms are now long extinct, but they are represented in historical time by the present-day horse-forms, with hoofs. (*From Prof. H. F. Osborn's " The Age of Mammals "—Charles Scribner's Sons.*)

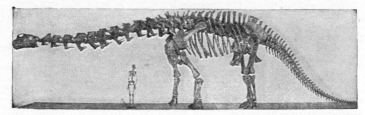

FIG. 4.—*Skeletons of the extinct Dinosaur Diplodocus and of a Man.* The brain of Diplodocus was a good deal smaller than the enlargement in the spinal cord opposite the hind-limb. Compare the bone plan of this reptile form with that of the horse (Fig. 3) and of the skeleton (Fig. 10). Note the heavy bones which go with a clumsy, weighty organism, and the long spinous processes of the middle vertebra, which give thus the stronger leverage for supporting the elongated head and tail. (*From Prof. H. F. Osborn's " Origin and Evolution of Life "—Charles Scribner's Sons.*)

the time when skeletal structures first appeared, down to the present day, there is a mass of evidence in support of the theory, and the evolution of many organisms such as that of the horse has been traced in great detail.

In the Vertebrates it is possible to trace, by fossil remains, the development from Fish to Amphibian and thence to Reptiles and the two warm-blooded classes of Vertebrates, the Birds on the one hand and the Mammals, including Man, on the other.

The fossil skeleton of the large Reptile Dinosaur (Fig. 4) is heavy and stout and is thus much more likely to be preserved than are the lighter skeletons of flying Reptiles and of the primitive Bird.

(ii) Evidence from Embryology

Then there is the *evidence of embryology*, that is, the development of the mammalian fœtus, the name given to the baby while it is growing in the mother's body before it is born. The *fœtus* starts its growth as a single cell, comparable to an amœba-type of animal. Rapid cell division follows, and after perhaps a week the fœtus looks very much as though it were going to develop into a simple kind of sea-anemone, with an inside digestive system and an outside skin. At the end of a fortnight its development suggests the possibility of it being a rather more mobile and complex type, such as a worm. It is then about the size of a pea.

At the end of four weeks, however, the faint appearance of a growing spinal column shows that it has definitely left the invertebrate class. Moreover, the development of four limb-buds which might turn into fins, of gill-slits in the neck and of a heart resembling that of a fish seems to suggest that some kind of fish is maturing.

The gill-slits, however, only persist for about a fortnight, after which lungs are seen to be developing. The animal is to be an air-breathing land animal, at any rate. The heart becomes four-chambered as in mammals, and the limbs show signs of joints, but are short and stumpy, and there is a tail. A small primitive type of mammal is suggested—a mole or hedgehog-like animal.

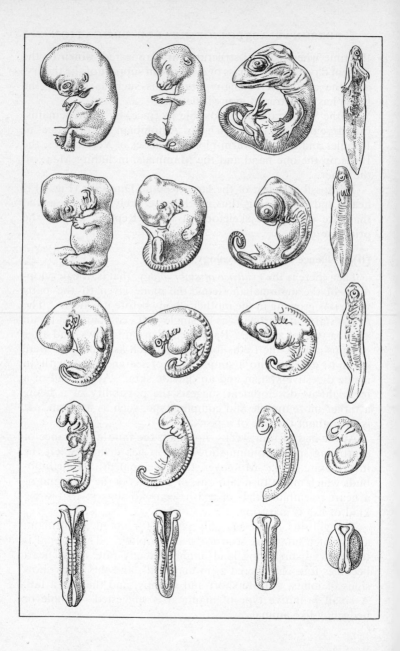

At the end of some eight weeks of development the fœtus is about the size of a large chestnut ; it has lost its tail, and its limb appendages, which might equally well have developed into hoofs or paws, have now definitely taken the latter alternative. At the end of four months the fœtus is about the size of a new-born kitten. It could now only develop into a monkey or a human infant : by the end of the eighth month it has passed all earlier biological stages and can only become a human baby.

Thus the individual tends to recapitulate during its development the developmental stages of its ancestors. It is, however, a fallacy to say, for instance, that the human embryo is at one stage a fish or at another a monkey. What it does is to pass through stages of having fish-like or monkey-like affinities. Analogously a tadpole, though not a fish, passes through the stage of having a fish-like tail and no legs. This is the zoological *Theory of Recapitulation.*

(iii) Evidence of Vestigial Structures

Vestigial structures in the body also offer evidence of evolution. Such structures have at one stage been useful, and are subsequently retained, though they have long ceased to be of service and may even be possible sources of illness.

The appendix, the inflammation of which causes appendicitis, is perhaps the best-known example of such a structure. In man it is a blind tube about the size of a finger, opening into the large intestine, and it appears to serve no useful purpose, whereas in the horse, rabbit and other herbivora it is a large and useful part of the intestine that actively helps in digestion.

FIG. 5.—*A collection of vertebrate embryos.* Each upright column represents the development of a single type—left to right, Man, Calf, Lizard, Newt—the earliest embryos being below and the latest above. The early stages are very like each other, and the animals become more unlike as they develop. In the first stage, the nerve-folds are closing to form the brain. Then the gill-slits appear. In land animals these close later ; in the newt and dog-fish feathery gills appear. The human tail and its gradual shortening are clearly seen. (*After Wells, Huxley and Wells.*)

The outer ear is of little use in man to collect sound. Some people can still move the muscles of the ear slightly, but in dogs and cats and horses, for example, the power of movement is still strong, and is useful to the animal.

The cat has a so-called third eyelid, which can sometimes be seen when the eye is half closed. In man all that remains of this structure is a small protuberance in the inside corner of the eye.

The number and distribution of valves in the human veins, that help the return of blood to the heart, is better adapted for an animal that walks on four legs than on two. Doubtless this distribution—comparative redundancy in the arms and too few in the legs—was settled at a biological stage before an upright walk was assumed. The tendency to get varicose veins of the legs is partly the result of this.

The saltness of the sea, when amphibians first crawled out of it, has been calculated, and found to be much less salt than now. It is therefore of interest that the salinity of the blood is calculated to be of the same strength of salt solution as was the saltness of the ocean when our remote ancestors first ceased to live, as it were, in a perpetual salt solution, and took to a land life.

(iv) Evidence of Existing Animals and Plants

A fourth source of evidence of evolution lies in *the classification of animal types*, which is not fundamentally an artificial scheme imposed by man, but the understandable outcome of the evolutionary relationship of all living forms. Man has interpreted, he has not invented, such classification. The fact that out of the whole wide variety of animal life, each species fits accurately into the scheme, and shows a lesser or greater relationship to all other species, could only be explained by some such theory.

The majority of stages through which the main stream of life has passed are to-day represented in the flesh by those species which have, metaphorically speaking, fallen by the wayside. While many species have developed and improved, many more have stayed at their same level of development. There are countless varieties of worms, of shell-fish, of mussels and fish that have found for themselves, as it were, a niche in the scheme of life. So also there are amphibians, such as frogs, reptiles as lizards, and mammals, each adapted to specific kinds of climate and food-supplying conditions. They have become adapted to their particular environment, and this remaining unchanged throughout the ages, so also have they. From amœba to mammal there is a vast array of these isolated remnants which have survived unchanged, and to-day shed light on the stages of that progress that has passed them by.

Similarly, there is the evidence of backward races, such as the Australian aborigines, who in level of intelligence and in way of life must correspond closely to primitive man. Their chief characteristic is lack of originality.

Man, then, is not an isolated animal. His emotions and fears come as does the salinity of his blood out of the distant but not wholly uncertain past. The appeal and emotional stimulus of chasing, hunting and hiding games for children and for adults should be noted

One of the difficulties about believing that *organic evolution* has taken place has been doubt about the age of the Earth. Was the Earth old enough to have allowed time for these gradual changes, for the evolution of any new type—plant or animal—is estimated to need at least 50,000 years.

The *age of the earth* can now be estimated by the decomposition of the radio-active elements Uranium and Thorium into Lead. If this decomposition has been going on at a regular rate, the amount of lead present in any rock determines the length of time that must have been needed for this accumulation. This enables geologists to estimate that the age of the Earth is at least five thousand million years, a much longer period than other evidence available suggested, and long enough, in fact, to support the whole theory of organic evolution.

Social Aspect of Health Education

The Social Aspect of Health Education is of equal importance with the personal aspect and must now be considered.

The health and well-being of the individual is closely bound up with that of the community in which he lives and here again can be seen evolution in the social care, for example, in the Vertebrates.

The bony-skeletoned Fish, for instance, produce many thousand eggs which are fertilised externally. There is little or no paternal care and few eggs reach maturity.

The Amphibians, of which the frog and toad are modern examples, were the first vertebrate land-dwellers. They lay relatively larger eggs with considerable yolk, on which the young feed in the early stages of life. The eggs however are without a protective shell and have to be laid in or near water. The jelly of, for example, frog spawn is a protection against enemies. Here a larger proportion of individuals reach maturity.

The Reptile, evolving from the amphibian, produced a new type of egg. This egg had a watertight covering which enabled the immature reptile to develop, as it were, in its own private water-pond, and thus made it completely independent of the need for an outside source of water.

The eggs also were relatively larger and allowed of greater development before hatching and so gave a better chance of survival to the young.

From the reptile stock the Birds evolved with their nesting habits and high degree of maternal care. This care however is matter largely of instinct and is not apparently learnt as in the Mammals.

A second warm-blooded line of Vertebrates emerged in the early *mammals*. They were hair-coated, which prevented over-rapid heat loss. The young developed inside the mother for the first period of life and were fed, after birth, by suckling, hence the general name of mammals. Far fewer young were born, which increased the individual's chance of reaching maturity ; and the development of a family life, the parents teaching the young, made for higher potential development of intelligence.

From family life developed the joining up of a number of families in the tribe for mutual protection, but still the strong dominated the weak, enslaving them.

It is only in this century that the ideal has really become

clear-cut that every individual rich or poor should have a chance of satisfactory health and of living happily, that no one should be penalised by having to live in insanitary houses, be short of essential food, places to play or of medical care in illness.

Hence develops the social aspect of Health Education with free education, prenatal and nursery school care, re-housing schemes, equal rationing of food in times of limited supply, and social insurance against illness, unemployment and old age.

The preservation and improvement of the race has now become the conscious endeavour of human communities. Ways and means of individual and social betterment are deliberately sought, studied and tested. Hence we have ante-natal care, infant welfare centres, child guidance clinics, special schools for children needing extra care, and wide provision for therapeutic work throughout adult life.

Bacteria and Viruses

" Hygiene is very roughly the process of making things difficult for germs," a journalist, Anthony Cotterill, has stated. Everyone experiences attacks of micro-organisms as a personal matter, as in catching a cold, and needs to know how to mini-mise its effects and to prevent it from being passed on to any-one else. There is also the need to understand how to use and co-operate with the public health services so that infections are dealt with by the individual and so are not broadcast to the community. Thus the problem of dealing successfully with infections is both personal and social.

While a number of micro-organisms do parasitise man, causing such illnesses as tuberculosis, diphtheria, and measles, many other forms are neutral to him, neither benefiting nor harming him, and many are beneficial and indeed essential to the balance of life. Most of the decay of organic matter—plant and animal—is brought about by micro-organisms, thus bringing the material of them into circulation again to be used in the growth of new generations of living things. It is micro-organisms that give flavour to butter, cheese and tobacco.

The parasitic micro-organisms that need to be considered are (i) Bacteria, (ii) Viruses, and (iii) Protozoa.

Bacteria are of two main kinds, the spherical shaped—the

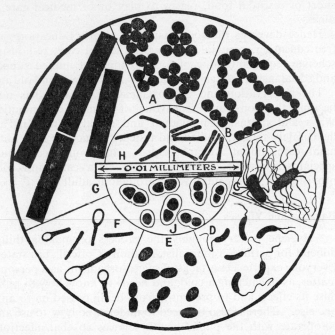

FIG. 6.—Diagram to show the *shapes of bacteria*, highly magnified. A, staphylococcus, common on all skin surfaces ; B, streptococcus, common in nose and throat. Both produce inflammation ; C. typhoid bacillus ; D, cholera bacillus ; E, plague bacillus ; F, tetanus bacillus, producing lock-jaw ; G, anthrax bacillus ; H, tubercle bacillus, producing tuberculosis ; I, diphtheria bacillus ; J, pneumococcus, one of many bacteria found in pneumonia. Each of the small divisions of the scale in the centre = $\frac{1}{1000}$ millimetre = $\frac{1}{25000}$ inch. (*From Campbell's " Readable Physiology and Hygiene "* —*G. Bell & Sons, Ltd.*)

cocci—and the rod shaped—the bacilli. Some have coil like appendages that help their movement in moisture. Bacteria have no proper nucleus and under good conditions—moist food, warmth and darkness—they increase rapidly by constant division. Thus, as a bacillus divides about three times in an hour (one into two, these two into four and the four into eight), at the end of eight hours, an ordinary night's sleep, there would, in favourable conditions, be over 16,000,000 offspring from one bacillus, and there would obviously be many more than one to start with. However, shortage of food and their own toxins tend to inhibit this rate of growth progressively.

Some bacteria, in adverse conditions, such as too much light, the presence of poison, or very high or low temperatures, go rapidly into a resistant resting condition by forming spores with thick firm walls. Such spores can be boiled, chilled or dried and still live. Anthrax spores have lived in a 1 per cent. carbolic acid solution for fourteen days, and have survived dry for at least fifteen years. Sunlight quickly kills spores, hence its disinfectant value.

Bacteria are breathed in and out at almost every breath. They exist in all unsterilised water and in foods and in top soils, giving the characteristic after-rain smell.

Some micro-organisms, the *filter-passing viruses*, produce typical effects as of measles, but they are so small that they cannot, owing to the properties of light, be seen through any ordinary microscope. Common cold, influenza, mumps, infantile paralysis and chicken- and smallpox are virus-caused diseases. Unlike bacteria, viruses cannot grow outside the body of a living animal or plant, and this, together with their smallness, has made research on them difficult. Viruses can be seen and photographed by using an electron microscope.

Some of the uni-cellular animals classed as *Protozoa* have adopted a parasitic mode of life in contrast to Amœba and Paramœcium, which are free-living. Malaria, amœbic dysentery and sleeping sickness are caused by such micro-organisms.

How micro-organisms invade the body, how their attacks are repelled and how healthy living and the knowledge gained from Science can help the body in its fight against them are among the problems to which Health Education should supply an answer.

CHAPTER II

BONES AND JOINTS

THE body moves about on a framework of lime, some two hundred and six bones, making up about 20 lb. of the body's weight, which give support, protect vital organs from injury, and give solid points on which muscles can pull to bring about movement. All the roughnesses, ridges and protrusions on bone surfaces that seem irregular and purposeless make a joining place for a particular muscle or muscles, the ridge giving a rather stronger and easier range of movement when the muscles contract.

Bone surfaces also are pitted with smaller and larger holes, some areas more so than others, as shown in the ends of the thigh bone, which are pitted more than the smoother shaft. Here blood-vessels enter and leave the bone tissue, so that live bone is a pale pink, not dry and yellowish, as in a preserved skeleton.

Bones are less dense in the interior, and their compactness of tissue, which can be seen in examining a skeleton, varies according to where, in use, the main strength or resilience will be needed. Thus *long bones*, those of the limbs, have compact smooth-surfaced shafts with comparatively open tissue, called cancellous, inside. This makes these bones lighter for the muscles to carry about and more resilient and elastic against shocks; they have, as we say, more " give " in them and so are the less likely to fracture. Red corpuscles are made in the cancellous tissue of the ribs, sternum and vertebræ—one example of the body's efficient packing arrangements.

Flat bones, as those of the skull, have two layers of compact bone matter with a layer of cancellous tissue in between. This makes the bony case all the better protection for the brain, because the cancellous tissue dulls the force of any blow so that the brain is the less jarred.

Many of the bones grow first and remain for the early years of life as *cartilage*, that is, gristle in meat. Cartilage is tough, elastic, bendable, semi-transparent grey tissue, without blood-

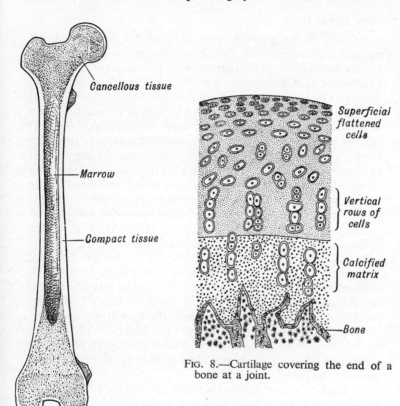

FIG. 7.—A long bone, the femur, cut lengthwise.

FIG. 8.—Cartilage covering the end of a bone at a joint.

vessels in it. The baby, because its bones are yielding, is born the more easily. Within this cartilage the bones have " growing points," from which increase in length and size takes place ; there are such points, for example, in the two ends of the thigh bone. Cells called *osteoblasts* have the power of laying down lime deposits in the cartilage tissue, thus gradually hardening the bone into its final adult form.

How Bones Grow

As long as the *growing points* or *epiphyses* have not closed up and finished growing, the child can continue to increase in height and width. Different growing points cease growth development at definite ages ; for example, the elbow at sixteen, the hand bones at twenty, the femur and the shin bone (tibia) between eighteen and twenty, the hip-joint at twenty-five, after which age the bone skeleton is fixed in shape and size. It is thus possible to tell whether a skeleton was over or under twenty-five, and if under, the approximate age, by the number of " growing points " closed up. Growing children who habitually assume bad positions tend to become fixed in the wrong posture. They should be taught sound posture habits so that they may maintain these habits into adult life.

The skeletal framework is made up of the skull, a jointed spine with a bony protective cage of ribs in front, and the *pelvis*, comprising the two hip bones and the bottom bones of the spine, the *sacrum*, which attain the greater strength by fusing to form a basin-like concavity above to take the weight of the abdominal organs. With the two thigh bones the sacrum makes an arch so that, with the two instep arches of the feet, the body weight stands on three arches. The characteristic of such arches is that the greater the weight above, the stronger and more firmly pressed together are the component parts of the arch.

The brain-case or *cranium* is made up of eight bones, joined by immovable finely-laced joints, that make altogether a dome shape, so that on the principle of the arch again, the vibration of a blow on the skull is distributed to lessen shock. The dome shape gives additional protection to the brain inside because blows tend to slip off the rounded surface. On the under surface of the cranium towards the back, there is an opening through which the spinal cord leaves the brain.

These cranial bones in a baby at birth are soft and still separated at points called the *fontanelles*. This allows for

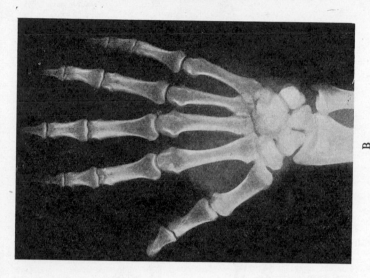

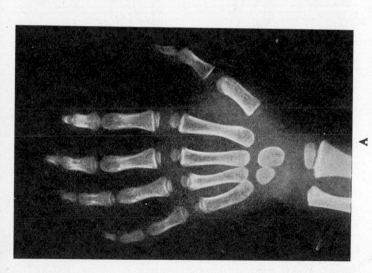

FIG. 9.—A. An X-ray photograph of the bones of a child's hand. It shows the epiphyses or growing points at the ends of the radius and ulna and of the phalanges. B. An adult hand. Compare the wrist bones in A and B. (By courtesy of Professor T. B. Johnston.)

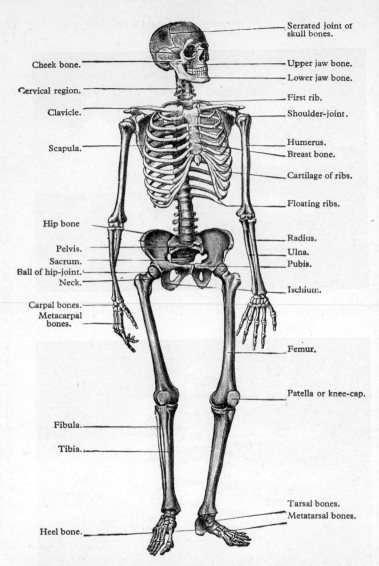

FIG. 10.—The skeleton. Note the similarity of plan of the arm and leg bones. Which bones correspond to which in the arm and leg? Compare the right and left forearms. In the right, the action of the pivot-joints at the elbow is shown.

greater elasticity in the baby's head in the process of birth, and for growth of the brain.

The *face* is made up of fourteen bones, of which one only, the lower jaw bone, is movable. The eyes are deeply set in bony sockets that protect them. A blow on the eye rarely causes injury except to superficial tissues round the eye, giving the characteristic bruises and blood-shot appearance of a black eye. Similarly, the hearing part of the ear is protected by being sunk to the inner end of a narrow bony canal in the bone of the skull.

The *spine* is made up, in the child, of thirty-three bones, called vertebræ, fitted one on top of the other, as reels of cotton might be, and with a hole down the middle of the column, as there would be down superimposed reels, in which the spinal cord from the brain lies thus well protected from injury.

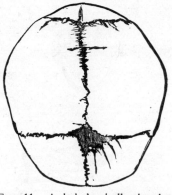

Each *vertebra* consists of a body to the front that takes the weight, the hole for the spinal cord behind the body, and the spinous processes—three of them—that protrude and on which muscles pull to get better purchase to turn,

Fig. 11.—A baby's skull, showing the incomplete joining up of the skull bones and the fontanelle or space between the bones at the front of the head. There is also a smaller fontanelle at the back of the head. They join up towards the end of the second year.

bend and steady the trunk. The spine is almost straight in a newly-born baby, but directly the child begins to sit and stand up the spine, looked at from the side, takes on its characteristic bends, that is, forward in the cervical or neck region, backward in the shoulder or dorsal region, forward in the lumbar or waist region and backward in the sacrum. These curves help, with other factors, to make the spine less rigid and more elastic to withstand shocks and jolts to the body. (See Fig. 13.)

There are seven vertebræ in the cervical region ; and the spinous process of the seventh cervical vertebra can usually be seen as a small prominence at the back of the neck, if the head is bent forward. These vertebræ are lightly made and delicate, having little weight comparatively on them.

The twelve dorsal vertebræ are progressively more heavily made, and to each of them is attached a pair of ribs. The five

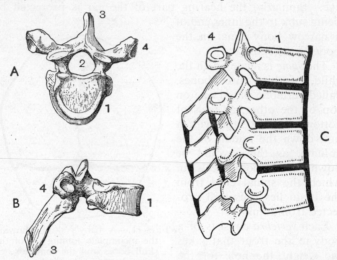

FIG. 12.—A, dorsal vertebra, viewed from above ; B, from the right side. 1, body ; 2, cavity for spinal cord ; 3 and 4, spinous processes on which muscles pull ; C shows how ligaments—shown in black—hold the vertebræ in alignment and yet allow elasticity. (C is from Eastwood's " Hygiene for Students and Teachers" — Edward Arnold & Co.)

lumbar vertebræ have more substantial bodies still. In an adult the five vertebræ of the sacrum join with each other, and with the two hip bones, as has been said earlier, form the pelvis. The coccyx is a rudimentary tail, movable on the sacrum in women, thus allowing a slightly larger aperture for birth.

The ten pairs of upper ribs slant downward and forward to join the breast bone or *sternum* in front, either directly or by an elastic cartilage connection. The two bottom pairs do not join up thus and are called floating ribs. The twelve pairs of ribs thus form a bony cage which protects the heart and lungs and yet is light in weight and elastic. In addition, each rib is joined to the rib immediately above and below it by bands of muscle, which, when they contract, serve to lift each rib outward and upward, thus enlarging the total chest capacity. Put your hands on your chest wall below your armpits and try this movement for yourself. (Fig. 45.)

The *shoulder girdle* comprises the right and left clavicle or collar bones, the upper arm bones (the humerus), and the scapulæ or shoulder-blades.

The *clavicle* keeps the chest wide so that the range of movement of the arm is increased. It is a bone in the body which is often fractured, for example, directly from falls in riding, or indirectly from falling forward and saving a complete fall by catching the

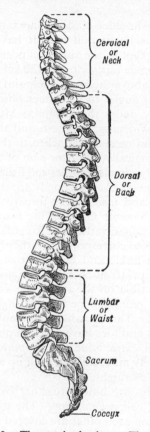

FIG. 13.—The vertebral column. The bodies of the vertebræ, which take the weight increasingly, become heavier towards the lumbar region, and the spinous processes (on which muscles to turn and bend the spine pull) are shorter and more sturdy. The forward and backward curves of the spine make for less rigidity, minimising jars and injury. If exaggerated, they detract from height.

weight on the heel of the hand. This jars and fractures the clavicle.

The shoulder-blade is an example of a bone that is purely for muscles to pull on. It has no protective value. If the arm is kept to the side, it is possible to feel the lower point of the *scapula* fairly close to the spine, whereas, if the arm is then raised above the head, the point will be found to have rotated at right angles to its former position, so that it is now almost directly under the arm-pit. Muscles that pull the shoulders back, widening the chest, and that move the arms and make the head erect are attached to the scapula.

Biologically, the *bone-plan* of the human limbs is that of all limbed animals, reptiles and fishes ; the single upper arm bone, the *humerus*, corresponds to the thigh bone or *femur*, the *radius* and *ulna* of the forearm correspond to the *tibia* and splint bone or *fibula* of the lower leg ; there are eight small *carpal* bones, rather like irregular lumps of sugar, in the wrist, and seven corresponding rather heavier *tarsal* bones that make up the ankle and back part of the foot and the heel. The actual protrusions called the ankle bones are the lower ends of the tibia on the inner side and the fibula on the outer side. In the palm can be felt five small long bones, the *metacarpal* bones. The foot has five similar *metatarsal* bones, and the fingers and toes have fourteen phalanges respectively. The leg has an extra bone in the *patella* or knee-cap that can be passively moved about both up and down and sideways, if the knee is straightened.

Bones are bound together by tough, strong grey bands of tissue, called *ligaments*. The touching surfaces of bones that move on each other are covered with smooth pads of cartilage, and lubricated by fluid *synovia*, just as a bicycle or motor must have its moving parts bathed in oil to prevent the moving parts from becoming hot from friction between them.

Types of Joints

Where a wide range of movement is needed, as at the hip and shoulder-joints, the *joints* are ball and socket in type, while the knee and elbow are hinge-joints, with no power of side-ways movement—but only of a bend and stretch movement as in opening and shutting a door. Actually it would be inconvenient if the knee joints failed to lock and had to be controlled by muscle contraction against giving way sideways or backwards.

If the hand is placed palm upwards on the desk, the raising of the forearm brings into play the hinge-joint at the elbow ; in doing this the radius lies on the thumb side of the arm from elbow to wrist, and the ulna, the upper end of which can be felt as the point of the elbow, is parallel to the radius on the little finger side of the arm. Besides bending up the forearm on the upper arm, it is also possible to rotate the hand so

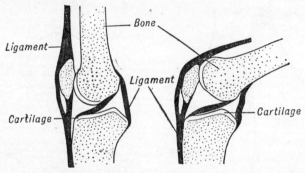

FIG. 14.—The ligaments of the knee in long section. The ligaments actually surround the joint, supporting it.

that the palm, which was up, faces down. In this position the radius has crossed over the ulna, and to do this the radius pivots on the ulna at the elbow and wrist. Thus we write with the palm down but take a plate or book that is passed to us with the palm up, to get the width of the fingers to help balance widely distributed weight. The pivot-joint is used in turning keys and wringing out clothes, to give two examples.

It is this joint, combined with the fine gliding joint of the wrist and the long delicate and flexible phalanges, that has made the hand and arm able to effect such minute and intricate varieties of work. The fact, too, that the thumb can move across the palm to touch the little finger has made a much larger variety of movements possible to the hand than

2

to the foot, and almost certainly had a great deal thus to do with the development of intelligence in early primate ancestors.

The leg bones are considerably heavier and more massive than are the arm bones. They are less adapted for delicate movement than for taking weight. The knee-joint, as noted earlier, has a more limited range of movement than the elbow. The tarsal bones are, relatively to the wrist bones, large, with the heel bone, in white races, standing out markedly for the attachment of the calf muscles that lift the heel. The tarsal

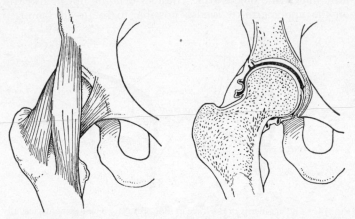

FIG. 15.—The hip joint, showing the ligaments and the ball-and-socket joint that they help to hold firm. (*After Knowles' " Man and Other Living Things"—Harrap.*)

and metatarsal bones fit together to form the arch of the foot on the inner border, a mechanical contrivance that makes for greater agility, and light and less tiring walking.

Finally, while the hip-joint socket is deeply set in the hip bone and deepened by cartilage to hold the rounded ball of the femur head the more securely in place, the socket into which the humerus fits in the scapula is a shallow concavity no deeper than the palm of the hand. Thus the hip-joint is solid and secure and rarely likely to be dislocated, but it has a limited range of movement, while the shoulder-joint is considerably less strong but has a much wider range of movement.

The hip-joint range is actually increased by the way in which the neck of the femur joins the shaft at an obtuse angle and allows the shaft to move clear of the pelvis. This neck is part of the arch of the pelvis and is liable to fracture, particularly in older people. It is to be noted that while it is

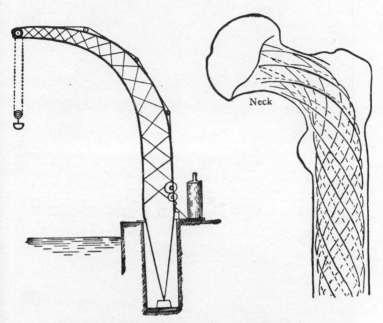

Fig. 16.—The arrangement of the " stresses and strains " in the strengthening tissues of the femur are similar to those of a weight-lifting crane. Thus the neck of the femur allows wide range of movement round the joint while keeping its weight-carrying strength. Note also the ball of the ball-and-socket joint. (*From Keith's " Engines of the Human Body "—Williams & Norgate, Ltd.*)

convenient to raise the arm till it is parallel to the ear, to be able to raise the leg thus, except as an acrobatic feat, would entail a loss of stability.

The pelvis in men is narrower than in women, so giving points of attachment for the sheets of abdominal muscle. Thus the female pelvis is better adapted for supporting weight

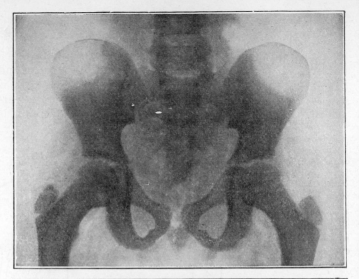

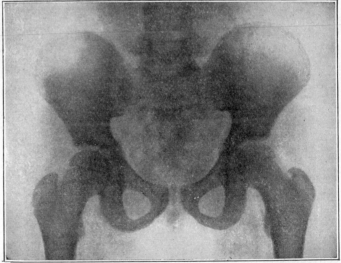

FIG. 17.—*Radiogram of the pelvis* of a boy aged 10 (above) and of a girl aged 11 (below), showing the marked differences in contour even *before* puberty. The girl's pelvis is already wider than that of the boy, and the femurs are set at different angles. Note also the differences in shape of the basin of the pelvis, as outlined by the hip bones in each case. In the boy's pelvis two epiphyses which have not united, can be seen obliquely above the head of each femur. (*From " The Primary School," by permission of the Controller of H.M. Stationery Office.*)

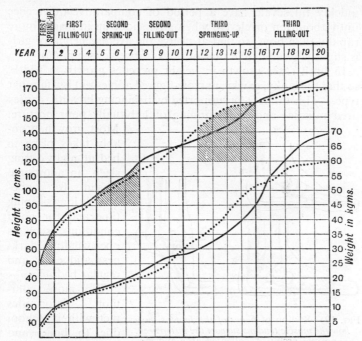

FIG. 18.—The growth curves for Height (cms.) and Weight (kgms.) in children show three " springing-up " periods followed by three " filling-out " periods, the shaded areas representing rapid growth—Boys : ——— continuous line ; Girls : ...... dotted line. The first " springing-up " period is associated with rickets, scurvy, digestive disturbances and infant diarrhœa ; from 2–7 infectious diseases such as measles, whooping-cough, and diphtheria are specially prevalent ; from 8–11 is often connected with the after-effects of infectious diseases and affections of the eyes, teeth, middle ear and the tonsils and adenoids ; from 11–15 postural defects show because of the rapid growth in height *before* the " filling-out " from 16–20 years of age.

as in pregnancy, but less well adapted for heavier muscular work and for weight lifting.

Finally, it should always be kept in mind that children are continually growing and changing, and that to grow rapidly is hard work for the body. This effort beyond normal should therefore be continually but unostentatiously taken into account. Growth also is irregular. Thus children grow quickly till seven, have a period of comparative quiescence until about ten or eleven, when girls shoot up in height more rapidly than boys, so that at twelve the average height of girls is slightly greater than that of boys of twelve (see p. 66).

In both sexes growth in height precedes growth in width, so that the lanky, gawky, narrow-figured adolescent is a familiar type. This tallness, unsupported by balancing breadth, causes tired muscles and the assuming of habitually poor posture.

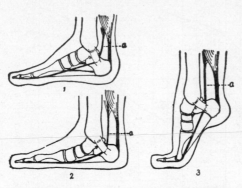

Most growth probably takes place in bed at night during sleep, an additional reason for adequately long sleeping time and for good conditions, such as open windows, darkness and early and regular bedtime.

The more common deformities met with in school due to bone and joint changes may be caused by after-effects of accidents, rickets (see Chapter VIII), tuberculosis (see Chapter XXIX) and infantile paralysis (see Chapter XXVIII).

FIG. 19.—Section of *bones of the foot to show how the muscle tendons support the instep arch.* 1, normal arch ; 2, collapsed arch and flat-foot ; 3, the corrective value of standing on the toes for flat-foot. *a*, tendon of muscle that flexes the toes and lifts the instep arch. (*From Drummond's " School Hygiene "— Edward Arnold & Co.*)

Flat Foot

Flat-foot is the giving way of the arch made by the foot bones, due to inheritance of foot shape, or long-continued standing, particularly in a hot, moist, enervating atmosphere, as a laundry, or the wearing of too heavy boots that inhibit the use of the natural foot-thrust of the back foot in walking. Often only one foot is flat, or one is flatter than the other. Flat-footed people may be recognised because they tend to walk with their feet turned out, and thus the weight of the body is taken along the inner border. If the feet are turned in, the main weight comes on the outer side.

In a normal bare foot, a space, where the instep is on the inner side of the foot, should not touch the ground in standing : in a flat-foot up to the whole sole touches the ground, according to the extent of the defect, the bones thus pressing painfully on the tendons, ligaments, blood-vessels and nerves usually protected by the arch.

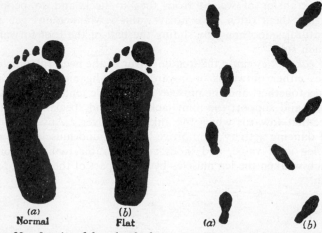

(a) Normal   (b) Flat   (a)   (b)

FIG. 20.—*Imprint of the sole of a foot* (a) with a normal instep arch ; (b) with a dropped arch and flat-foot.

FIG. 21.—(a) Correct *economical walk*, the feet pointing straight forward ; (b) incorrect and tiring walk, with the feet turned out. Method (b) shortens the stride for the same output of energy. If the two methods are tried, the relative loss of foot agility in (b) becomes obvious.

Massage for the foot and lower leg muscles, exercises, such as heel raising with toes touching and heels parted, and walking on the toes along a straight line on the floor, are of value, as are also country dancing and skipping. Æsthetic dancing, in which the feet must be turned out, is likely to be harmful.

Arch supports are of little value because, in the long run, they tend to inhibit the patient from using his own foot muscles.   They are not a substitute for exercises to strengthen the feet.   Children, some fifty years ago, used to be taught to turn the feet out in walking, which shortens the stride proportional to the output of energy.   Actually the most economical way of walking is with the feet pointing straight forward ; the heel should touch the ground first, but, in an easy elastic walk, the transfer of weight from the heel to the ball of the foot should be smooth and noiseless.   High heels make for a jerky transfer of weight from toes to heel, and so people wearing them often have noisy walks.   Mannequins get an unnatural smoothness by sliding the ball of the foot forward at each step.

Weak ankles cause the treading over of the heel stiffening of shoes either outwards or inwards.   The ligaments that join bones together, and the muscles and muscle tendons that surround and support the joint lack tone, and specially on one side, that towards which the ankle goes over.   Any jumping and dancing activity to improve the all-round muscle tone of the leg is of value, and shoes are preferable to high boots, which weaken the leg muscles by doing part of their work for them.

Chapter III

MUSCLES

MUSCLE tissue has the power to contract and so draw nearer together parts of the body, to which the particular muscle is joined. Such muscles as those that move the arm or leg are under the control of the will, and are termed *voluntary muscles*, and their tissue is striated.

There are also muscles that move continuously without our being able to decide mentally that they shall do so, and these are called *involuntary muscles*. Except for the heart muscle their tissue is unstriated. The walls of the 36 feet of the digestive or food canal, and of the blood-vessels, consist mostly of this involuntary muscle, as does the iris, the coloured part of the eye which reacts to light. Tripe, which is the stomach and intestine of the cow, is involuntary muscle tissue.

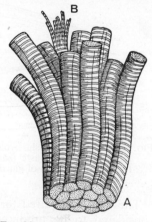

FIG. 22.—A bundle of *voluntary muscle fibres*, cut across transversely, A. Lean meat is such muscle tissue. One bundle has been further split up to show smaller muscle fibrils, B.

Voluntary muscle tissue is the red flesh that is eaten as lean meat. It is arranged in bundles of fibres, which can be seen when meat is carved by cutting it across horizontally. The fibres consist of myriads of microscopic, long slender, striated muscle cells, each of which has the power of closing up like a concertina. Between these fibres pass the smallest kind of blood-vessel, called capillaries, which supply through their very thin walls each muscle cell with food and oxygen.

Food is a fuel which provides the energy to enable cells to contract, just as coal is a fuel which we burn to provide energy in the form of heat. There are some two thousand capillaries in a cubic millimetre of muscle tissue, a volume about twice the size of a pin's head.

In among these muscle cells there are also the end organs of nerves connecting the muscle with the spinal cord and the brain. When it is decided to pick up a book, for example, the mind and brain can thus send the impulse to the appropriate series of muscles—not just one—to contract in due order and degree and to take the book.

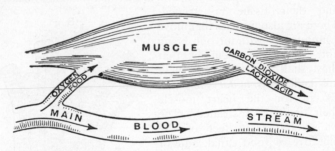

FIG. 23.—Diagram to show the supplies that the blood brings to any muscle, and the waste that it carries away after contraction. The food is in the form of glucose sugar.

The energy required for all muscular contractions is now considered to be produced by sugar together with oxygen both in solution in the blood plasma. Similarly, petrol-driven motors get their energy for movement from oxygen and petrol. Starchy foods, such as bread and potatoes, which form the bulk of the average diet, are turned by the chemical process of digestion into animal sugar or glucose. The liver and the muscles also store animal starch, glycogen, and this is rapidly turned by enzyme action into sugar when wanted for muscular work. This glucose in solution is taken round the body by and in the blood to the individual muscle cells.

All the body cells, not just the muscle cells, are constantly equalising their chemical content, which is always being healthily upset. For example, a cell needs oxygen or food and absorbs these from the moving blood stream ; waste products result from the cell's activity and these are discarded into the blood to be replaced again by food and oxygen. This chemical interchange is more rapid in rate at some times than at others. It is more rapid during running, for example, than during rest or sleep.

Osmosis and Diffusion

This interchange of materials goes on, partly at least, through the process of *osmosis*. If a pig's bladder, filled with salt or other crystalloid solution, is immersed in water, water is drawn inwards, even until the bladder bursts, and the solution is progressively diluted. This occurs because the bladder tissue is a *semi-permeable osmotic membrane*. Analogously, if a cell is surrounded by a strong solution, water is drawn out to the stronger surrounding solution, and the cell contents shrivel up. Cell membranes are semi-permeable too. This effect is used in " salting " of pork.

In the body, such extreme variations would be harmful, but osmotic exchanges, of water and selected dissolved substances, are continually occurring, as the blood and lymph move in the tissues. Waste matter (lactic acid and CO_2) is given up and oxygen and food are absorbed. Each animal cell, in fact, comprises a number of continually changing osmotic surfaces, both on the surface of and within each cell.[1]

Materials also move from cell to cell and from capillary to cell by *diffusion*. If a single crystal of permanganate of potash is dropped into a beaker of water and left unstirred, the pink colour will, in a matter of days, diffuse through the water so that the water becomes a uniformly pale pink. This is brought about by the constant bumping of water molecules against each other and against the coloured permanganate of potash molecules. The same process is an important one in the body cells because this is one way in which the mixing of substances in solution takes place.

---

[1] How colloids with larger molecules and fats enter the individual cell is not fully understood. Enzyme action is possible.

The mechanism of contraction is complicated ; each muscle cell appears to contract, squeezing itself up, and, in doing this, a certain amount of glucose is turned into lactic acid. The oxygen supply turns about four-fifths of the lactic acid back

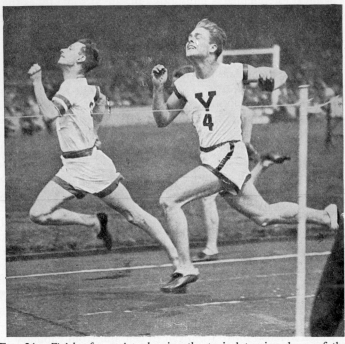

FIG. 24.—*Finish of a sprint*, showing the typical turning down of the corners of the mouth, and straining of the neck muscles, of acute oxygen shortage. Note also the hamstring tendons of the nearer runner's left leg, and the contracted calf muscles of his right leg. His shadow shows that he is off the ground. (*Photograph by Central News, Ltd.*)

into glucose, so that, by this economical chemical arrangement, part of the waste matter of contraction, the lactic acid, can be thus used and re-used in the muscle. Roughly, the other fifth of lactic acid combines with oxygen to form carbon dioxide (CO_2) in solution and water. These chemical changes produce heat (Fig. 98).

When, however, we walk quickly, or run, or crank up a car, or make any continued vigorous series of movements, oxygen cannot be brought fast enough to the muscle cells to oxidise the lactic acid as it is produced. Thus lactic acid accumulates in each muscle cell which has been contracting, and there is an increasing feeling of fatigue. This shows as an increasing urge to stop the movement and as actual pain in the muscles. Any hockey or football player knows the feeling.

In local fatigue, such as in running (Fig. 24), the pain in the muscles rapidly subsides as oxygen reaches the muscle cells in sufficient quantity to change the lactic acid back into glucose. In the course of a normal day's activity, however, fatigue products tend to accumulate throughout the body and a period of relatively prolonged general rest, lying down as in sleep, is necessary for these to be similarly dealt with.

As a result of vigorous muscular effort, the blood also gets charged with carbon dioxide in a much stronger solution than normal, and the nerve centre in the brain that excites quicker and deeper breathing is stimulated by this. We become aware of breathing and, as we say, " out of breath," until the balance of carbon dioxide and oxygen in the blood is again equalised.

How Leverage Helps Movement

The principles of leverage are used when bodily movements are made by the contraction of muscles. A lever is a rigid bar that moves freely on a fixed point, the *fulcrum*, so that if the *effort or power* is applied at one point, a weight can be moved at another point on it. Thus, if a poker is pushed across a bar of a grate under a tightly lodged coal, the bar becomes the fulcrum, the coal the weight, and the downward hand pressure of the person poking, the effort. The fulcrum is similarly between the effort and the weight in see-sawing, in the nodding of the head on the spine, in weighing with a pair of scales, and in opening a box with a chisel. Such levers are of the *first order*.

When the weight is between the effort and the fulcrum, the lever is called a lever of the *second order*. An example is

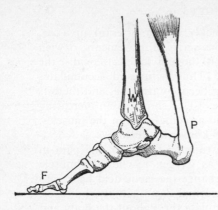

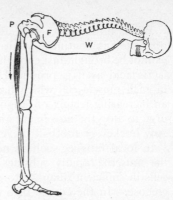

Fig. 25.—The raising of the body on the toe. The toe on the ground is the fulcrum (F), the weight of the body is concentrated at the ankle (W) and the calf muscles supply the power (P) at the heel.

Fig. 26.—The motion of the body on the hips. The hip-joints form the fulcrum (F), the contracting muscles at the back of the legs and thighs the power (P) and the trunk is the weight (W).

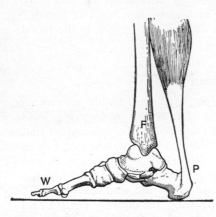

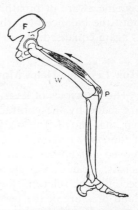

Fig. 27.—Tapping with the toe on the ground. Lift one foot and tap, and the effort is from the calf muscles (P), the fulcrum is the ankle joint (F), and the ground offers resistance (W).

Fig. 28.—Lifting one leg off the ground. The hip-joint is the fulcrum (F), the leg is the weight to be moved (W), and the extensor muscles from the shin bone to the hip are the power or effort (P).

a wheelbarrow. A nut-cracker is a double lever of this second order ; a crowbar when used for lifting a weight, one end of the crowbar being on the ground as the fulcrum, is another example ; a door which is moved by force by the door knob is another ; the body raised on the toes is an example in which the toes are the fulcrum, the weight of the body is concen-

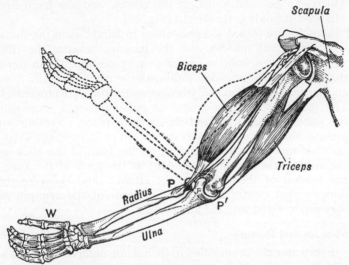

FIG. 29.—The raising or bending of the forearm is an example of a lever of the *third* order. The elbow-joint is the fulcrum (F), the contraction of the biceps gives the effort (P), and the forearm and hand, plus anything held, is the weight (W). This mechanical arrangement gives quick rather than strong movement, unlike levers of the first and second orders. The triceps is the antagonistic muscle to the biceps, extending the arm at the elbow.

trated on the tibia and the effort or power, which lifts the heel, is supplied by the calf muscles (Fig. 25).

In a lever of the *third order* the effort is exerted between the weight and the fulcrum. Coal- and sugar-tongs are examples of double levers of this order. The head of the tongs is the fulcrum, the coal or sugar is the weight and the effort is supplied by the hand of the person using the tongs.

This type of lever gives less mechanical advantage than

do those of the first and second orders in moving heavy weights, but it is a type much more used in the body than any other, because it allows quick, agile movement. In the raising of the forearm by the biceps muscle, in front of the humerus, the elbow is the fulcrum, the tension exerted by the biceps muscle into the forearm just in front of the elbow, which can be readily felt, is the power, and the hand and whatever it holds is the weight (Fig. 29).

Muscles are joined to bones either in bands, as in the sheet-like abdominal muscles and the muscles between the ribs, which give slow wide movement, or by *tendons*, tough fibres that exert all the muscles' pull at the one point on the bone and so make for quicker, stronger and more deft movement. The tenseness of muscle tendons passing over a joint help the joint ligaments to hold the joint in place. Tendons of muscles that move the fingers can be felt in front of the wrist ; the tendon of Achilles, which raises the heel, at the back of the ankle ; the hamstring tendons at the back of the knee ; the tendon of the biceps at the elbow ; and those of the muscles that contract the chest in front of the arm-pit, as they are inserted into the humerus.

Muscles and Posture

Every muscle or muscle-group has an *antagonistic muscle* or group, each, on contracting, producing the opposite movement from its antagonist. Thus there are muscles to bend the fingers and hand up and others to stretch them out, muscles to bend and to extend the leg, to contract and to expand the chest width, to part the knees, fingers and toes and to press them each together.

Muscles that bend the body up, thus generally working with gravity, are called *flexors*, while those that stretch out the fingers and toes and enable the body to stand upright are called *extensors*. On the whole, the flexors are stronger than the extensors, hence some difficulties about maintaining a good posture.

Resting muscles are not fully relaxed. The tension of the skeletal muscles is known as *muscular tone*, which is maintained by the constant equal pulling of antagonistic muscles all over the body. A cold shower stimulates and tightens up the muscles generally, and gives a feeling of extra alertness and briskness, whereas a prolonged hot bath, or staying for long in a hot moist greenhouse atmosphere, slackens the general tenseness of the muscles and makes for lethargy and unwillingness to initiate effort.

In training good posture, the cultivation of a good " *habit* " *length of muscles*, is of great importance. The posture that the body habitually falls into when posture is *not* being thought about consciously, is the result of this habit length of muscles. When any position is held, or any movement is made, impulses keep on streaming out from the brain and spinal cord along the nerves concerned to cause the muscles to contract just the required amount and possibly to continue to do so. It is rather as though, along these nerves, a path leading to the particular movement becomes worn. It

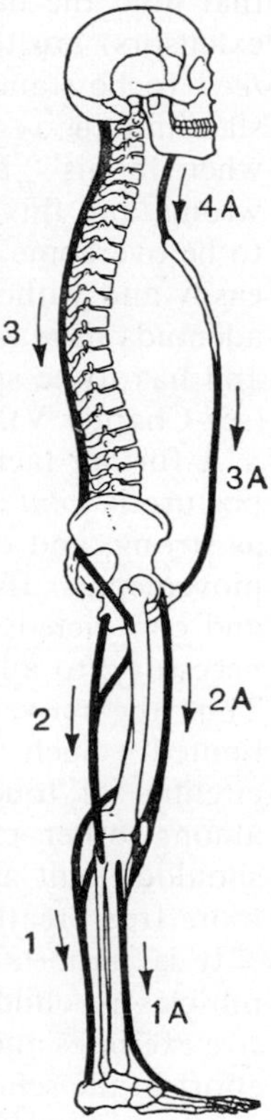

FIG. 30.—Diagram showing the action of the chief muscle-groups which keep the body erect.
Muscles which tend to keep the body from falling forward—1, muscles of calf ; 2, of the back of the thigh ; 3, of the back.
Muscles which tend to keep the body from falling backward—1A, muscles of the front of the leg ; 2A, of the front of the thigh ; 3A, of the abdomen ; 4A, of the front of the neck. The arrows show the direction in which these muscle-groups act. Note their antagonistic arrangement.

becomes increasingly easy for the nerve to convey just that impulse and for the muscles to respond, and soon there is a habit[1] of holding the head on one side, of sitting in a particular way, of standing badly or well, or throwing a ball or of walking with a particular action.

An adolescent who habitually stoops and has a poked head, has, as the result of lack of training, overgrowth, or

[1] These are examples of conditioned reflexes, see Chapter XVI.

lack of confidence or effort, taken to a "habit" length of muscles, so that muscles that contract the chest and bend the head forward are too short and strong, while those that hold the back and head erect, and widen the chest (the extensors) are too stretched and weak. Such an adolescent *feels* to be standing wrongly and to look conspicuous, when standing in a good posture, and inconspicuous and right, when in his "habit" length posture. He feels right when wrong, and this psychological factor is definitely one that has to be overcome even after the correct posture can be assumed easily and without effort. Similarly, an adenoid child, whose adenoids have been removed, feels right with the mouth open and has to be specifically taught to breathe through the nose (see Chapter V).

A further factor to be taken into account in training good posture is *joint stiffness.* The body needs to be agile as well as strong, and over-strong muscles make for slow ponderous movement. If muscles get, from "habit length," too short and contracted, they cannot then stretch out passively when necessary, to allow complete contraction of their antagonists. Thus the movement possible at a particular joint becomes limited. Such much-used exercises as quick single arm circling, or touching the toes with the knees straight, aim, among other effects, at stretching the muscles round the shoulder-joint and the hamstrings respectively, thus allowing more free breathing and lighter walking and running.

It is important then to train good "habit lengths" of muscles in children and adolescents both by definite corrective exercises and by the influence of a continually high tone of effort in the school.

The *value of organised physical training and games* is not just corrective, however. It should (i) encourage free and un-hampered growth, (ii) prevent as well as correct poor posture, (iii) give a positive standard of economical easy posture in standing and walking, and (iv) train agility and deftness of movement, thus lessening confidence-destroying clumsiness.

Games also should give the child the chance to learn and practise courage, the power to hold on as well as other people, to see the value of co-operation and to work with a group, to use initiative on occasion and yet to be willing to support and obey a leader with loyalty. Such effects should be attained by appealing to the strong play spirit that is in all children. The work should not be dull or be made a medium for a high-handed overbearing manner. If people doing exercises do not want to co-operate, the exercise will have but little value.

A *good standing posture* should be easy and effortless, otherwise it is unlikely to be maintained as a habit. The body should be at its full height, with no exaggeration of the lumbar curve, the chest high, the abdominal muscles reasonably retracted, the knees braced back and the weight should be on the balls of the feet as well as the heels, the feet being turned out only to the extent that the closed fist's width can just be touched down between the toes. Such a

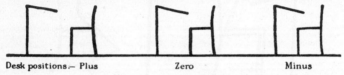

Desk positions.— Plus   Zero   Minus

FIG. 31.—The plus position is the more comfortable for reading, the minus position for writing.

posture is economical of nervous and muscle energy, giving a feeling of mental as well as physical readiness and quiet confidence, which is not that apparent over-confident aggressiveness that is often the result of inward fears and self-doubt.

How to Sit

Everyone should, in *sitting*, sit well back on the seat so that the pelvis and almost the whole length of the thigh is supported by the seat. The sacrum should touch the chair back in sitting and the seat should be such that the whole of the thigh to within a couple of inches of the knee is supported. Desk seats that are only 10 inches wide are not satisfactory. Flat-topped tables are preferable to desks because these allow practical constructive work to be done at them. The sloping desk suggests an undue proportion of book work.

A chair of good shape, separate from the desk, is preferable to a fixed desk, both for posture and for room-cleaning facility. It is of interest to everyone that better mental work is done when the body is sitting upright to a table than when lounging in an arm-chair, because in the upright position the big blood-vessels of the trunk can convey blood about the body and to the brain the more freely.

No desk, however satisfactorily fitted to a particular child, can be otherwise than harmful to posture if periods of con-

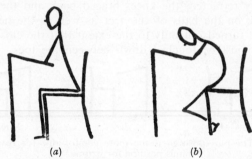

(a)　　　　　　　　　　(b)

FIG. 32.—(a) Economical good *writing position*, with the chair drawn up under the desk, the seat fully supporting the thigh, the feet firmly on the floor, not dangling, and the shoulder weight partly supported by the left arm. (b) Uneconomical bad writing posture. The chair is too far from the desk, and the thighs unsupported. The trunk is cramped and not erect. The chest is contracted, producing round shoulders and increased likelihood of respiratory diseases.

tinued sitting are too long. Tired children, in writing, tend to lean forward so that the chest wall is against the desk edge, which causes pain in the heart and impedes its action detrimentally.

A tired sitting posture means that the eyes are brought too near to the work, causing eye tiredness and loss of interest, and the abdominal organs that in an upright posture are free and unhampered, are congested. This happens in that commonly recurring tired posture in which the child slips the pelvis forward on to the seat until the weight is on the end of the spine. A poked head, also, results.

From the view-point of health and posture, it is a reprehensible practice to make children sit, as a means of bolstering up discipline, with " hands behind " or " hands on heads." The former conduces to the slipping forward of the pelvis on the seat, while the latter confirms and even teaches the holding of a hollow-chested, poked-head position from fatigue.

The only antidote for such harmful sitting posture is to have shorter periods of continued sitting, and very much more

FIG. 33.—Effects of different *sitting postures for reading*. 1, good posture. The chair back is shaped to fit into the lumbar spine. In 2 and 4 the trunk has slipped forward, so that the weight comes increasingly on the end of the spine and the chest and abdominal organs are cramped. Part of the bad effect of 4 is due to the too low chair. In 3, though the body is well back on the seat, the lungs and viscera are probably impeded. (*From Drummond's " School Hygiene " — Edward Arnold & Co.*)

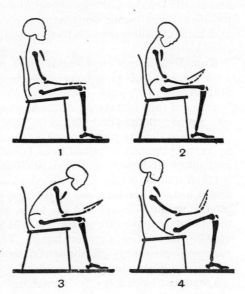

frequently repeated vigorous *relief drills*, for perhaps one or two minutes on end, interspersed during the longer sitting periods, all the windows and doors being wide open. The movements should consist mainly of jumping variations in place (if noise does not distract other groups), trunk bending downward and knee-springing, since these stretch the hamstring muscles shortened by prolonged and unnatural sitting. Arm stretchings alone, are of considerably less value.

Round Shoulders

Round shoulders is the name given to exaggeration of the dorsal curve backwards of the spine. Mechanically it is the result of the heavy weight of organs being in front of and so all pulling on the movable spine. It is caused by overgrowth, particularly if accompanied by poor feeding, too little sleep and fresh air, and overwork out of school hours. Lack of efficient posture training, prolonged sitting in ill-fitting desks, and in the overheated enervating atmosphere to be found in too many classrooms, short-sight, general low muscular tone, and lack of will-power and self-confidence also conduce to round shoulders.

Round shoulders are possibly more prevalent in girls than boys, because girls grow in height earlier than do boys. They also have more out-of-school work to do in helping in the home, and they metabolise calcium, which hardens the bones, less completely than do boys, which may increase the incidence of postural defects for them. The deformity is accompanied by varying degrees of poked head,[1] contracted concave chest, protruding abdomen, and very often the weight in standing is taken mainly on the heels and the knees are bent. Height also is lost. Therefore, one of the first points to work at is to get the weight forward and the knees braced. In any event, this point is a posture matter on which teachers should be insistent in training a correct habit. The attaining of habitual good posture is greatly helped by living in a community where a high standard is assumed.

Treatment consists of stretching contracted muscles, strengthening the weak ones, the extensors, and giving a feeling of right posture, but little ultimate good will result unless the child *wants* to improve, and this attitude must probably come from the teacher's interest and standard.

It is partly for this reason that the wearing of *shoulder straps*, supposed forcibly to pull the shoulders back, is of very doubtful value. The straps also cut into the arm-pit, and the wearer holds the shoulders forward to ease the strain, thus actually

---

[1] If in standing the coat or blouse collar can be felt touching the back of the neck, the head position must be correct and not poked forward.

using and strengthening the very chest-contracting muscles that are already too strong. Actually the direction " shoulders back " is rarely used now, as it conduces to making too pro-

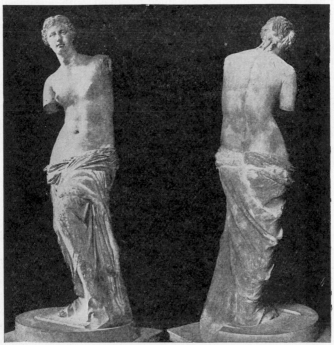

FIG. 34.—*The Venus di Milo statue* shows the effect of standing with the weight " on one leg," the right in the statue. The right hip is over-prominent and the pelvis, as judged by the hip bones, is made uneven. This causes a lateral curve in the spine with the convexity to the left, (see back view). The shoulders also are uneven and height is lost. Habitually to stand thus, particularly during adolescence, from tiredness and overgrowth, or lack of will power, readily causes a spinal curvature that becomes permanent, unless treated by remedial exercises. (*Photographs by Alinari and Giraudon.*)

nounced a waist curve. " Make yourself slender," or any direction to stretch up to the full height, has taken its place. Hump-back is due to collapse of the bodies of the vertebræ. One cause may be tuberculosis. Its incidence is decreasing.

Hollow Back

Hollow back is an exaggeration of the lumbar curve forward. Unlike round shoulders, it may be allied with an upright self-respecting posture, but there is always a loss of height, and the lack of support of the abdominal organs by the pelvic basin makes for ultimate pain and weakness. Overgrown girls carrying younger children, or paper boys carrying a heavy tray slung in front from the shoulders tend to show it. Infants told to walk " like soldiers " produce a hollow back from misplaced over-effort. " Hips firm " was dropped because it produced hollow back. Any form of touching the toes with the knees straight, which makes the lumbar curve concave forward instead of convex, helps to correct hollow back.

Lateral spinal curvature (viewed from the back, not the side) results from overgrowth without compensating nurture, long-continued standing in a poor posture, cramping desks, flat-foot, if one foot is the more affected, and rickets. It may be accompanied by degrees of round shoulders and hollow back. Perhaps the commonest cause in children, and one that the teacher can help to prevent, is that of standing " on one leg," that is, with the weight in standing more on one leg than the other. This often repeated during growth tends to make prominent the right hip, the inclination being to rest more on the right than on the left leg, and often the left shoulder is raised. The Venus di Milo statue viewed from behind shows this.

Growing children, and all children are this, should not be expected to stand for long periods, such as in school assembly or for singing. Walking or running is actually less tiring and conducive to fatigue postures than is continuous standing, because of the alternate contracting and relaxing in walking against the continued contracting of muscles in standing.

All these spinal deviations, if untreated when they first appear, tend to permanent deformity owing to the continued unequal pressure on the inter-vertebral pads of cartilage, which finally become unalterably wedge-shaped, with a consequent deformity of the spine in that region. Such deformities are closely correlated with muscular tone. If tone is high, if games are played, if the child sleeps well, is fed nourishingly and gets plenty of tonic outdoor life, sunlight and bracing cold, such deformities are the less likely to occur, though their possibility cannot of course be entirely eliminated.

It is difficult sharply to divide *muscular fatigue* from mental fatigue. Chemically, the increasing difficulty in getting a muscle to move when it is fatigued is due to the clogging up of the nerve endings in the muscle by fatigue products made by contraction. The brain, which originates the impulse to the muscles to contract, and the nerve along which the impulse travels, are relatively unfatigued, but the stimulus cannot be conveyed to the muscle tissue. A rest, which enables the blood to convert and to remove the excess waste, partially balances matters.

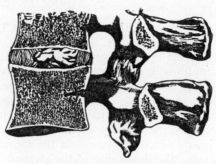

FIG. 35.—Section through lumbar vertebræ, showing an *inter-vertebral disc of cartilage*. The cartilage is elastic, and thus allows of movement of the vertebræ. These discs are compressible, so that at the end of an active day most people are slightly shorter than on first getting up.

Muscular fatigue shows itself independently of the person's feeling of tiredness by increasing slight inaccuracy and spoilt work (see Chapter XVII).

Chapter IV

BLOOD AND CIRCULATION

ALL the interchanges of food and waste in the body that are continually going on with every breath taken or movement made take place through a liquid medium, that is, the blood and the lymph.

The heart pumps the blood round a closed system of vessels, the arteries, capillaries and veins, and so back to the heart, which is situated in the thorax between the two lungs under the lower end of the sternum with the point rather to the left. Actors who clasp their left side to emphasise sentiment are clasping the stomach, not the heart at all.

The heart is a hollow muscular four-chambered pump, which has the power to squeeze itself up so that all the blood in it is pressed out into the vessels and round the body. Then it relaxes, so that blood can run in again. This it does seventy to eighty times a minute in an adult at rest. The two top chambers, called *auricles*, contract first and press the blood into the two lower chambers, the *ventricles*.

Used venous blood enters the right auricle, having been collected up from the veins, and when the auricles contract this blood is forced into the right ventricle ; from here it is propelled into the pulmonary arteries leading to the lungs. In the lungs it takes up oxygen from the air and gives up carbon dioxide, and comes back to the left auricle bright red and charged with oxygen and ready to go round the body ; it is squeezed from here into the left ventricle, whence it leaves the heart by the *aorta*, the largest artery of the body, which soon divides up into arteries to the head, arms, legs and viscera of the abdomen. The left ventricle, because its contraction has to be strong enough to send the blood all over the body, has thicker and more muscular walls than the other

48

three heart chambers. The *pulse*, taken by pressing the fingers (not the thumb, for there is a pulse in that), on any large artery, as that at the thumb side of the wrist, is a record of the wave effect on the blood made by the left ventricle as it contracts.

The blood in the heart is prevented from being squeezed backwards by a system of *valves*, that are mere flaps of skin against the heart wall, as the blood flows from auricle to ventricle, but when the ventricle contracts become bellied out with the pressure of blood, so that they fit together and prevent any blood from passing back into the auricle. Thin tough cords attached to the inner heart wall hold the ends of the flaps so that they fit together. Similarly, working valves, but without cords, prevent blood from regurgitating backward from the left auricle into the lungs. If these valves become defective owing to strain or infectious disease, a doctor, in testing the heart, can hear the

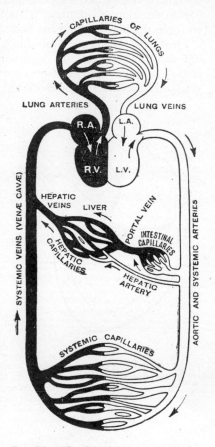

FIG. 36.—*The Circulation of the blood.* R.A. and L.A.—Right and left auricles ; R.V. and L.V.—right and left ventricles. The hepatic artery and vein carry blood to and from the liver. The significance of the portal vein is discussed in connection with digestion. The " black " vessels show those carrying deoxygenated blood, the " white " oxygenated blood.

sounds of regurgitating blood, and this means that the heart has to do more work than it should normally at each beat to force the blood round the body.

The heart sounds are " lub-dub " followed by a rest, that is, the auricles contract, the ventricles contract and the heart rests. In infants the heart-beat may be 140 a minute, but this gradually decreases throughout life.

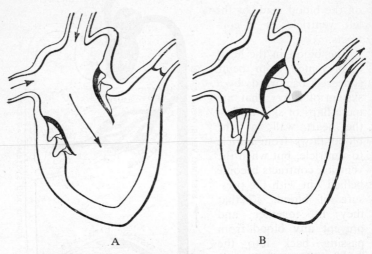

A   B

FIG. 37.—*How the valves of the heart act.* In A, the heart is relaxed, and blood flows freely from the auricles to the ventricles, the valves being flaccid. Note, however, that those leading from the ventricles are closed. In B, when the ventricles contract, the tough cords that hold the valve flaps are stretched and the flaps fit accurately together. Blood is thus forced out of the heart.

Arteries are vessels with thick elastic muscular walls the resiliency of which helps to force the blood along them. " A man is as old as his arteries " refers to the gradual loss of this elasticity. The blood in an artery is oxygenated (except in the artery that takes de-oxygenated blood from the right ventricle to the lungs), and always it flows away from the heart. If a large artery is cut, blood spurts out in rhythmic jets, and if vigorous pressure is not put on the heart side of the wound immediately, death follows from loss of blood—in the case of the large thigh artery in 90 seconds and in the upper arm artery in 120 seconds only.

Arteries are usually well protected by bones so that they are the less likely to be injured. The brachial artery can be felt on the inner side of the humerus deep under the biceps muscle; the femoral artery is on the inner side of the thigh; the two arteries of the wrist are on the inner sides of the radius and ulna respectively, and the finger arteries travel up the sides of the fingers (see Fig. 165, p. 147).

The larger arteries branch off into smaller and smaller vessels until they merge into the thin-walled *capillaries*, or hairlike vessels, which form a network all over the body, except in cartilage. The muscles and organs contain a sponge-like mesh of capillaries, and in them the blood, because of the increasing drag on the

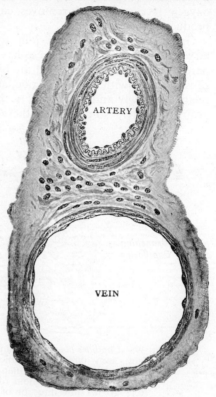

FIG. 38.—Transverse section of a small *artery and vein*. The artery has stiffened yet resilient muscular walls, the contraction of which helps on the flow of blood. The vein walls are thin and comparatively flaccid, and do not actively hasten the blood's flow. Magnified about 250 diameters. (*By permission of Sir E. Sharpey-Schafer.*)

sides of the vessel walls, flows more slowly, and through the very thin capillary walls the business of the blood is done.

By osmosis and diffusion, the blood delivers the food and oxygen it carries, and removes carbon dioxide and waste products.

Gradually the capillaries join together into increasingly larger vessels, the *veins*. These have thin flaccid walls compared to those of arteries, and the blood, now " impure " because charged with carbon dioxide, and darker coloured, flows relatively slowly and pulselessly in them. The flow is mainly against gravity ; so as a help, there are at frequent intervals

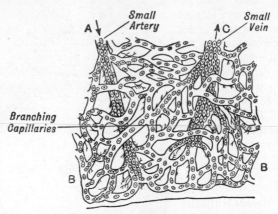

FIG. 39.—*Capillary blood-vessels* in the web of a frog's foot, seen through the microscope. The small artery (A) breaks up into many branching capillaries (B) ; which eventually join to form the small vein (C) ; arrows show direction of flow.

little flaps of skin, the *valves*, that, as in the heart, lie limp against the vessel wall as long as the blood flows towards the heart. If for any cause, such as lengthy standing, the flow is retarded, the flaps fill with blood and come into position, thus preventing further back flow.

In *varicose veins* these valves are over-strained, due to prolonged standing, to the wearing of tight garters or knickers, or to continued pressure on the big veins of the trunk, as in chronic constipation or in pregnancy ; thus they degenerate and fail to function. Prevention by sleeping with the foot of the bed raised 3 or 4 inches to facilitate back flow of blood at night is of value, as is resting during the day with the feet up. Treatment by injection of quinine into the degenerated veins is now used successfully as a partial cure.

As the flow of blood in the veins is slower, there are roughly two sets of veins, a deep and a superficial, to each set of arteries. The veins finally join up to pour their blood into the

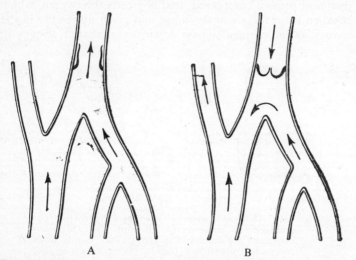

A   B

FIG. 40.—*Diagram of veins*, A, with valve open; B, with valve closed. By pressing on a superficial vein, the knotting at the valves on the side *away* from the heart can quickly be seen. It is such valves that deteriorate in varicose veins.

right auricle. Muscular contractions help the venous flow by squeezing blood out and along them, whereas arteries cannot be so compressed. Thus, while used blood is squeezed out of a muscle, oxygenated blood can continually come in to take its place.

The Fluid Medium—The Blood

Blood is made up of a colourless salty-tasting *plasma*, in which is dissolved or carried a number of differing amino-acids, gases, mineral salts, urea and other substances, and in which float red and white corpuscles. There are about ten pints in the body.

The *red corpuscles*, red in mass but yellow individually under a microscope, are bi-concave discs of a smallness that 5,000,000 are contained in a drop of blood the size of a pin's head. In such a drop there would be about 10,000 white corpuscles. The red corpuscles have in them a substance *hæmoglobin*, an iron and protein compound, that is greedy for oxygen, which is taken from the air in the lungs and given up readily in the tissues, as the corpuscles pass down the capillaries, usually in

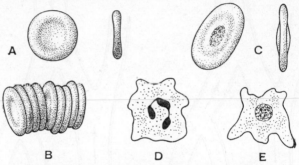

FIG. 41.—The *red corpuscles* are regularly shaped and arranged in rouleaux (A, B and C). The *white corpuscles* are amœboid in shape (D). E is a white corpuscle from frog's blood. (*From Hentschel and Cook, " Biology for Medical Students "—Longmans.*)

single file. In the mass the red corpuscles tend to fit themselves together in rouleaux rather as biscuits might.

A red corpuscle may travel as much as a mile in a day, and it is estimated that a drop of blood circulates round the body at rest, and back to the heart again in 15 to 25 seconds. Red corpuscles are not strictly alive because they have no nucleus, and it is because of this lack that their life is only about six weeks. They are made in the bone marrow and destroyed in the spleen, and the liver uses their waste matter to colour the bile and urine their green and yellow.

The hæmoglobin of the red corpuscles very readily unites with the gas, *carbon monoxide*. This gas is given out from motor exhausts, is present in ordinary coal-gas and may be generated by stoves or geysers with faulty flues. It is also absorbed in small but increasingly harmful quantities in inhaling tobacco smoke. It is the "fire damp" of mines. Carbon monoxide prevents the red corpuscles from taking up oxygen, thus leading to dizziness and *malaise* and, if sufficient is inhaled, to unconsciousness and death.

There are at least six different kinds of *white corpuscles* or *leucocytes*, which are colourless, relatively formless masses of protoplasm with a nucleus, and capable of active movement, rather like the amœba. They are considerably larger than red corpuscles. Their work is to protect the body against disease germs. Directly a wound is made in the skin, additional white corpuscles are summoned to the site to resist the germs of sepsis, that are always present on the skin, when they try to make entry.

White Blood Corpuscles

Some white corpuscles appear to give out granules that paralyse the germs, after which others, called *phagocytes* or eating cells, engulf and eat the quiescent germs. The bacteria, however, give out toxin or poison that if strong enough kills the white corpuscles, which are, as it were, pushed into the rear rank by other white corpuscles, who go on fighting. The dead bodies of white corpuscles are got rid of as pus, or matter. The application of an antiseptic, such as iodine, helps the fight by making conditions less favourable for the invading germs.

If the battle is prolonged, and the patient suffers disquiet and pain, inflammation has occurred. Hot applications, such as fomentations, are then applied to draw more blood to the part and so hurry on and shorten the fight. Some white corpuscles have the power to pass through the thin capillary walls into the surrounding tissues, others probably manufacture antitoxins to counteract the specific poisons or toxins that germs make.

Opsonins present in the plasma are a kind of sauce to the white corpuscles. They make the corpuscles more active and the germs less powerful. The opsonic index

3

of an individual's blood can be measured for specific diseases. *Agglutinins*, also present in the plasma, cause germs to stick close together, thus helping the white corpuscles to attack.

The body is protected from excessive loss of blood at injury by *the forming of a clot* over the site of the wound. In the blood-plasma is a protein, *fibrinogen* or fibrin, that on exposure

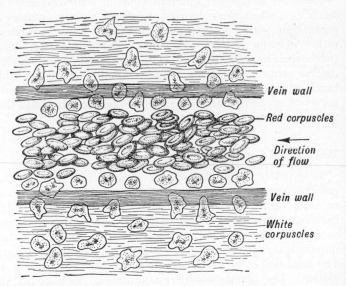

Fig. 42.—The *migration of white corpuscles* from a small vein. The arrow shows the direction of flow. It is to be noted, in contrast, that in a capillary the red corpuscles can usually pass only in single file.

to air rapidly takes the form of a network of jelly strands, which catches the corpuscles in it and tends to dry up, stopping the bleeding and protecting the injured part, until eventually new skin has grown together beneath it. *Blood platelets*, which are smaller than either kind of corpuscle, appear to be concerned with clotting and with the production of immunity.

The Work of the Lymph System

In addition to the blood transport system, there is also a system of *lymph-vessels and glands*, permeating all the tissues. Lymph is a colourless watery fluid, that very obviously does not possess so much power to clot as does blood, as is seen when the skin is grazed slightly and lymph and not blood exudes. Capillary vessels form a network among cells, but the cells are actually bathed in lymph. To it, by osmosis, is delivered up much waste material to be finally taken away by the blood-stream. In the course of the lymph-vessels are enlargements, the *lymph-glands*, through which the lymph flows. In these glands, poisonous matter collected from the tissues is rendered harmless, and white corpuscles, that are made here, are added to the lymph stream. They are examples of ductless glands (see Chapter XV).

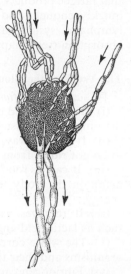

FIG. 43.—*A lymphatic gland and lymph-vessels.* Arrows show direction of flow. The many valves give the beaded look to the vessels.

There are specially numerous groups of lymph-glands under the arm-pit, in the groin and down the front of the neck. Sometimes, if there is a septic injury on the hand, the lymph-glands in the arm-pit become hard, painful and swollen. They are having more toxin than they can deal with comfortably. Poisons from decayed teeth may drain down to the lymphatic glands in the neck, causing pain and swelling and eventually even tubercular abscess if the gland becomes too much overtaxed. Such swollen glands should never be rubbed or poulticed, for to do so only tends to disseminate and stir up the poison there. It has been said that the difference between the circulation of the lymph and of the blood is comparable to the difference between stagnant marsh water and a river flowing between banks.

The frog has lymph hearts, but in man the circulation of lymph is maintained by movement in the vessels caused by muscular contraction, and helped by valves in the lymph-vessels. Any active exercise, as skipping, stimulates lymph movement, and this adds to the general feeling of well-being, because a comparatively stagnant lymph circulation means that fatigue products, such as lactic acid, are not being removed quickly enough, and a heavy lethargic feeling results. The lymphatic system also enters largely into digestion and absorption (see Chapter VII).

The Work of the Blood

To sum up, the *functions of the blood* are these :

(i) It takes round oxygen in the red blood-corpuscles from the lungs to the tissues ;

(ii) It brings away, dissolved in the plasma, carbon dioxide to be got rid of from the lungs and skin ;

(iii) It carries food to build up tissues and to serve as fuel to maintain the body temperature and to supply muscles with energy ;

(iv) It removes waste products of muscular contraction, such as lactic acid and urea ;

(v) The white corpuscles defend the body against harmful organisms and their toxins ;

(vi) Fibrinogen causes blood to clot ;

(vii) The blood conveys material from which glands prepare their secretions, internal and external ; and

(viii) It distributes and equalises heat all over the body, acting as a hot-water pipe system.

It is essential to recognise that the blood is continually having its chemical balance disturbed, whereon it rights itself only to be disturbed again ; every breath, every meal, every movement does this in some degree.

The Heart

The heart rests briefly after each beat, but its most complete rest is obtained in bed. The horizontal position of the body allows the heart to do its work more easily in not having to work against gravity, and gradually slows down its rate of beating by as much as from five to ten beats a minute. Sitting slows the rate slightly, while standing gives a faster pulse, and rapid exertion will increase its rate by twenty-five or more beats a minute. The test of heart muscle tone is to note the speed with which the pulse becomes normal again after specific vigorous exercise. Thus, roughly, if the pulse is not back to its normal rate at the end of five minutes, the heart muscle is definitely less efficient than it should be.

The heart muscle, as all other muscles, only maintains the strength and resiliency for which a daily normal demand is made. Thus anyone who ordinarily lives a sedentary sub-active physical life at office work, and on a holiday starts on the first day a heavy mountain climbing expedition, is likely to get a strained, that is dilated, heart. The muscle, asked to stand the unusual strain of pumping six or seven gallons of blood through it in a minute, instead of about a gallon, is a little like old elastic, and may be over-stretched by the effort. This is more likely to occur after than before thirty, for young muscle tissue is the more elastic. Reasonable training and regular moderate exercise helps to avoid the danger of straining the heart.

The supply of blood to the different organs varies according to use and stimulus. The arteries are controlled by nerves, and havè, as it were, stop-cocks that can order their bore to dilate, as occurs in sudden blushing, or to contract, as in people who go pale with anger, pain or cold. Such stop-cock mechanism, however, is not mainly influenced by such emotions or cold.

Mental work increases the supply of blood to the brain, while during sleep the supply is less. To read a detective novel last thing at night is to keep the brain working and so well supplied with blood and over-active for sleep. After a heavy meal there is an extra supply of blood to the stomach walls, and this is not the time for attempting mental work. When playing foot- or net-ball, additional blood is drawn to the leg and trunk muscles. The use of any part of the body, in fact, entails an automatic increase in its blood supply.

Fainting

Fainting is unconsciousness due to lack of blood in the brain. This shortage may result from shock, heart strain, hæmorrhage or severe pain. Some people are apt to faint as a result of prolonged standing : walking does not induce fainting.

Fainting in women, owing possibly to looser corsets and the robuster value that is placed on positive health, is less prevalent than formerly. Heroines of the more modern novels more often react to emotional shock by being reflexly sick than by fainting. Anyone who feels faint should lean forward with the head between the knees to get the blood back to the head. The onset of a faint can often partly be controlled by the will not to give way.

To restore a person who has fainted, lay the patient down flat, lifting the legs to help the return of blood to the brain, undo tight clothing, open windows and doors, and send away crowding spectators. Only after consciousness has returned should a stimulant be given. Black coffee is better than alcohol, and sal volatile is useful. Treat for shock by keeping the patient warm and quiet, but avoid fussing.

Anæmia

Anæmia is a condition in which there is deficiency in the number of red blood corpuscles or of hæmoglobin in the actual corpuscles. There is thus difficulty in getting oxygen to the tissues, and an anæmic person becomes breathless on slight exertion. The hæmoglobin content of the blood can be measured, and, in anæmia, may be only 80 per cent., or even as low as 60 per cent. of the normal.

Red blood corpuscles are manufactured in the bone marrow and after three weeks destroyed in the liver, and in normal health a balance of supply is maintained.

Anæmia may be caused by too little iron due to faulty diet, by excessive destruction of red corpuscles, as in malaria, or by interference with the manufacture of corpuscles in the bone marrow. This last may be because of toxins given off from bacterial action, for example, from some chronic inflammation such as an abscess or from the organisms that cause rheumatism. Anæmia is also associated with shortage of Vitamin C in the diet.

Sedentary living (with late hours), too little sleep (possibly in a stuffy room), too little fresh air, sunlight and exercise, and the presence of decayed and neglected teeth, all conduce to anæmia.

The cause must be found and treated. An iron tonic is usual, but treatment by medicine is often only an adjunct to the drastic and often unwelcome reform of bad health habits. Change to a healthier environment, relief from worry, the stopping of carious teeth, and a diet of nourishing, well-cooked food of satisfactory vitamin content are all useful.

Heart Disease in Children

Acquired Heart Disease in children is often an after-effect of rheumatism, chorea or scarlet fever, and so-called valvular disease of the heart results.

Inflammation of any of the four valves may cause thickening so that the opening of the valve is narrowed or *stenosed*, and the free passage of the blood through the heart is obstructed. When, for example, the mitral valve is affected the patient is said to have *mitral stenosis*.

Inflammation may also damage the heart valves so that a valve does not close completely and blood flows the wrong way, that is from a ventricle *back* into an auricle. This is termed regurgitation.

Fortunately the heart has the power of *compensation*, that is of adapting itself to these impaired conditions so that, in a good proportion of cases, the one-time patient can go through life without continuing to experience any symptoms of the defect.

(See Chapter XXX—Rheumatism).

CHAPTER V

THE LUNGS AND BREATHING

AIR is a mixture of colourless gases. Everyone has seen the effect of its movement in a flickering candle-flame, and felt it when walking or cycling against the wind. Its pressure is roughly 15 lb. to the square inch and is exerted equally in all directions. In blowing up a tyre or a football, air is forced in till the pressure inside is greater than the pressure of the air outside.

Chemically, air is roughly one-fifth oxygen, four-fifths nitrogen. It also contains small varying quantities of carbon dioxide and water vapour. Floating about in the air are dust (particles of wool and cotton fibre, road grit, soot, skin scales), and bacteria, harmless and harmful. A beam of sunlight shining into a room lights up only the larger particles of dust which continually float around us (see Fig. 163, p. 411).

How the Lungs do their Work

The active constituent of air that nearly all living things must have is oxygen. Three minutes without it is sufficient to cause death. The body continually needs to take in fresh oxygen and to give up carbon dioxide. *The lungs*, where this interchange between the blood and air takes place, are two spongy bags that fill up the chest or thorax cavity. The thorax is divided from the abdominal cavity below by the *diaphragm*, a concave sheet of muscle, that is, dome-shaped, attached to the bottom of the sternum and all round the lower ribs, the rib cartilages, and the vertebral column. The remains of sheep's diaphragms can often be seen in the carcases in butchers' shops.

When it contracts the diaphragm gets flatter, pressing down on the abdominal organs, the liver, stomach and intestines, below it. It is impossible to lie flat on one's back and breathe in without the abdominal muscles rising, and this is due to the diaphragm that is pushing the abdominal contents forward and upward.

62

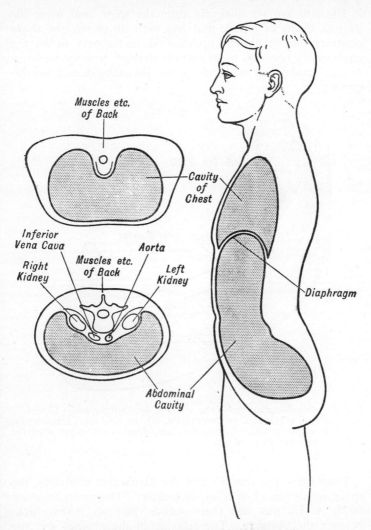

FIG. 44.—*The body cavities.* (*After Campbell.*)

3*

The ribs are set obliquely from the spine, and when the narrow sheets of muscle that join each rib to the one above contract, they lift the ribs up, each one on the next, so that the chest cavity becomes wider and the sternum is raised forward. It is possible to put the hands on the ribs each side and feel this effect.

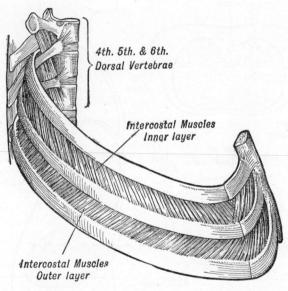

FIG. 45.—The diagram shows the *sheets of intercostal muscles* (2 and 3), some of which can, on contracting, lift the ribs apart transversely, thus widening and enlarging the chest, whereas others can draw the ribs together to expel air.

Thus when the ribs lift and the diaphragm contracts, the space inside the chest is made greater. The pressure of air inside it is thus less than outside, and air rushes in to balance the pressure. The relaxing of the muscles and the contracting of antagonistic intercostal and abdominal muscle, squeezes the lungs and forces the air out again. This drawing in of air by the piston action of the diaphragm is characteristic of mammals. The frog, having no diaphram muscle, has to swallow at each breath, a less efficient method.

Through all this the lungs are quite passive. They are enclosed in serous lubricating membranes, the *pleura*. Compare the synovia in which joints work, and the engine oil of a motor-car. Pleurisy is a condition of inflammation of the pleura which causes the production of too much fluid and sharp pain on breathing.

In judging chest capacity, it is the difference between the measurement of the chest when inflated and when deflated that is important. If the chest circumference is taken around the widest part with the chest first deflated, that is, after breathing out, and then with the chest completely inflated, after breathing in, a difference of from 2 to 3 inches shows a fair amount of chest mobility.

The Larynx and Voice

Air should be drawn in through the nose, where it is cleaned, warmed and moistened ; it passes down the back of the throat to the *glottis*, the opening at the top of the *larynx*, or voice-box, which can be felt high up under the chin. The glottis has a small stiff flap, the *epiglottis*, that is usually open, but, in the mechanism of swallowing, guides the food smoothly to the glottis dividing the bolus like a ship's prow, thus preventing food from passing down into the lungs (see diagram, p. 92).

Across the cartilaginous larynx or voice-box stretch the *vocal cords*, two curtains of tissue, not cord-like, which are relaxed and leave a wide opening in quiet breathing, but which are tensed up by connecting muscles, to leave only a narrow slit, when words are spoken with voice. Whispers are sounds formed in the mouth only, by the lips and tongue, without the force of breathed-out air behind them.

The larynx in man is bigger and more prominent than in woman, and the vocal cords are longer and so give a lower tone. Low tones, for men and women, are less tiring for continued speaking, as in teaching and preaching, than are shrill ones. Physical training commands, particularly, should not be high-pitched. Much loss of voice in inexperienced teachers is due to faulty over-effortful voice production.

The air passes from the larynx down the *trachea or windpipe*, which can be felt, with its incomplete cartilaginous rings that stiffen it, minimising the possibility of suffocation by compression. It divides into two stiffened tubes, the bronchi, one

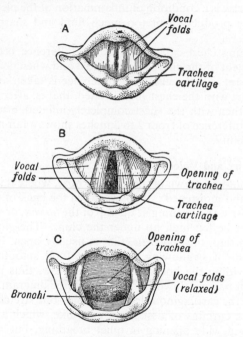

FIG. 46.—Three laryngoscopic views of *the larynx and vocal folds* with the glottis almost closed: A, as when singing a high note; B, during easy breathing; and C, during the taking of a deep breath.

to each lung. These divide again and again until they end in millions of tiny air-sacs, called *alveoli*, with transparently thin walls, through the substance of which pass numberless capillary blood vessels.

The branching of the bronchi has been likened to the branching of a tree, with the leaves representing the alveoli.

The smallest branches—the bronchioli—are of a diameter only wide enough to allow a fine needle to pass down them.

All these air passages are ringed with involuntary muscle fibres that regulate the amount of air that passes down them, more or less, so that all parts of the lung tissue are used.

Better than deep breathing exercises is vigorous activity —running and skipping—that makes the runner out of breath and the breathing quicker and deeper so that all parts of the lungs are filled with fresh cool air.

So thin is the membrane between the air in the air-sac and the blood passing through the capillaries, that the interchange of oxygen and carbon dioxide can readily take place here. The lung surface shows the body's economical packing. The surfaces of the alveoli if spread out flat would cover an area half the size of a tennis-court, and the capillaries bringing blood to this relatively immense surface, put end to end, would be long enough to stretch across the Atlantic for 3000 miles. This relatively large area enables the body quickly to get extra oxygen to the tissues for vigorous movement. Contrast the slowness of the snail with its relatively tiny lung.

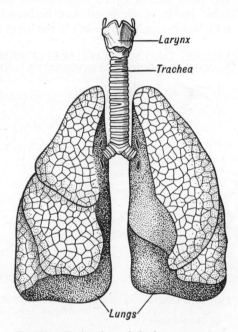

FIG. 47.—Front view of *the larynx, trachea and lungs*. Note the space in the left lung into which the heart fits.

In quiet *tidal breathing*, some 30 cubic inches are breathed in and out. In breathing in as deeply as possible, a further 100 cubic inches of air, spoken of as *complemental air*, can be added. In breathing out as deeply as possible, the complemental and the 30 cubic inches of tidal air can be expelled and a further 100 cubic inches, called *supplemental air*, that is, roughly 230 cubic inches of air in all, can be breathed out. There must still, however, always be left in the lungs some 120 cubic inches

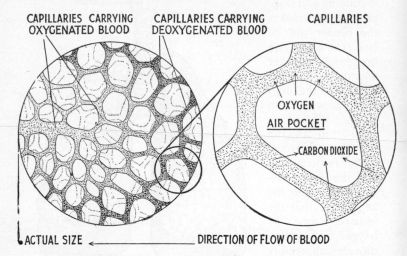

CAPILLARIES CARRYING OXYGENATED BLOOD   CAPILLARIES CARRYING DEOXYGENATED BLOOD   CAPILLARIES

OXYGEN
AIR POCKET
CARBON DIOXIDE

ACTUAL SIZE ⟵————————— DIRECTION OF FLOW OF BLOOD

FIG. 48.—Diagram to illustrate the exchange of gases in the Air Pockets of the Lungs. (*From " Looking at Life," by Clark and G. Buckland Smith—Dent.*)

of *residual air* that cannot normally be expelled, but it is sometimes partially forced out, as when one is " winded " by a fall, which causes discomfort until the air-balance has righted itself again.

The air in the lungs is continually moving to and from the alveoli and being mixed up, so that the air taken in one breath is unlikely to be the same air that is breathed out in the breath immediately following. Thus though the amount of residual air is constant, the content of it is continually changing. The quiet breathing rate is about eighteen times a minute.

The walls of the respiratory passages are lined with mucous membrane, which is covered with hair-like *cilia*, that keep up a constant ordered rhythmical movement of themselves, with the force directed from the lungs towards the mouth and nose. Thus any foreign particles that are not caught by the nasal mucous membrane, when they get on to the mucus-lubricated cilia are moved back toward the nose, rather as if they were on a moving staircase.

A cold causes clogging of the cilia with extra mucus, which the body tries to get rid of by sharp reflex blasts of air, a cough or a sneeze. Germs that penetrate to the alveoli are likely to be killed by the white corpuscles. In spite of the work of the nose and cilia, it is possible to tell that a man has worked in a mine or lived in a city by the deposit of black particles that make the lung tissue look darker than normal.

Droplet Infection

The air breathed out at each breath has less oxygen and more carbon dioxide than ordinary inspired air. Were it not that green plants in the light continually take carbon dioxide from the air and give out oxygen, the proportion of these gases in the air would be rapidly altered. Exhaled air is also warm and full of droplets of moisture, as can be recognised by breathing out on one's hand or on the cold desk surface. On a frosty day these droplets condense in the cold air and little clouds mark each breath. In these droplets of moisture, that everyone continually breathes out, are the micro-organisms of colds, or of any kindred infection that anyone in the room may happen to have.

In an unventilated room, inverted cone-shapes of hot, moist, breathed-out air rise from each person to mix, cool and descend again to be re-breathed. Open windows allow this used and possibly germ-laden air to be carried away and fresh cool air to take its place. In a closed room full of people, or in a crowded bus or train, the air will tend to be breathed and re-breathed, and the relative amount of moisture and of droplets containing germs gets continually higher. There is markedly too much moisture in room air when it is seen to condense on the cold window-panes and run down the glass.

Most common colds and influenza infections are caught

thus indoors from breathing in infected droplets or dust in sufficient doses. Thus if an infectious patient were visited and the visitor sat in a current of air between the open window and fireplace, and some feet from the patient, he would breathe in a smaller dosage of germs than if he sat near the patient in a room with a closed window and no fireplace.

Air can be breathed in through either the nose or the open mouth, but the healthy way to breathe for quiet tidal breathing is both in and out through the nose. The bones inside the nose are folded over like scrolls to make a larger area

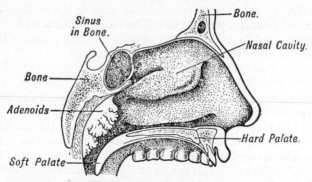

FIG. 49.—Position in which *adenoids* grow when they occur. They readily block the passage of air from the back of the nose to the throat, thus causing mouth breathing. Note the scroll-like, mucus-covered bones, over which air passes, in the nose.

of warm viscid mucous membrane over which air must pass on its way to the lungs. The back of the two nasal passages, which are divided by the septum, opens into the throat above the soft palate, which can be felt with the tongue by following the hard palate back till it feels soft.

Communicating with the nasal cavities are mucus-lined spaces in the facial bones call *sinuses*. These make the bones lighter for their size and probably improve the voice tone. It is because of the possibility of forcing up infective material, such as mucus laden with bacteria, into these cul-de-sac sinuses, that vigorous nose blowing and douching by sniffing fluids up the nose are practices now looked on with some doubt.

If breathing is done through the mouth, the air is not warmed and cleaned, and the cold air continually strikes on the teeth, the contrast between hot and cold tending to crack the enamel. Only after active exercise, when the body is trying to rid itself of carbon dioxide rapidly, should breathing be done with the mouth open.   Note the characteristic oxygen-shortage expression of runners at the end of a sprint (see Fig. 24, p. 34).

Adenoids

If a child, through continually catching colds, or sleeping, mouth open, gets into the habit of breathing with its mouth open, there is a tendency for the too - little - used nasal passages to become stopped up by the growth of *adenoids* at the back of the nose, above the soft

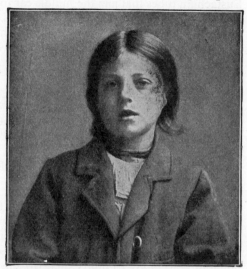

Fig. 50.—The expression typical of a child with adenoids.

palate. These feel like soft, grape-like masses of tissue, and a child having adenoids ceases to be able to breathe except through the mouth, and presents an increasingly characteristc physical appearance.

The mouth is habitually held open, and the vacant expression thus produced is enhanced because the loss of tone in the muscles between the lip musculature and the lower eyelid, causes the eyelid to ride up over the eyeball, giving a characteristically veiled appearance.   The bridge of the nose, that should develop from a baby to an adult-form nose at about five years of age, fails to develop through lack of use ; it remains depressed and the nose is over-*retroussé*.   The voice is toneless.

A child with adenoids constantly catches colds, and does not get as much air into the lungs and oxygen round the body as would a normal breather, and so is slow and dull in development and often pale and pasty in complexion.

This dullness is accentuated by the deafness that results from the adenoids pressing on and partially closing the two Eustachian tubes that join the middle ear to the throat, opening into it just at the back of the nasal passages. Adenoids tend to disappear of themselves at puberty, but their disabling effects persist throughout life. Early treatment is essential.

The Tonsils

With adenoids, *tonsils* are coupled. These are two masses of lymphoid tissue that can be seen, if the mouth is held open widely, at the back of the throat, the uvula of the soft palate pendulous between and in front of them. The tonsils act as scavengers to the alimentary canal and respiratory tract. They partly atrophy by ten years of age.

In many people they are healthy, but if, as the result of colds, after-effects of infectious disease, bad teeth or a tendency to rheumatism, they become septic, it may be considered necessary for them to be enucleated, that is, completely removed. Underlying causes of tonsil and adenoid defects are (i) faulty diet, (ii) unsatisfactory housing, (iii) bad hygiene of the mouth and nose and dental disease. Such conditions must be remedied.

One reason among others for the removal of persistently septic tonsils is that septic matter has a tendency to make its way up the Eustachian tube to the middle ear, causing the formation of an abscess with accompanying pain and possibly permanent deafness. Defective tonsils are also connected with the onset of rheumatism (see Chapter XXX).

A mouth-breather, after an operation for the removal of adenoids, feels right with his mouth open, and has to be trained by breathing exercises and the incentive of personal interest in his progress to breathe through the nose, as well as to say *m*, *n* and *ng* through the nose. Children who have handkerchiefs, and are encouraged to use them properly, are the less inclined to become mouth-breathers. Infants' schools can do valuable health work by setting a tone that demands

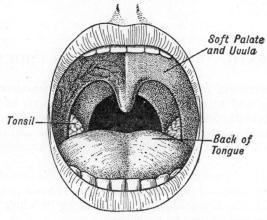

Soft Palate
and Uuula

Tonsil

Back of
Tongue

FIG. 51.—View of the back of the throat, showing the tonsils. When examining the throat, the child may be told to say " Ah " to get the tongue flat.

that each child shall have a handkerchief or rag, and use it. A child with the upper lip covered with mucus may well be considered a reflection of and on the school standard.

CHAPTER VI

VENTILATION—SUNLIGHT AND SMOKE

THE problems of ventilation were at one time considered to be chemical, and to depend on the relative amounts of oxygen and carbon dioxide in the air, but they are now recognised to be physical, and to relate to the problem of allowing the body to lose heat continually without being uncomfortably chilled.

In solid substances, such as metal, heat is distributed by the heat of one particle heating the next one. Thus a poker with one end in the fire gradually gets hot along its whole length. This is termed heating by *conduction.*

Gases and liquids expand when heated, becoming lighter so that they tend to rise, and thus the place of the heated air or liquid is continuously taken by cooler gas or liquid, that is in its turn heated. In this way currents, called convection currents, are set up, and this method of heating is termed heating by *convection.* Note that the outlets for air are usually at the top of a room, and windows on the whole are opened at the top to let the heated rising air escape. Hot-water pipes heat the air in a room by convection.

The sun, gas, coal and electric fires heat by *radiation*, that is, the objects round are heated without the heating of the intervening air. This is the healthiest form of heating.

How the Body Loses Heat

The temperature of the body is normally about $98 \cdot 4°$ F., whereas the air temperature in a dwelling-room is usually kept at from $55°$ to $60°$ F. Thus the body is considerably warmer than the air around it, and to be comfortable must keep on losing heat. This is done by the continual breathing out of warm air from the lungs and by loss of heat from the skin's surface, five-sixths of the body's lost heat being lost thus.

74

The *skin loses heat* in two ways : (i) by convection, that is, by heating of air next to it which rises to be replaced by cooler air which is again heated ; and (ii) by the evaporation from its surface of perspiration. The fact that liquids use heat up when they evaporate can be recognised elsewhere : for example, hot water splashed on a stocking feels cold as it dries : scent, which evaporates quickly, feels markedly cool on the skin as does petrol.

All over the skin surface are openings of sweat glands, popularly known as pores. The tissue just below the skin is richly supplied with blood, and capillaries interlace the coiled-up reservoir of the sweat glands (see Fig. 81, p. 150), which extract water, with some salts dissolved in it, from the blood. Thus the gland gradually becomes fuller until the sweat escapes on to the skin, where it dries up or is soaked up by clothing. The acid smell of sweat is due to the 2 per cent. of urine salts in it.

Even when the body is quiet or the weather cold, perspiration is always being exuded, but not quickly enough for visible beads to form, as happens after vigorous movement, or when in an over-hot atmosphere, as a hot-house or a cinema.

Heat is generated in the body by slow combustion, that is, the oxidation of food, and by muscular movement. Hence the body temperature would rise above $98 \cdot 4°$ F. if the surplus heat were not got rid of. To effect this, more blood goes to the skin, which becomes flushed and warm, and perspiration takes place, that is, the sweat glands empty and re-empty themselves. The extra heat is lost by the drying up of this moisture. Normally, about one pint of water is lost in a day by perspiration. This is often increased to five or six pints by moderate exercise on a warm day.

Heat is also lost through the mucous membrane which lines the air passages. This is kept taut and stimulated if cool dry air is breathed in. Its lymph circulation is active, bringing anti-bodies to destroy invading germs, the lymph being rapidly re-absorbed and drained away. Oxygen is readily absorbed through the capillary walls in the membranes, allowing satisfactory oxygenation of the blood. Heat and moisture are got rid of in breathing out.

If, however, the air breathed in is hot and moist, as in an ill-ventilated room, evaporation from the respiratory membranes lining the lungs is slow ; the membrane is flaccid and comparatively clogged ; the lymph moves sluggishly upon it. The blood obtains less oxygen, germs are not destroyed efficiently, and resistance to the attack of cold and other germs is lessened.

When loss of heat is too slow, foods making heat in the body, carbohydrates and fats mainly, are used up over-slowly. Their incompletely metabolised products circulate in the blood as harmful toxins, instead of being of use. The whole rate of metabolism of the body is in fact affected adversely by a hot stuffy atmosphere that prevents heat loss.

Ill-effects of a Stuffy Room

The *ill-effects of a stuffy room,* then, are due to the physical properties of the atmosphere, (i) too high a temperature, (ii) too much moisture in the air, (iii) too little movement, and (iv) to the presence of a high proportion of infective bacteria from breathed-out droplets.

If the *temperature of the air* is too high, there will not be enough difference between the temperature of the body and that of the air to enable the body to heat the layers of air next to the skin so that they rise and give place to fresh layers of cooler air.

If there is too much *moisture in the air*, so that the air is too near saturation-point, the sweat cannot evaporate and thus allow heat to be lost. Nor can heat and moisture be lost from the mucous membrane lining the lungs.

Any *movement of air* in a room helps loss of heat by changing the layers of air next to the skin so that cooler dryer air can take up heat and moisture from the skin. Though open windows are much preferable as a means of keeping the air moving, an electric fan is sometimes the only practicable method. Note the use of fans in heated restaurants, and how they give a feeling of freshness in an atmosphere that would otherwise be hot and stagnant.

Emphatically, the oppressiveness of a stuffy room is not due to the chemical properties of the air, lack of oxygen or too much carbon dioxide. Mountain health resorts at high altitudes, as in Switzerland, have, because of lack of barometric pressure, a considerably less proportion of oxygen than is present at sea-level.

In submarines, where the air is kept cool automatically by the surrounding water, the air may be so short of oxygen and so highly charged with carbon dioxide breathed into it that a match cannot be lighted, but the men notice no ill-effects. They automatically breathe more deeply, and so take in more oxygen at each breath.

In the stuffiest room in London, says Dr. Leonard Hill, there would not be enough carbon dioxide present to be injurious. In every ordinary room there are always crevices round doors and windows where some air can enter and leave, sufficient to prevent the accumulation of carbon dioxide in harmful quantities and to ensure sufficient oxygen.

A Viennese, Professor Flugge, experimented by placing a man with his body in a vitiated air chamber and his head outside where he could breathe fresh air. The man felt all the restlessness and ill-effects of being in a stuffy room. When, however, his head only was in the stuffy chamber and his body was in fresh air, he felt no ill-effects at all, although he was breathing vitiated air.

The air of a stuffy room has no characteristic smell any more than has fresh air. Any smell that a room has is due to the things or people in it, stale unwashed bodies and dirty clothes, and dirt-infiltrated furniture, carpets, curtains and wall-paper. Clean people who wash adequately and wear clean, frequently changed underwear, do not make a room atmosphere smell.

The ordinary dry-bulb thermometer measures only the temperature of the air, and not its relative cooling power due to movement and moisture saturation. Dr. Leonard Hill's *Kata-Thermometer* is an instrument to measure such cooling power, that is, it shows how rapidly a warm body is cooled by air at different temperatures and moving at varying rates. The optimum reading would vary, at different temperatures, according to whether sedentary or active work was being undertaken. A lower temperature and more air movement would be better for active than for sedentary work.

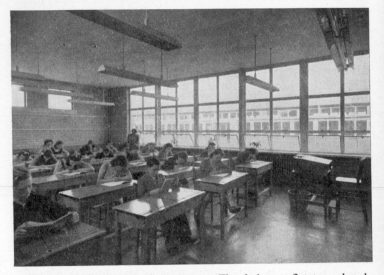

FIG. 52.—A modern school classroom. The desks are flat topped and light to move and the chairs are not fixed to the desks. Light comes from the left and the artificial lighting is "Daylight" in type. The radiator is inconspicuous. The ventilation is by hoppers with Chaddock windows swinging on a central pivot. (*By courtesy of Mr. H. V. Lobb, F.R.I.B.A.*)

Ventilation and Heating

The problem of ventilation is therefore a quite separate one from that of heating, with which it has in the past been to some extent confused in school planning.

The best type of ventilation is provided in a classroom which has a relatively large number of windows that will open, and in which the air can be introduced and diffused upward by a generous use of hopper-shaped openings. Chaddock windows, which swing vertically on a central pivot and can be opened with reference to the prevailing wind, are valuable for quick mass ventilation in recess and for opening on milder and hot days.

A large opening produces less sensation of draught than a narrow one, for through a sash open 6 inches the same volume of air is being drawn into a room as if the sash were thrown up a couple of feet. Thus the speed with which the air enters the 6-inch opening will have to be relatively greater and is the

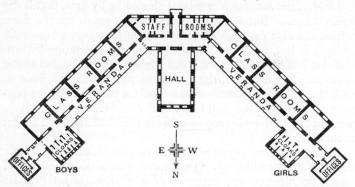

Fig. 53.—Plan of *a Staffordshire or Pavilion type of school.* The two classroom wings can be built as shown, at an angle, or continuous with the staff-rooms, that is, at right angles with the hall. Note (i) the cross ventilation between classroom and veranda ; (ii) the convenient central isolation of the hall ; (iii) the placing of the building in relation to the sun ; and (iv) the covered way to the offices. (*Adapted from Clay's " Modern School Buildings "—B. T. Batsford, Ltd.*)

more likely to be noticed as a draught. Similarly, if a paper is held in front of a fire to draw it up, one hears the roar of the volume of air because the same amount of air is being drawn through the narrowed space up the chimney.

Windows should be of a type that can be opened easily, quickly, and without noise ; noisy cords that break and stick should be taboo. A system of fresh-air corridors with cross ventilation possibilities, as in the *Staffordshire type of school,* has much to recommend it, as also have French windows that open on to the playground.

It should be possible if there are, as in the Staffordshire type of schools, windows on two sides of the room, to adjust the open windows so that the air is changed and kept fresh and odourless without any child having to sit in front of an open window. He should not, for example, have to sit near a sash opening where he would get chilled by a direct current of air. Constant, small, stimulating draughts of air on the skin are preferable, for they do not produce an over-rapid loss of heat.

Ideally, the *heating* of a school should be by fires, that is, by radiant heat. But as the effects even with gas or electric fires, which are also expensive, are over-local (one part of the class being too hot, another chilled), some form of heating by hot-water pipes has to be used. All pipes heat the air, but in the most satisfactory kind, the hot pipes pass under the floor so that the heated air comes up and warms the feet. Pipes running round the room tend to make for cold feet and hot heads, which is bad for resistance to colds in the head and for efficient mental work.

A fire in a living-room always helps ventilation by making a draught up the chimney. The chimney of a bedroom should never be blocked up, because, even if there is no fire, air currents passing over the chimney top tend to lessen the presure of the air over the chimney and draw air out of the room. This should be in addition to open windows (Fig. 159).

Artificial Ventilation

Early in this century it was the fashion to build the *central hall type of school*, in which the classrooms, in one or two storeys, enclosed the hall. This plan made cross ventilation difficult, and to meet the problem, an artificial system of ventilation, called the *plenum or propulsion system*, was installed. In this system the air was drawn from high up away from ground dust into the school by an electric fan, cleaned and moistened by passing through a damped screen of jute or coke, warmed by passing over hot-water pipes and carried by shafts to the classrooms, so that it entered by hopper openings at from 6 feet up, passed round the room and out by an opening low down, and so by shafts to the main outlet.

The system had several defects : (i) The windows, though made to open, had to be kept closed, thus setting the children a bad example since they saw the wrong thing—the windows shut—in school, and were more likely to remember and copy what they actually saw than anything they might be told about the value of open windows. (ii) The machinery was noisy and was fairly costly to run. (iii) The air, artificially moistened, cleaned, and warmed, had a dead physical level, that is, it was depressing instead of stimulating physically, as natural air is.

The *ill-effects of living in a stuffy atmosphere* are cumulative. There is increasing languor and unwillingness to make any effort, loss of mental alertness, a tendency to yawn, to experience headaches, drowsiness and even to feel faint.

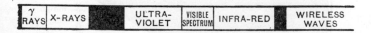

FIG. 54.—From the scale diagram, it can be seen how comparatively short is *the range of the visible spectrum of light*. The gamma, X-rays and ultra-violet rays give shorter waves, whereas the infra-red and wireless waves are relatively long. The ultra-violet rays tan the skin, forming vitamin D, but do not give heat. It is the infra-red rays that supply the heat associated with sun- and other light.

People who habitually live in an over-heated and moist atmosphere tend to have little resistance to colds and lung infections, such as tuberculosis, and to lack that vitality that makes activity in the healthy animal seem worth while. This may lead to lessened appetite and weakened digestion with its accompanying poor complexion and tendency to anæmia and defective muscular tone.

Teachers should be alert to these facts so that if a class is restless, fidgety and disinclined to concentrate, the possibility of inadequate ventilation being the cause should jump to mind. The success of any system of natural ventilation depends on the health-conscience of the teacher, who must see that windows are opened and be sufficiently public-spirited to consider the class needs first. A lazy teacher, with a dormant health-conscience, can render the best-planned system valueless by not opening windows. The reward is coughs and colds (not only to the teacher, unfortunately) and a restless class that must be driven to work with undue expenditure of emotional energy.

Values of Sunlight

Allied to the problems of ventilation indoors are those raised by the effects of *sunlight and smoke* out of doors. Ordinary white light, when passed through a prism, splits up to make the coloured spectrum of red, orange, yellow, green, blue, indigo and violet rays. The same range and arrangement of colours can be seen in a rainbow.

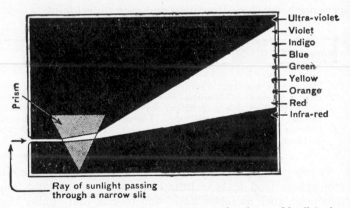

FIG. 55.—Diagram to show how *a prism* can break up white light into the band of colours called the visible spectrum. (*From Campbell's " Readable Physiology and Hygiene "—G. Bell & Sons, Ltd.*)

At the red end of the spectrum are *infra-red rays*, invisible but felt as heat, and beyond the violet ray are *ultra-violet rays*, invisible but affecting the body, as in sunburn. If a body, such as a poker, is heated in the fire, it is at first hot but looks no different. It is giving out invisible infra-red heat rays. As the heating continues it becomes red-hot and gives out rays from the red end of the spectrum. Continued heating may make it white-hot, that is, the light given off is white, a combination of all the visible rays of the spectrum. Compare the white light given off by incandescent gas mantles and new electric light bulbs, as against older bulbs, the light of which looks more orange.

One of the many *values of sunlight* is that it acts on green chlorophyll, enabling plants, as noted earlier, to take in carbon dioxide from the air, which combines with the water absorbed by the roots to make carbohydrates (starch and sugar foods). Actually, in eating meat or fish, transformed grass or plankton is consumed, for the growth of both of which sunlight has been an essential factor. What may be called a carbon cycle occurs when, for example, we eat potato, which is mainly carbo-hydrate; it produces energy and the waste product, carbon dioxide, is breathed out; this carbon dioxide is absorbed by green plants by the help of sunlight and remade into carbo-hydrate, to be again eaten. Without sunlight, in fact, there would be no life.

Apart from thus sustaining life, sunlight kills the resistant spores of bacteria, hence the value of hanging bedding and upholstery in the sun to air. Sunlight on the skin increases the germ-killing and resistive power of the blood by stimulat-ing the white corpuscles, and it actually causes an increase in the blood of iron, calcium, phosphorus and iodine, without the taking of any medicines or change of diet. Sunlight also makes for a cheerful bouyant outlook and is mentally stimulating.

Sunlight prevents and cures rickets and some forms of tuberculosis. It is surmised that the epidemic of respiratory illnesses that occur at the end of every winter in February and March is partly due to the length of time that has elapsed since the summer and the lack of prolonged doses of sunlight. In tanning or sunburn pigment is laid down in the deeper layers of the skin. The process should be gradual, and the degree of tanning is an index of the amount of benefit obtained from the sunlight.

Sunlight in excess is a powerful though delayed poison which may cause severe sun-burn, fever, headache and malaise, so, while sun-bathing is of value, prolonged sudden exposure by city people on short holidays is harmful.

Children should have chances of going about with a minimum of clothing in summer. Tuberculous children in Swiss sanatoria, after being gradually tanned, can safely be allowed to play and work in the snow, wearing only boots, a loin-cloth and a hat. These children are found to be markedly resistant to infections such as chicken-pox and measles.

Classrooms can be glazed with " *vita glass*," which, unlike ordinary glass, lets through the short ultra-violet rays. Most

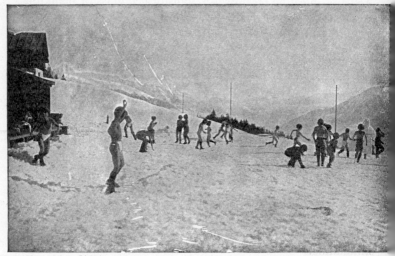

FIG. 56.—Children dressed only in loin-cloth and boots snowballing in front of an Alpine sanatorium. (*From Campbell's " Readable Physiology and Hygiene "—Edward Arnold & Co.*)

clothes, except artificial silk, stop these rays, and as at least a sixth of the body's surface needs to be exposed for ultra-violet rays to do most good, school children in rooms with vita-glass windows would need to wear less than normal clothing to benefit fully. Vita-glass windows must be as thin as possible and be kept clean. The cost of vita-glass is somewhat higher than that of ordinary glass.

It is estimated that practically all children are slightly anæmic towards the end of the winter from shortage of sunlight.

Open-air classrooms and schools, school camps, and physical training and games taken out of doors, all encourage an appreciation of fresh air.

Artificial sunlight, the dosage of which can be controlled, can be applied by a mercury-vapour lamp. The eyes must be protected by goggles, and dosage regulated to avoid sun-burn and to induce gradual tanning. The value seems to be largely in its general tonic effects when allied to other forms of treatment.

The Effects of Smoke

Sunlight then is essential to health, and yet *smoke* is allowed to hang over industrial areas, screening sunlight and making for lessened community health, when actually such screening could be avoided were public opinion informed and strong enough to demand effective legislation.

Smoke from factories fouls the air, as does the lighting of thousands of smoky domestic fires all over the country daily. Legislation to control factory smoke does exist, but is not always put into force. In Oldham there was recently found to be a deposit of soot of 960 tons per square mile per annum, whereas in Malvern the deposit per annum per square mile was only 69 tons. This soot, when it is in the air, cuts off available sunlight ; the evaporation of water is hindered, and the cold dampness of the atmosphere increases. Thus people are kept indoors for recreation instead of being tempted out for exercise and fresh air.

There is an immense waste of the by-products of coal in this soot which could be put to profitable use. Vegetation cannot grow without light and under these soot deposits. Lettuces and cabbages of the same batch of seed were grown at increasing distances from the centre of Leeds. The plants reared in the industrial smoky districts were puny, and they increased uniformly in size the farther out from the city centre that they were grown. The fabric and stone-work of buildings is continually eaten into by deposits of soot chemicals. Smoke damage costs £50,000,000 per annum in Great Britain. In addition, black smoke-coated buildings absorb light and make cities darker and send up lighting costs.

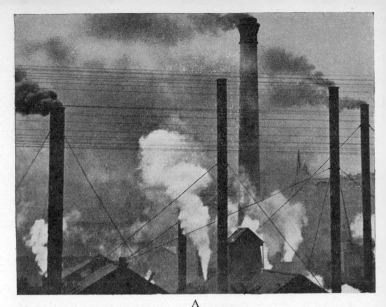

A

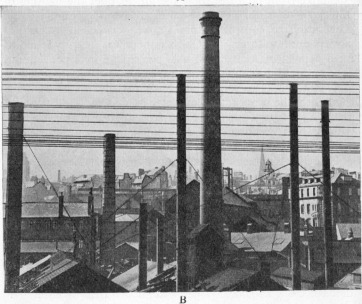

B

FIG. 57.—A, an industrial city showing the ordinary pollution by smoke; B, the same view taken during a bank holiday. (*Photographs by courtesy of W. Stevens and the National Smoke Abatement Society.*)

Everyone in cities, in fact, has to pay for this smoke by extra washing, both household and personal, extra painting and decorating, and artificial light, and by rates and taxes for renovating public buildings. In addition, it is estimated that the loss due to burning raw coal is in Great Britain alone £80,000,000 per annum.

Excessive smoke could be prevented by making illegal the use of any but smokeless fuels, such as hard smokeless coal or anthracite, gas, electricity, oil or gas coke. The present Government scheme for unification of electric power supplies throughout the country will, when completed, reduce the price of electricity per unit, and should make its use more common. In New York nothing but smokeless fuel may be used ; the buildings are white and the city gets sunlight, much of which would otherwise be cut off.

Apart from using smokeless fuels, however, the fitting of well-designed furnaces and domestic fire-grates saves coal and prevents smoke, by more complete consumption of the fuel. In institutions it also pays to have a man who understands management of the furnace because of the saving of fuel thus effected.

Chapter VII

DIGESTION OF FOOD

The myriads of cells of which the body is made are continually altering, being worn away and renewing themselves, making movements, using energy, and then being clogged with fatigue products and giving to the body as a whole the familiar sensation—hunger—that calls for more material to carry on all this activity.

Essential Food-stuffs

Energy cannot be created out of nothing, and it is the food eaten that supplies power for all work and activity. Food-stuffs include body-building material, the *proteins*, which repair waste and make for growth. Meat, fish, egg-white, cheese, fruits and vegetables are among foods supplying these.

The *fats* and the *carbohydrates* (sugars and starches) produce energy and warmth when eaten. Fats are contained in butter, milk, egg-yolk, fat of meat, bacon, while some mainly carbohydrate foods are bread, cakes, biscuits, chocolate, milk puddings, potatoes and bananas.

Body-regulating foods, as *vitamins* and *mineral salts*, supplied mainly by red and green vegetables, fruits and salads, are also needful for *metabolism*, the name given to all the chemical processes that go on in the living body, both building up and breaking down of tissues.

Besides these the body needs *roughage* or ballast, supplied by indigestible fibres of vegetable and fruits, which make bulk in the intestine ; and it also needs plentiful supplies of *water*. In touching the skin, protein is touched ; the desk wood is cellulose, to man an indigestible form of carbohydrate ; the teeth are calcium-phosphate. Calcium is another name for lime.

88

How Food is Digested

The alimentary or food canal is a muscular mucous-membrane-lined tube, 36 feet long, extending from the mouth to the anus. The food, as it is squeezed along, is broken up, mois-

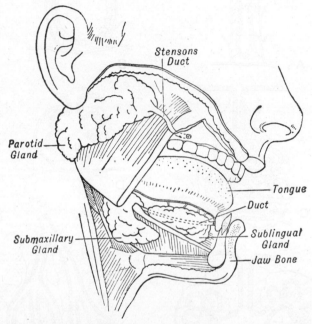

FIG. 58.—Three of the six *salivary glands*. They secrete ptyalin, an enzyme that changes starch into sugar. The parotid glands are those first affected in mumps. It is by the secretion of these glands in dogs that Prof. Pavlov judged the strength of learnt or conditioned reflexes. (Fig. 96.)

tened, and mixed with chemical fluids, so that the insoluble parts are made soluble. Then, when it has been converted from a variety of solids on our plates into a liquid form, it is absorbed into the body and any waste eventually excreted.

Taste and smell excite appetite and warn the body, though not always correctly, against harmful foods. The smell and sight and then the taste of food excite the flow of *appetite juice*

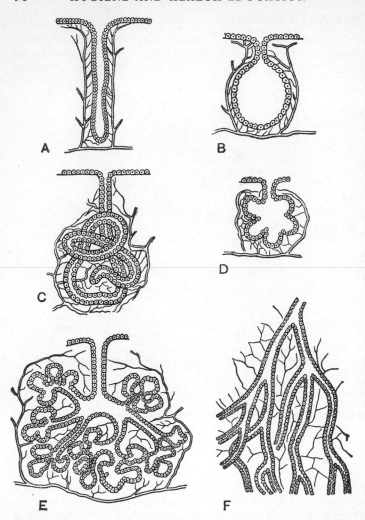

FIG. 59.—Types of *glands having ducts*, from which the substance manufactured in each one, such as mucus, sweat, saliva, gastric juice, fat, is secreted. Note the blood-vessels that encircle the gland walls. From these the gland cells take out the special materials they need from the blood.

in the stomach, which continues for about ten minutes, after which the urge for food becomes less and less. In the mouth the food is cut off by the front and ground up by the back teeth, the while being moistened by alkaline *saliva*. This is secreted by three pairs of glands, of which the best known probably are the parotid glands, which swell up in mumps.

A *gland* is an organ whose chief work is to manufacture, and to secrete or excrete some specific fluid.[1] Some glands do this by means of a special tube or *duct*; thus the sweat glands excrete sweat, the salivary glands secrete saliva, the liver bile. Other glands secrete not by a duct, but by depositing their secretion into the blood as it flows through them. These are termed endocrine glands (see Chapter XV). (The saliva contains a ferment, *ptyaltn*, that begins the breaking up of starch into sugar. Note the proverb, "Bread tastes sweet to a hungry man.")

Enzymes

A *ferment or enzyme* is a substance that assists in the breaking down of chemical compounds very rapidly. For example, in a laboratory this could be done only by a long and laborious series of chemical processes. A well-known enzyme is that in yeast, which splits sugar into alcohol and carbon dioxide. Enzymes are not alive, and they can continue working when out of the body. Each is specific, that is, it will only break down a particular compound, as in the body starch or protein. Enzymes help in all putrefaction, and their action is utilised in such industries as tanning, brewing, and vinegar and cheese-making.

The bolus of food is tipped to the back of the throat, the epiglottis closes the trachea opening and the muscles of the gullet grasp the bolus and squeeze it down to the stomach, a muscular bag situated high up on the left side of the abdomen, close under the diaphragm, and holding, when extended, about two litres. The fact that the food does not fall into the stomach by gravity enables trick performers at fairs to swallow when upside down. Thus in taking pills, once the pill has got to the back of the throat so that the gullet muscles can grasp it, there

---

[1] The lymphatic "glands," so called, are an exception to this.

is no difficulty about swallowing it. On the whole, a rather larger pill is easier to swallow than a very small one, because the larger is the more readily grasped.

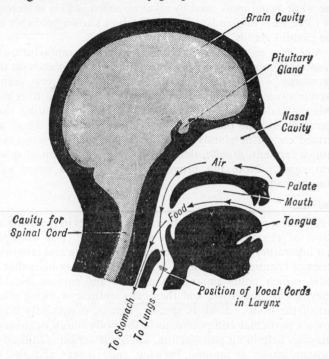

FIG. 60.—Diagram showing *cavities of the head*. The passages for air and food cross in the pharynx. The flap that is silhouetted immediately above the passage to the lungs is the epiglottis, which guides food away from the pharynx and into the gullet. (*From Campbell's " Readable Physiology and Hygiene "—G. Bell & Sons, Ltd.*)

The Work of the Stomach

The stomach walls are made up of three layers of involuntary muscle tissue, contracting in different directions, and lined with a membrane pitted with glands to secrete *gastric juice*. The muscles keep up a rhythmic wave of contractions, usually three waves starting to a minute, but sometimes there may be as many as six waves.

The food is fairly quiescent in the top part of the stomach, the *fundus*, a kind of hopper to supply the lower *pyloric part*. Gastric juice is poured out on to the part of the food mass next to the stomach wall, which is worked downward so that a fresh layer of the mass comes next to the wall continually. Inside the mass the saliva can go on changing starch into sugar, but directly acid gastric juice reaches the food this stops, because ptyalin only acts in an alkaline medium.

Food impregnated with gastric juice is passed to the pyloric lower end of the stomach, where it is churned round with considerable vigour, so that the semi-solid food eventually takes on the consistency of thick cream and is called *chyme*. The meat course, which is mainly protein, is thus better eaten before the pudding, because it can pass the more quickly to the pylorus, and be digested there while the starchy pudding can continue to digest the more slowly in the fundus (see Fig. 62).

The pyloric end of the stomach is closed by a round sphincter muscle such as closes the anus and iris. Through this the food, as it becomes semi-liquid, is spurted out in jets to the small intestine. If food is bolted in lumps, the juices cannot get beyond the outside of each lump, which stays too long in the stomach, giving pain and possibly flatulence.

Gastric juice contains *hydrochloric acid* (manufactured partly from the common salt eaten), and certain ferments, of which the best known are *pepsin* and the *rennin* which causes milk to curdle. In an acid medium pepsin breaks down proteins into more soluble peptones, which, in the duodenum, are further changed to *amino-acids* and are ultimately absorbed into the blood.

The ·2 per cent. of hydrochloric acid is sufficient also to kill cholera and other germs that are taken into the stomach, whereas in the rest of the alimentary canal the juices are alkaline, in which medium most bacteria live readily.

Extreme fatigue, as that of doctors and nurses during an epidemic, or the nervous person's fear of catching disease, can inhibit the flow of gastric juice and so deprive a person of

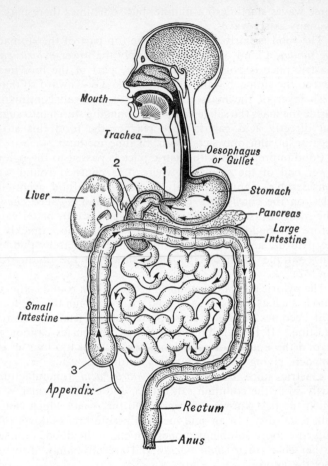

FIG. 61.—General view of the alimentary canal, the liver being turned up. 1, the pylorus, or valve between the stomach and duodenum; 2, opening of the common duct of the liver and pancreas into duodenum; 3, valve between the ileum and first part of large intestine. Large intestine consists of ascending colon, transverse colon, descending colon, and rectum leading outside. (*From Paul's " Domestic Economy.*")

its protective powers. This seems to be some kind of confirmation of the popular view that people who are afraid of catching infection make themselves by their fear the more liable to be attacked. Bovine germs of tuberculosis that are

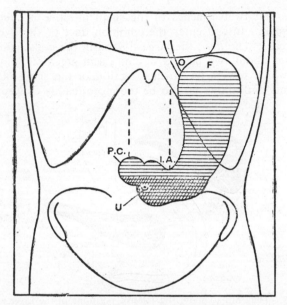

FIG. 62.—*The position and shape of the moderately full human stomach*, as revealed by X-ray photography after a meal mixed with oxy-chloride of bismuth, which is opaque to X-rays. O, gullet (œsophagus) ; F, fundus of the stomach (containing air) ; PC, pylorus of stomach opening into the small intestine. This is the part of the stomach where the more vigorous mixing of the food occurs. U shows the position of the umbilicus (navel) on the surface of the body and the dotted lines the position of the backbone. (*From Hurst's " Constipation and Allied Intestinal Disorders "—Oxford Medical Publications.*)

present in infected milk, because they are wrapped in a protective film of fat, are unaffected by the gastric juice and reach the alkaline safety of the intestine, there possibly to multiply and cause tuberculosis infection later.

4*

The *gastric juice*, in addition to (i) beginning the digestion of proteins, (ii) makes milk clot, (iii) simplifies cane sugars and (iv) digests away the nitrogenous envelopes of fat globules.

The Liver and Pancreas

The first twelve inches of the small intestine is called the *duodenum*. Into it enter the common duct of the liver and pancreas. The *liver*, the largest gland in the body, (i) manufactures about two pints a day of viscid green secretion, the *bile*, which lowers the surface tension of the small intestine contents and allows fats to be the more readily emulsified so

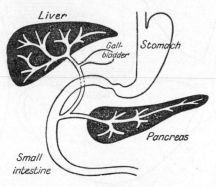

FIG. 63.—Diagram to show the relative positions of the Liver and the Pancreas in relation to Stomach and Duodenum. (*From Eastwood's "Hygiene for Students and Teachers"—Edward Arnold & Co.*)

that the ferment *steapsin* in the pancreatic juice can split the fats into fatty acid and glycerine; (ii) extracts urea and uric acid-protein waste products which are later excreted by the kidneys ; (iii) changes sugars to glucose which is stored as glycogen ; (iv) neutralises toxins ; (v) manufactures fibrinogen, which promotes clotting of blood, and heparin, which prevents blood from coagulating ; (vi) breaks down hæmoglobin ; the pigments thus made are excreted in the urine and fæces, hence their colours. Bile is stored in the gall bladder until needed for digestion.

The *pancreatic juice* contains, besides (i) the ferment that splits fats, ferments (ii) to change starch into malt sugar, and (iii) proteins and peptones into amino-acids, in which form they are readily absorbable. Thus the pancreas completes the work of digestion. It is helped by the *intestine juice*, secreted from the intestine walls, that acts mainly on carbohydrates and peptones.

An internal secretion, *secretin*, from the lining of the intestine, starts the flow of the pancreatic juice when food from the stomach is ready to pass on to the duodenum. In the substance of the pancreas is made *insulin*, an internal secretion which is taken directly into the blood (see Chapter XV). Its presence regulates the amount of sugar in the blood, which is normally about ·1 per cent. Lack of insulin causes diabetes.

The Small and Large Intestine

The *small intestine* is about 20 feet long. It is a muscular tube richly supplied with blood-vessels and lined with a mucous membrane. The inner surface is folded and wrinkled up, an arrangement which increases the area in contact with the food, and slows the rate of movement through the intestine. Finger-shaped *villi* protrude from the surface like the pile of velvet, 10,000 to a square inch. In each of these villi there is a vessel called a *lacteal*, which absorbs the broken-up fats into the lymph system, the lymphatic vessels emptying themselves into the *thoracic duct*. This lies deep in the body cavity against the ribs, and empties these absorbed fats direct into the left subclavian vein and so to the heart for distribution.

Sugars and converted starches and proteins are absorbed into the blood capillaries which join up to take this blood, venous but richly laden with food, to the liver. Here the vein —the Portal—breaks up into capillaries again, so that the liver can change sugar into glycogen that it stores up in itself. The side-tracking of the main part of the fats which the liver does not want, to the thoracic duct, is thus skilfully arranged (see Fig. 36).

The muscular intestine walls keep on squeezing the semi-liquid food along, so that every particle comes in contact with digestive juices and then with the folded villi-covered intestine wall, through which food is absorbed. This progressive movement is termed *peristaltic action*. The absorptive surface of the small intestine, stretched out flat, would cover at least 50 square yards, about the floor area of an ordinary classroom. The main work therefore of the small intestine is to absorb the digested food into the blood and lymph systems.

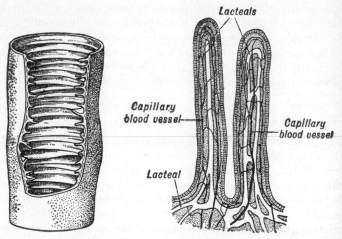

FIG. 64.—A part of the *small intestine* laid open to show the folds of mucous membrane. These greatly increase the absorptive surface.

FIG. 65.—Two *villi*, magnified 100 diameters. They protrude from the inner surface of the intestine, 10,000 to a square inch.

By the time the food reaches the *large intestine or colon*, a 6-foot long tube, digestion is virtually finished. There are few bacteria in the small but many in the large intestine, and these act on the unabsorbed residue ; water is extracted, and fæces, coloured by bile from the worn-out corpuscles, are excreted.

On an average a meal takes ten seconds to get down the gullet to the stomach, stays four to five hours there if hard to digest, ten minutes or less if easy ; six hours later the food begins to pass into the large intestine, and from ten to twenty-four or forty-eight hours later the residue reaches the rectum.

Constipation

In a healthy person, evacuation should not be a matter of continual concern any more than micturition is. Some people's rhythms of evacuation are not 24-hour rhythms, but shorter or longer. Missing an evacuation should not mean immediate recourse to an aperient. The rhythm should have a chance to right itself.

A frequent cause of constipation is delay in going to relieve the bowel immediately the reflex stimulus to do so is felt. Delay until the stimulus is no longer felt blunts the reflex and causes constipation. It is preferable, if the habit can be trained, for the reflex to be felt immediately after breakfast daily, and enough time should always be left free so that such functions can be attended to without undue hurry. The taking in of food into the stomach at breakfast tends to stimulate peristaltic movement throughout the length of the intestine and so to excite evacuation of the bowel.

Diets to prevent constipation must contain sufficient (i) bulk of food and roughage, (ii) foods containing vitamins (see Chapter VIII) and (iii) water, six to eight pints a day. Reasonable exercise is useful, so that the tone of the abdominal muscles and thus of the intestines is tense rather than flabby, reflecting the abdominal wall tone. Carious teeth help to produce constipation, both because food is not fully masticated and because poison from them is swallowed.

Aperients alleviate but do not cure constipation. If an aperient must be taken, cascara, which, however, loses its effect if taken regularly, is less harmful than such a medicine as castor oil, which has an after-constipating effect. Liquid paraffin as an aperient interferes with the absorption of calciums and phosphates and of vitamins. Hence its regular use is to be condemned. Fortunes have been made from selling aperients, for it is easier to take a dose than to have the determination to alter bad health habits.

CHAPTER VIII

FOODSTUFFS AND CHOICE OF FOODS

SENSIBLE eating to assuage hunger should be a source of satisfaction and an occasion for sociability and civilised habits. In the past, perhaps, too much emphasis has been laid on the culpability of greed and the gentility of a small appetite. While a tendency to be greedy has to be inhibited as a part of nurture, hunger-urges for particular foodstuffs, that come upon every healthy person at times, are now recognised to be physiologically sound. In the words of an old song: " A little of what you fancy does you good."

Active, healthy children do need a great deal of readily absorbable sugar ; after an active game or a long walk, an adult may be conscious of wanting chocolate, sugar having been used up in the muscles in movement ; people living in an institution where the diet is deficient in fresh foods, tend involuntarily to choose salads when out to tea ; and a craving for chops and steaks shows a protein hunger which buns and biscuits will not satisfy.

Children, adolescents and young people up to the age of twenty-five should not be made ashamed of a vigorous appetite. They are growing, and if they are using energy in vigorous work and play, they must have ample food to make all this possible, just as a fire must have coal to give out warmth. It is better for the community as for the individaul to eat well and work hard than to eat little and work half-heartedly. People over twenty-five need progressively less food as growth has stopped by then. Diets must be mixed both for interest and health, and related to climate, age, work done, whether sedentary or active. Many health problems arise unnecessarily from ill-balanced diets, and no one food is perfect.

100

Proteins

Proteins form the bulk of the body tissue, and a supply of proteins in food is necessary for repair, and for growth, particularly for children and for pregnant and nursing mothers. From proteins digestive juices, enzymes and hormones of the endocrine glands are made. Shortage results in poor physique, stunted growth and lack of energy, resource and initiative. Protein is also used to produce energy.

Proteins are made up of groups of amino-acids, of which there are some twenty. Each protein, when eaten, is broken up into its specific amino-acids in the food canal, and distributed by the blood-stream to the tissues, there to be resynthesised into the protein of the consuming animal. The proteins of beef, mutton, pork, fish, fowl, crab are all distinct.

Proteins are classed as First Class or Second Class.

First Class proteins are those containing all the amino-acids necessary for life and growth. They include most proteins of animal origin, milk and its products, egg, lean meat, fish, poultry. They tend to be expensive and to be omitted from children's diets in times of economic stress. (The subsidised free milk in schools aims at ensuring, among other nutrients, a supply of First Class protein, regardless of the parents' means. Everyone should have some complete protein in the diet every day. Green leaves supply First Class protein, but too large a bulk needs to be eaten to make them a satisfactory sole supply per man.

The Food Yeast (*Torolopsis ulitis major*) gives First Class protein, as well as " B Complex " Vitamins. It has a pleasant nutty flavour. It grows on a mixture of molasses and ammonium (nitrogen supplying) salts. It is a relatively cheap source of First Class protein, because, unlike cattle and sheep, it does not dissipate energy on movements as they do. Soya bean and Brazil nuts also supply First Class protein.

Second Class proteins are chiefly of vegetable origin, such as gluten of bread, zein of maize, legumin of peas and beans, most nut proteins and gelatin (an animal protein) from bones. They repair muscular waste, but lack amino-acids essential for growth. On the whole they are more difficult to digest but are cheaper than complete proteins.

Protein waste is excreted as urea and uric acid by the kidneys and skin.

The special value of lean meat is probably due to the stimulating action of the *extractives* present in addition to its protein. These extractives are drunk in commercial beef extracts and in beef-tea, little if any protein being present in the liquid. Any sediment is protein. They do, however, supply riboflavin and nicotinic acid (pages 109 and 110).

Carbohydrates

Carbohydrates—the sugars and starch—contain carbon, hydrogen and oxygen only. They are fuel foods and from

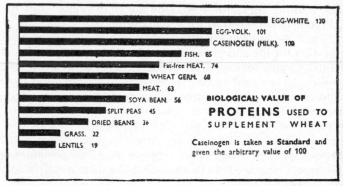

FIG. 66.—(*From Plimmer's " Food Values at a Glance "—Longmans.*)

them heat and muscular energy are liberated during the process of slow combustion with oxygen from the lungs. Compare the quick combustion of petrol in a motor or of coal in a steam engine, when energy, which results in movement, is liberated. Carbohydrates are easily digested. They are of vegetable origin and hence cheap.

Natural sugars, such as those contained in fruits and honey, are absorbed in their natural form, but the more complicated cane and other sugars and the starches have to be broken down by digestion to glucose (also known as dextrose or grape sugar).

Starch needs careful cooking to burst the hard envelope in which each grain of starch is encased. This is necessary to allow the digestive juices to get to the carbohydrate (Fig. 163).

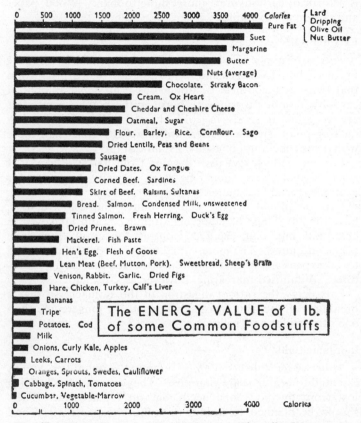

FIG. 67.—(*From Plimmer's " Food Values at a Glance"—Longmans.*)

Babies until they cut their teeth have not got ptyalin in their saliva to digest starch, and should only have natural sugar, such as lactose of milk. To feed them on solid food too early leads to acute digestive disturbances. In times of hardship children may tend to have too large a proportion of carbohydrate in their diet, for bread, jam and potatoes, which are cheap, are mainly carbohydrate, and a fat, flabby child with little power of resistance to infections, results. Plant cellulose is a form of carbohydrate indigestible to man. Wood, paper and cotton are examples.

Fats and Oils

Fats also supply heat and muscular energy. They are made up of carbon, hydrogen and oxygen, but in such a proportion that twice as much heat is supplied as if an equal amount of carbohydrate or protein were burnt in the body. Hence fats are economical foods in cold climates. Fats with a low melting-point, such as butter, are more digestible than those with a high melting-point such as mutton fat.

For the body to get its full value from its fat intake, it is essential that starch should be eaten as well. Consider, for example, bread and butter.

Fats of animal origin, such as butter and fish liver oils, have the advantage of supplying vitamins A and D as well as heat and muscular energy. Contrast olive oil, chocolate, beans and nuts. The more valuable fats, such as butter, tend to be expensive, so that children often get less useful substitutes. Vitamised margarine, however, is satisfactory.

Fats delay the rate of digestion in the stomach, so that a breakfast of bacon is more satisfying for a longer time than one of porridge and rolls.

Inorganic Salts

Mineral constituents of food in minute quantities are as essential to health as are vitamins. They are continually being lost from the body and need constant replacement. Diets should be planned to include calcium, phosphates, iron and iodine and, if these are present, other necessary minerals are unlikely to be absent. Valuable minerals are too often thrown away in cooking water. Steaming, as against boiling, conserves minerals.

Calcium is the chief constituent of bones and teeth. It controls the heart rhythm, blood clotting and response to nervous stimuli. Shortage results in nervous excitability, lessened

FOODS RICH IN
CALCIUM (LIME), PHOSPHORUS AND IRON

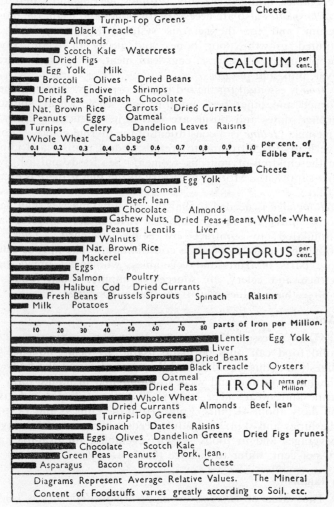

FIG. 68—(*From Plimmer's "Food Values at a Glance"—Longmans.*)

muscular activity and, possibly, in chilblains, asthma and skin diseases. Foods rich in calcium include milk, cheese, green vegetables, oranges, egg yolk, sardines, herring and watercress.

Phosphates also are necessary for bones and teeth, the blood serum, and for the nervous system. Deficiency leads to stunted growth, poor bones and decay of teeth. Food supplying it are cheese, egg, lean meat, nuts, whole wheat, liver, milk and potatoes.

Iron is essential for the red blood corpuscles. Liver, kidney, corned and other beef, mutton, egg, whole wheat, spinach, prunes, dates and raisins are rich in it. Deficiency leads to anæmia. *Iodine* is a constituent of the thyroid gland. Shortage leads to goitre and to cretinism, deaf mutism and idiocy in the children of goitrous women. Sea foods and fish liver oils supply it. More is necessary in the diet if there is excess of fat.

Roughage is needed so that the intestinal muscles shall have some mass to squeeze along. Involuntary muscles are stimulated to contract by being stretched. Lack of roughage tends to produce constipation. The fibrous cellulose parts of fruits and vegetables, wholemeal bread, figs, lettuce and celery are sources of supply. Such foods, of course, have value apart from that as roughage.

Water

Water is essential for the whole metabolic process. Dry solid food can only be made usable by being liquefied in digestion ; this liquid " food " is carried round the body by the blood serum, and waste is eliminated in liquid form as urine and sweat. The body is 70 per cent. water and gives off daily about $4\frac{1}{2}$ pints, 3 pints from the kidneys and $1\frac{1}{2}$ from the lungs and skin. An adult needs sufficient water a day in beverages and in foods—green vegetables, for example, are 90 per cent. water to balance this loss.

Vitamins

The value of *vitamins or accessory food factors* is (1) to produce and maintain perfect health and optimal growth and (2) to prevent and cure specific deficiency diseases.

Vitamins, except vitamin D, are of vegetable origin and are only present in animal foods because these animals are herbivorous or have preyed on herbivorous animals. In a normal diet vitamins are present in quantities too minute to make any contribution to the energy supply of the body, as do sugars and starches, nor are they present in sufficient bulk to make up the cell structure as does protein.

Partial shortages probably cause general ill-health, proneness to infections, poor development and industrial inefficiency over a period. Extra supplies are needed for hard physical work, during pregnancy and lactation, for growth and during convalescence. The five main classes of vitamins are A, B, C, D, and E, and they are not interchangeable in a diet. Vitamins K, P and F are also known.

Vitamin A

Vitamin A is growth-promoting and it keeps the skin and mucous membranes all over the body healthy. If there is shortage, the mucus membranes tend to dry up and become horny, so that bacteria can multiply unchecked. Thus vitamin A protects the body against infections—colds and respiratory disease—and helps in the healing of wounds. It promotes vigour and stamina.

A *shortage* of vitamin A shows as night-blindness (which causes many road accidents), skin lesions, retardation of bone growth and the upsetting of the formation of the enamel and dentine of the teeth. Dull, listless eyes with muddy whites suggest partial shortage. The dimness of sight associated with fasting is probably due to vitamin A shortage. Chronic shortage causes stone of the kidney, gastric ulcer and catarrhs.

The *absence* of vitamin A causes hardening of the cornea of the eye—xerophthalma—and much preventable blindness, for example, in India.

Vitamin A is fat-soluble and is allied to *carotene*, a yellow pigment that occurs, markedly, in green leaves, and gives the yellow colour to carrots, marrow, egg yolk, tomatoes and apricots, to quote some examples. It takes three to four days for carotene to be converted into vitamin A in the liver, where it is stored.

Carotene is present in the foods mentioned above—a $3\frac{1}{2}$-oz. helping of "greens," for example, supplies enough vitamin A for a day—and also in fish liver oils, fatty fish such as herrings, summer milk products, egg, fat of meat, apricots and peaches, fresh, dried or tinned, and in prunes. It is absent from vegetable fats such as olive oil, chocolate and nuts. Prolonged cooking destroys vitamin A, therefore it is not present in dripping and lard.

The body cannot use more than a daily optimal amount of vitamin A ; more than this amount affords no additional protection. There are, however, no ill effects from over dosage. Exposure to light destroys the vitamin. Hence milk should be stored in the dark. For this reason, also, fish liver oils are put up in dark glass bottles.

The *Vitamin B Complex* includes some nine different factors, three of which are of practical importance.

Vitamin B_1 (Aneurine)

Vitamin B_1 (Aneurine) or Thiamin is necessary for neuro-muscular efficiency and for satisfactory growth and the maintenance of normal weight and health in adults. It partly controls carbohydrate metabolism.

A *shortage* of vitamin B_1 shows as loss of appetite and indigestion, accompanied by apathy, loss of initiative and irritability. There is also diminished ability to do heavy muscular work owing to the rapid onset of fatigue. An early symptom is the slowing down of the heart beat. Slight neuritis and neuralgia may also be associated with shortage of this vitamin. There is a parallelism between the symptoms of vitamin B_1 deficiency and of neurasthenia.

The *absence* mainly of vitamin B_1 produces the fatal general neuritis—*beri-beri*—which means " I cannot " and so describes the disease. Indians, feeding chiefly on rice, who take to European polished rice, the outer layers of which—the part which contains vitamin B_1—have been removed, contract beri-beri ; but can be cured rapidly by eating whole, or unpolished, rice again. A small tax on polished rice, thus putting it out of the reach of the poorest people, would save many lives in India. Pigeons, if offered both, will choose polished rather than unpolished rice, and eventually show symptoms of polyneuritis. This can be cured by a diet of whole rice.

Water-soluble vitamin B_1 is present in yeast and yeast extracts, such as Marmite, and in the husk and germ of cereals and the wholemeal foods that supply these (" Bemax " is germ of wheat). It is also present in dried peas, beans and lentils, nuts, green vegetables, egg, carrots, tomatoes, pork, liver, kidney, potato and egg yolk. Limited quantities are found in milk and lean meat.

The amount eaten needs to be directly proportional to the amount of carbohydrates in the diet. Thus, manual workers and active children need relatively more than do sedentary workers. Vitamin B_1 cannot be stored in the body. It withstands freezing, canning and ordinary cooking if soda is not added.

It is not present in polished rice, sago, tapioca, sugar, jam, or white flours and bread, biscuits or cakes made from white flour. It can be synthesised and so added, for example, to white bread, to " vitamise " it.

Vitamin B_2 (Riboflavin)

Vitamin B_2 or G (Riboflavin) has to do with preserving the characteristics of youth. A *shortage* stunts growth in youth and tends to premature aging in adults. There is unhealthiness of the skin and mucous membranes, cracks at the corners of the mouth and discomfort of the eyes and eyelids. The best sources are yeast, summer milk and cheese, egg-white, fish roe, liver, kidney, lean meat and meat extracts, and green vegetables. Hence a well-balanced diet for other essentials is likely to supply all the vitamin necessary. Riboflavin is decomposed by sunlight, and withstands ordinary cooking. Overdosage has no harmful effects.

Vitamin B_3 and B_4 appear to be necessary for growth, while B_5 maintains the body weights. A diet supplying other vitamins of the B Complex will supply these vitamins.

Vitamin B_7 (Nicotinic Acid)

Vitamin B_7 (Nicotinic Acid or Niacine), which occurs in all living cells, has also been named PP that is " pellagra preventing." Pellagra is now thought to be a multiple deficiency disease related to other factors of the B Complex. Nicotinic acid is particularly concerned with keeping the skin healthy, with the health of the intestine and of the nervous system, and in preventing anæmia. The more fat there is in the diet, the more vitamin B_7 is needed proportionally. If the digestion of fats is poor, it may be that more of this vitamin is wanted.

A *shortage* produces skin eruptions and digestive disturbances. The *absence* is associated with the fatal disease, pellagra, which has been summarised as diarrhœa, dermatitis, and dementia. It occurs in districts of Roumania, Italy, Egypt, and in the cotton states of U.S.A., where the poorer workers live on diets with practically no fresh foods and no milk. In the U.S.A. the incidence of pellagra rises to a peak in June, just before fresh vegetables are available, and by September it has nearly disappeared. Pellagra is often associated with a diet of maize. A diet in which " first class " protein is included is a preventive. Thus the elimination of pellagra is chiefly an economic problem.

Nicotinic Acid (B_7) is present in yeast and yeast products, in lean meat and meat extracts, whole-grain cereals, liver, kidney, egg, mushrooms and pea-nuts. White flour, polished rice, fruit and vegetables and milk are relatively poor sources of supply.

It seems probable that a considerable fraction of our supply of vitamin B_1, Riboflavin (B_2) and Nicotinic Acid (B_7) is synthesised by bacteria in the large intestine. Hence food may affect our supply of these vitamins, not only by the amount it contains but also by the influence on the synthesis of the vitamins by these bacteria.[1]

Vitamin C (Ascorbic Acid)

Water-soluble *Vitamin C (Ascorbic Acid)*, in the minute daily proportion necessary (7/1000 gram), keeps the connective tissues healthy. It cements the body cells rather as mortar holds

[1] Vitamin B_{12}, isolated in 1948, is highly active in curing pernicious and other forms of anæmia.

the bricks of a house together ; hence it is needed for normal health, for healing wounds and fractures, and for the formation of the teeth, bones and red blood corpuscles. It helps resistance to infections. Extra supplies are required in illness and during growth periods. There is no danger of overdosage.

A *shortage* produces lassitude for no obvious reason, sallowness, imperfections of the teeth, unhealthy gums, anæmia and susceptibility to infections. Prolonged shortage seems to conduce to acute rheumatism and tuberculosis.

Vitamin C is richly present in black currants, strawberries, rose hips and in citrus fruits such as oranges, lemons and grape fruit, as well as in pineapple, tomato, swede, potato, and raw green vegetables, particularly parsley, cabbage and watercress. A large proportion of the vitamin in tomatoes, apples and oranges is in the skin or peel. Gooseberries and raspberries give moderate supplies. Pears, plums, bananas, grapes, peaches and cherries supply only a limited amount, as do meat and milk.

Vitamin C stands quick cooking, but prolonged cooking in an open pan oxidises and destroys it. Half the vitamin content is lost in the cooking of green vegetables. Heating to a high temperature without oxygen, such as in careful tinning, does not destroy the vitamin, particularly if the fruit is acid ; hence the value of tinned tomatoes, pineapple, grape fruit, strawberries and currants as sources of supply. It is absent from plum jam, twice-heated milk, stewed fruits, dried seeds and artificial fruit jellies.

Young fruit and vegetables, fresh cut from the garden, contain more vitamin C than do those that are kept for any length of time. " Old " potatoes and dried vegetables retain little vitamin C. Bottle-fed babies may be in danger of not getting enough vitamin C, particularly if the milk is pasteurised. Orange, rose hip or black currant juice counteracts this.

Vitamin C is stored in the super-renal capsules, eye lens, liver, spleen, kidneys and muscles.

Allied to vitamin C is *Vitamin P* which is present in red pepper and in lemon. It has to do with the permeability of the blood-vessels.

The *absence* of vitamins C and P causes scurvy, a disease not of the skin but of the whole system, which, if not checked by a change of diet, is fatal.

Vitamin D

There are two forms of Vitamin D.

Vitamin D_2 or Calciferol does not occur naturally, but is made by irradiating with Ultra Violet Rays the vegetable sterol Ergosterol, which is found only in plants, especially in fungi, for example, ergot (from which it takes its name), and in moulds and yeast.

Vitamin D_3 is formed naturally just under and on the skin surface and hair or plumage of animals and birds by the action of the sun [1] on the animal sterol Cholesterol.

(Vitamin D_1 is a name no longer used.)

Vitamin D_3 is found in egg yolk, butter and in fish liver oils.

Animals obtain vitamin D in two ways :

(i) By eating food containing vitamin D ;

(ii) By direct action of the sun on their own skin. Birds for instance, remove oil from the preen gland and spread it over their feathers as they preen them. The oil is thus exposed to the sun and part of it is activated to vitamin D_3 which is eaten in subsequent preenings.

Similarly the washing of fur by cats, dogs and rabbits, and the apparent hunting for fleas by monkeys is a way of getting activated vitamin D_3 by licking.

Fat that is sweated out on to the skin's surface in sunbathing, is activated to vitamin D_3 and as the sweat dries is absorbed. Hence immediate swimming after sun-bathing is inadvisable.

How vitamin D_3 gets into fish liver oils is not clear. Possibly the oils contain new anti-rachitic vitamins as well as D_3.

Milk is an extremely valuable source of vitamin D_3. This is not because of the actual amount present, which is relatively small, but because the anti-rachitic value of the vitamin is greatly enhanced by being given in milk. Cattle spend a good deal of time licking each other and it is probably thus, from the sun-irradiated natural oil of their hair, that the

[1] Artificial sunlight from an ultra-violet ray lamp acts as does natural sunlight.

vitamin D_3 of milk is derived. Summer milk products—including butter and cheese—contain much more vitamin than do winter products. The milk sugar, lactose, helps in calcification, whereas cane sugar and starch lack this property.

Vitamin D regulates the metabolism of calcium and of phosphates, stimulates growth in height and ensures strong teeth and bones. In this, vitamin D is associated with the work of the Parathyroid glands (see Chapter XV).

Shortage of vitamin D leads to less efficient absorption of calcium from the food as it passes through the intestine. Absence results in the deficiency disease—Rickets.

Rickets

Rickets is a disease of infancy in which the bones remain comparatively soft and yielding so that the chest may become " pigeon-shaped," the legs bowed or knock-kneed, or the spine curved. The forehead may take on a characteristic squareness, and there may be small body protuberances like beads on the ends of the ribs. The rickety child's muscles are flabby ; the general resistance and vitality are lowered ; and, until about seven, the child is often retarded mentally. Bone deformities may remain after the active rickets has subsided. Rickets is never found in the sunny tropics and is associated with darkness, smoke and fog ; so much so, indeed, that on the Continent it is known as " English disease." It is, fortunately, much less prevalent than it was.

A child who is being treated for rickets must have (i) a correct balance of calcium and phosphates in the diet, as well as (ii) vitamin D to regulate the use of these minerals. There must be no excess of carbohydrates. In addition to a correct diet and sunlight, (iii) he must have chances of physical activity without which the other agencies will fail.

In adults, a gross shortage of vitamin D results in *osteomalacia*, a disease in which there is a loss of bone calcium.

Overdosage of vitamin D in the form of Calciferol is possible, but if the supply is obtained from the food eaten in a well-balanced diet, there is no danger of excess.

Vitamin D can be stored in the body tissues. It is not easily destroyed by heat and milk loses none by boiling or by pasteurisation.   Tinned and dried milks also retain it.   Many foodstuffs can be irradiated to increase their vitamin D content.

Vitamins A and D are not supplied by margarine made from vegetable oils such as palm kernel, olive, cotton seed and linseed oils, or nut butters, but they are present in margarines

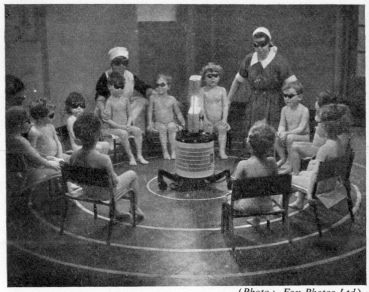

(*Photo :   Fox Photos Ltd.*)

FIG. 69.—Children receiving artificial sunlight treatment, which has the same good effect as does natural sunlight by supplying ultra-violet rays.   The goggles protect the mucous membrance of the eyes. The marked rings regulate the position of the chairs and the intensity of light received.   A mercury vapour lamp is used.

made from beef-suet fats.   Margarine is now required to be reinforced with vitamins A and D.

Vitamin E is present in whole wheat germ and leafy green vegetables, with small amounts in milk and eggs.   Lack of it, as, for example, from eating white flour, may produce lowered fertility and tendency to abortion.   The lack of it has the effect of producing sterility in rats.

Vitamin K is necessary for the initial stages of blood clotting. It is present in spinach and other green vegetables, tomato, liver, peas and rose hips, so that a normal mixed diet probably supplies it.

How Food is Safeguarded

Foods may be *adulterated* so that a poor product looks better than it is and the buyer is deceived. Colouring matter is put into butter (it is prohibited in milk), eggs are browned, wooden seeds and turnips are put into strawberry jam, inferior cake is coloured to look bright yellow as if it contained eggs, and white bread flour is bleached and adulterated. Meat may be tainted or come from a diseased animal, but the sale of such meat is prevented by supervision by Government inspectors.

Trichinosis is a painful parasitic worm infection acquired from eating pig meat. Hence the Order (1932) that all food refuse for pigs must be well boiled. The curing of bacon and the roasting of pork destroys any trichinella but the eating of infected sausages, especially if made from old pigs which are no longer profitable to keep alive, can be a source of infection. Cheap sausages, brawn and meat pies should be eaten with caution, especially if highly seasoned, which may only be to disguise the taint.

The Ministry of Health is responsible for seeing that food is what it pretends to be and that healthy sources only are used. Margarine, for example, must be labelled with the name of the contents on the top, bottom and sides in a set-sized lettering, to prevent fraud. Bread and tea must be sold by weight, and any animal or vegetable food may be seized if " diseased, unsound, or unwholesome," and destroyed on a magistrate's order, and a penalty inflicted.

Food may have preservative added which enables the vendor to sell it over an extended period, as good, but the amount of preservative must now be stated on the container label. Food should be kept in cold storage in hot weather, but frozen food loses taste and so is the less appetising. Tinned and sterilised food keeps well and is little trouble to serve in emergency, but it is relatively expensive, and the taste and food values, such as vitamins, may be lost.

Dehydrated foods, that is, food from which water has been removed, are less bulky and weighty and are preserved from decay because bacteria and moulds cannot grow without water. Thus shipping space, packing materials and refrigerating plants are saved. Eggs, milk, fruits, vegetables and meat are among the foods that can be dehydrated. Taste and vitamin content are maintained.

Food in shops should not be exposed to the dust and flies of the street. *Flies* breed on manure and carry germs, such as of typhoid. They should be kept off food by covering it with muslin, by the use of electric fans making for coolness, and by the greater use of wire-screen doors into food shops.

In the home contamination by flies should be combated by keeping food in cool, north aspect rooms, or out of doors in the shade in a narrow-mesh wire safe, and by the early removal of decaying animal and vegetable refuse. Earth closets and ashpits should be frequently emptied, for flies breed there. The decorating and repainting of old houses does much to disturb flies waiting in cracks and other winter haunts for the summer breeding season. " Kill that fly " is a slogan which, unlike many, has nothing but good in it as far as health preservation is concerned.

Shell-fish, oysters and cockles may be contaminated by sewage that is deposited in sea water in too large quantities locally ; such contamination may cause typhoid.

The carrying out of sanitary regulations in detail depends on the integrity and keenness of the sanitary and other Ministry of Health and Local Authority officials, but the more public opinion is organised against food frauds and profiteering and in favour of vigorous enforcement of safeguards, the better will such work be done. " Unfortunately there are many comparatively ignorant and financially impotent buyers who have to buy cheaply and who will have less knowledge of how to recognise and resist such imposition." Food is a commodity of which it may with reasonable truth be said that " the best is the cheapest."

Further, housewives should be trained to recognise and demand the foods that are of good quality and have vitamin and the other nutritional values.

Vitamin.	Found richly in :—	Little or none present in :—	Stands cooking. Stored in body.	Positive values.	Effects of partial and complete shortage.
A Related to Carotene.	Summer milk products, fish liver oils, egg, carrot, green vegetables.	Olive oil, lard, chocolate, nuts.	Stands ordinary cooking; stored in liver ; light destroys.	Growth ; stamina ; protects mucus membranes from bacteria ; helps healing.	P.S. infections, colds, stunted growth, night blindness, poor enamel and gums, horny skin. C.S. eye disease and blindness ; stone.
B_1 Aneurine or Thiamin.	Whole cereal, liver, egg, yeast, green vegetables, Bemax and Marmite	White flour, polished rice, sago, sugar, butter.	Stands ordinary cooking, baking soda destroys it; not stored in body.	Carbohydrate metabolism ; growth ; work of nervous and digestive systems and adrenals.	P.S. loss of appetite and vigour, fretfulness, apathy, indigestion ; poor growth. C.S. beri-beri, i.e. general neuritis.
B_2 or G Riboflavin	Yeast, meat extracts, egg, cheese, liver, whole meal bread.	Sugar, white bread.	Sunlight destroys; stands ordinary cooking.	Preserves characteristics of youth.	P.S. stunted growth, premature aging, cracked lips, rough skin, eye inflammation.
B_7 or PP Nicotinic acid or Niacine.	Yeast, meat extract and lean meat, liver, pea nuts, whole grain.	Fat meat, butter, white flour, sugar.	Stands ordinary cooking.	Healthy skin and general metabolism.	P.S. stunted growth, skin eruptions and digestive upsets. C.S. Pellagra.
C Ascorbic acid.	Rose hips, black currants, raw green leaves, oranges, lemons.	Vegetable oils, nuts, dried vegetables, grapes.	Only stands cooking without oxygen.	'Cements' body cells together ; anti-infective.	P.S. lassitude, sallowness, poor teeth and gums, slow wound healing ; low infections. C.S. scurvy.
D_2 Calciferol D_3 Cholesterol (Sunlight on skin can supply it).	Fish liver oils, summer milk products, egg, liver,	Vegetable oils, nuts.	Stands ordinary cooking. Stored in body.	Controls calcium- and phosphorus metabolism.	P.S. decayed teeth, slow healing of fractures, lymphatic gland enlargement. C.S. rickets.
E Tocopherol.	Green vegetables, whole cereals.	Cod liver oil, yeast.	Stands cooking.	Regulates reproduction, connected with pituitary.	Lack in rats produces sterility.
K Menaphthone	Green vegetables, tomato.		Stored in liver.	Helps blood clotting.	Undue bleeding.

Summarising Table of Chief Vitamins : P.S. signifies partial, and C.S. complete shortage.

Chapter IX

MILK AND OTHER BEVERAGES

On the whole people tend to drink too little liquid, as plain water or as infusions. *Tea, coffee and cocoa* all contain a stimulant, caffeine, which, taken in moderation, acts quickly on the brain and nervous system without after-effects of depression such as follow alcohol. Tea and coffee, especially, stave off the effects of nervous fatigue and allow impulses to flash to and fro in the nervous system more rapidly than normally. By reducing the resistance to the passage of nerve impulses at the synaptic junctions they ward off sleepiness and produce a feeling of alertness (see Chapter XVI).

Half a pint of freshly made tea, two or three times a day, is harmless, but tea that is left to stew contains tannin, which is constipating and retards digestion, particularly of meat. It follows that a meat tea, especially if the tea is strong, is of doubtful physiological value.

Coffee is more expensive than tea, and if properly made is a stronger stimulant. Taken with milk it is something of a food. Its moderate use is harmless. Children, up to sixteen or so, do not need stimulants such as tea and coffee.

Cocoa boiled, so that the grains of starch are broken up, is preferable, because, though it contains less stimulant, it supplies fat and starch and a little protein ; and, particularly if made with milk, it is a useful food. Unboiled, most of the starch is lost in the sediment at the bottom of the cup.

Aerated waters are sometimes pleasanter to drink than ordinary water. A better thirst-quenching drink, however, is still-lemonade made with the juice of fresh lemons, which gives vitamin C and mineral matter. Chemical lemonade powders, coloured possibly with aniline dyes, are of no value and may be harmful.

Water

Water must be obtained from a pure source. In big towns a safe supply is assured. In the country, deep well water, such as comes from the second impervious layer, 140 feet or more down, is safe. Shallow well water, which taps water from the first impervious layer, may be contaminated by adjacent cesspools and farmyard drains, particularly in wet weather, when the soil is the more likely to be waterlogged.

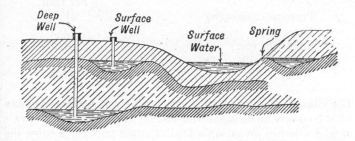

FIG. 70.—The darker shading shows layers impermeable to water such as rock or clay. Hence it can be seen why springs cease to flow after a spell of dry weather and why deep well water is harder but less likely to be contaminated than is surface well water.

Shallow well water is liable to be contaminated by typhoid fever germs, infected water having percolated into the well.

An artesian well is one bored through a series of strata to water-bearing strata enclosed between two impervious layers. It taps uncontaminated water collected on hill tops many miles from the well itself. The fountains in Trafalgar Square are supplied with water collected on the North Chiltern Hills which is tapped by an artesian well. Deep well water tends to be hard, that is, to contain dissolved in it lime and other mineral matter, which it absorbs as it passes through the soil. Very hard water may produce a tendency to constipation, but very soft water is popularly considered to induce decay of teeth, through lack of calcium.

5

Milk

Milk is glibly spoken of as " a perfect food." Human milk is a complete food for the baby, and cow's milk a valuable factor in children's dietary, but once a child is past the teething stage, bulk as well as liquid food is essential. An adult would have to consume uncomfortable quantities of liquid to get a sufficiency of the solids that milk supplies, if milk were his only food.

Cow's milk is made up of :

	Per cent.
Protein (casinogen)	4
Fat	3·5
Sugar (lactose) . . .	4·5
Mineral salts	·7
Water	87·3

The vitamin content of milk varies widely, however. Human milk contains more sugar and less fat and protein than cow's milk, so that in preparing a feed of cow's milk for a baby, the milk must be diluted with water and have lactose added. A little citrate of soda added to cow's milk helps the digestion of protein. A baby is much better, however, if fed naturally.

A continual controversy exists about milk. On the one hand, it is a food of great value for growth, but, on the other, it is easily infected and then becomes a source of danger.

Value of Milk

As an accessory food its value for growth has been proved by numerous experiments, of which that arranged by Dr. Cory Mann is one of the most striking in results. Groups of boys in an industrial school, all fed similarly on an adequate mixed diet, were given, in addition to this diet, one group one pint of milk a day, another a portion of water-cress, another biscuits, another dried casein (milk protein), another butter, another vegetable margarine, while a control group had no addition to its diet (Fig. 71).

Heights and weights, tendency to catch infections and to suffer from minor ailments, and intellectual levels were noted

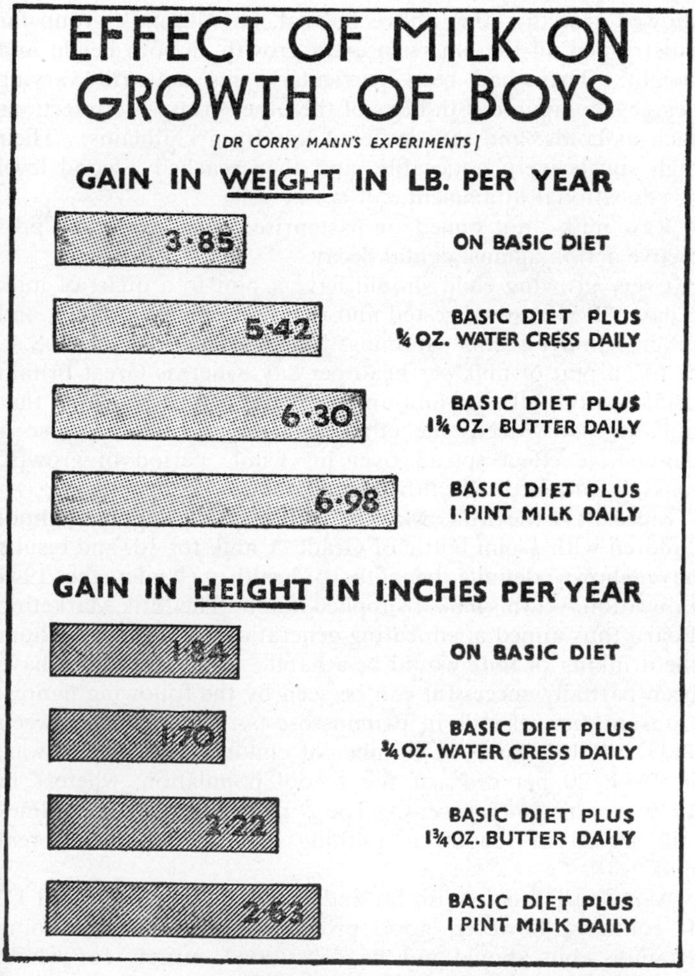

EFFECT OF MILK ON GROWTH OF BOYS

[DR CORRY MANN'S EXPERIMENTS]

GAIN IN WEIGHT IN LB. PER YEAR

3·85 — ON BASIC DIET

5·42 — BASIC DIET PLUS ¼ OZ. WATER CRESS DAILY

6·30 — BASIC DIET PLUS 1¾ OZ. BUTTER DAILY

6·98 — BASIC DIET PLUS I. PINT MILK DAILY

GAIN IN HEIGHT IN INCHES PER YEAR

1·84 — ON BASIC DIET

1·70 — BASIC DIET PLUS ¼ OZ. WATER CRESS DAILY

2·22 — BASIC DIET PLUS 1¾ OZ. BUTTER DAILY

2·63 — BASIC DIET PLUS I PINT MILK DAILY

(By permission of the Controller of H.M.S.O.)
FIG. 71.

over from two to three years. No groups were retarded in regular growth, some (the water-cress and butter groups) showed growth rather above normal, but the milk group far outstripped all the others in extra growth, in both height and weight. They had been particularly resistant (in varying degrees) compared with boys of the other groups, to infections such as colds, and they suffered less from chilblains. Their high spirits were noticeable, and they reached a good level of educational attainment.

Raw milk—not boiled or pasteurised—has a marked protective action against dental decay.

Every growing child should have a pint to a quart of milk a day. It is easily digested and rich in first-class protein, and in growth-producing vitamins. The populations of U.S.A. drinks a pint of milk per head per day, whereas Great Britain drinks only half that amount per head. It is probable that milk not only feeds the child immediately, but has also a cumulative effect spread over his whole period of growth, making for sturdier health throughout life.

Since 1934 the Milk Marketing Board has supplied school children with $\frac{1}{3}$-pint bottle of Grade A milk for $\frac{1}{2}$d. and results have shown definite benefits to health. (Under the 1944 Education Act this milk is supplied free.) The Milk Marketing Board thus aimed at educating generations of adults in whom the drinking of milk would be a habit. That these aims have been partially successful can be seen by the following figures. Consumption of milk in Britain rose by 18 per cent. between 1933 and 1939 and the number of children taking milk was, in 1934, 20 per cent. of the school population, whereas in 1939 it was 66 per cent. The " malted milk " sometimes still served in schools is nothing like so valuable as real milk.[1]

Skim milk has lost its fat and most of vitamins A and D. It contains, however, good protein, sugar, salts and some vitamins, but should not be substituted entirely for whole milk. Milk protein is the cheapest form of first-class protein.

---

[1] From July, 1940, expectant and nursing mothers and children under five have been able to have one pint of milk either at half the current price or, in necessitous cases, free.

Dangers of Milk

The two *sources of danger in milk* are from dirt in production and from tuberculosis in cows.

Milk, after all, is supposed to be drunk direct from the mother by the calf. If the mother were healthy he would get it sterile, warm and fresh. When milk is milked into a clean but unsterile bucket, by the milker's clean but unsterile hands, in an open cow-shed with dust and flies about ; when it is put into a milk churn to be collected possibly by motor, shaken up, warmed over-much perhaps, entrained with more possibilities of station dust getting into it, and finally distributed at the door in open jugs a hundred miles from where it was milked, there are obviously many chances of infection, particularly as milk is an almost perfect culture medium for many kinds of bacteria.

Even with clean methods of handling and cooling milk, the bacteria count per cubic centimetre tends to increase rapidly ; if the milker's hands or buckets be dirty or if manure be allowed to get into the milk, the rate is greatly increased. Machine milking makes for cleaner milk. The quick multiplication of bacteria in milk soon makes it become sour and so unsaleable, or if sold, unusable. Such diseases as scarlet fever and paratyphoid can be spread by infected people milking or handling milk, or by the washing of utensils in infected water. Cow-sheds should be whitewashed, and be light and airy, and the cows be pastured rather than fed in sheds.

Milk must be cleanly produced and distributed, but equally important, cows must be healthy. Hardy cows that live and are milked out of doors are not so likely to get tuberculosis, " a bedroom disease," as are those kept in stalls. The germs of tuberculosis may be present in the milk of a tuberculous cow. Such infected milk drunk in large enough doses will infect human beings. Children are markedly susceptible to bovine infections of tuberculosis, which show in the joints, bones and glands specially. The bacillus of the bovine form is different from the human bacillus, which is present, for example, in tuberculosis of the lungs and is passed from person to person by droplet infection or by inhaling infected dust.

This bovine tuberculosis in children results in loss of happiness, crippling, prolonged illness and death, and causes great expense both to the individual and to the community. And it is preventable. It is far easier and cheaper, actually, to inspect cows and to have sanitary cow-sheds built and thus to prevent bovine tuberculosis, than to pay for sanatoria and to effect what may after all be only partial cures. Vested interests and public ignorance of possibilities stand in the way of such preventive measures.

The feeding of a child on milk from one cow only, formerly advocated, is doubtful, because if the cow becomes tubercular large regular doses of germs will be absorbed, thus increasing the likelihood of infection, whereas, with mixed milk, it is likely that smaller and less regular doses of germs would be taken.

The bacteria in milk, not all of which are harmful, can be effectively destroyed by boiling, but in the process the milk's taste is altered and its value lessened ; for example, some of the albumen, casein and fat forms a skin on the surface and some of the vitamin content is probably destroyed. Therefore it is preferable to buy raw milk from healthy cows, if it has been carefully handled and bottled.

The Marketing of Milk

The Ministry of Agriculture and local authorities are responsible for issuing licences to milk vendors, who undertake to supply milk of tested bacterial purity and cleanliness, and for seeing that a set standard is maintained.

Under the *Milk (Special Designations) Order*, 1936, there may be sold : (a) Tuberculin Tested Milk, (b) Accredited Milk, and neither of these milks may be treated by heat. Also controlled by the order are (c) Tuberculin Tested Milk (Pasteurised), and (d) Pasteurised Milk.

A large proportion of the milk used in less populous areas is (f) Raw Milk.

To sell (a) *Tuberculin Tested Milk* the following conditions must be fulfilled : (1) each cow must undergo and pass the tuberculin test every six months ; (2) no cow may be added to the herd until this test has been passed ; (3) reactors or diseased cows must be isolated from the herd ; (4) a register of the cows must be kept and the herd kept separate from other cows ;

(5) milk samples taken before delivery to the consumer must contain no coliform bacillus in one-hundredth of a millilitre, and must satisfy a methylene blue reduction test. (Coliform bacilli are normal non-toxic inhabitants of the intestine.

For the production of (b) *Accredited Milk* the cows are not tuberculin tested, but must be examined every three months, and diseased cows or any suspected of being tuberculous must be removed from the herd. Other conditions and tests for bacterial content of the milk are similar to those for Tuberculin Tested Milk.

Milks Treated by Heat (and this includes 95 per cent. of London's milk) must comply with the 1923 Milk Order.

Milk is pasteurised by being kept at between 145° F. and 150° F. for at least thirty minutes, and then cooled rapidly to not more than 55° F. By this treatment both bacteria and their resistant endospores are killed. The main alteration of the nutritive value of the milk is some loss of vitamin C, which can be made up by including orange, tomato, or swede juice, or other acid fruit juice in the diet. Boiling of milk causes more loss of food values than pasteurisation. Milk is not boiled in being pasteurised.

Pasteurisation kills both tuberculous and also other milk infections. In Toronto, milk has, since 1915, been compulsorily pasteurised and no case of infectious disease has been traced to milk since.

(c) *Tuberculin Tested Milk* (*Pasteurised*) must be produced and delivered under the same conditions as for raw Tuberculin Tested Milk. A sample must not contain more than 30,000 bacteria per millilitre.

(d) *Pasteurised Milk* samples must not contain more than 100,000 bacteria per millilitre.

Pasteurised milks must be labelled as such, and must not be heated more than once. Unless the milk is preserved from further contamination, pasteurisation is a waste of time and money; pasteurised milk must therefore be distributed in bottles.

(f) Raw milk from uninspected herds and with bacteria content unchecked, is sold freely, except for general Ministry of Health regulations as to the adding of colouring matter, water, and as to cleanliness. There must be 3 per cent. of fat and $8\cdot7$ per cent. of solids in milk. Tuberculous cows may be compulsorily slaughtered and the owners compensated. Milk sold in bottles is not necessarily a " designated " milk.

Dried Milk must reach a certain legal standard of content, and the tins be labelled with its milk equivalent. *Condensed milk* often has sugar added, which helps it to keep ; it retains its vitamin C. Unsweetened brands need more heating and lose vitamin C. Do not buy tins with bulges, for the contents are probably not in good condition. For household use condensed milk should be bought in small tins, so that once opened the milk can be quickly used up. Babies can be fed on diluted condensed milk in an emergency, but if it is used regularly a shortage of vitamins will eventually be felt.

CHAPTER X

DIETS AND SCHOOL FEEDING

AN important function of our food is to supply energy for movement and heat to keep the body temperature some 40° F. to 50° F. above our surrounding temperature.

The capacity of food to supply energy is measured by its capacity to produce heat, the unit of which is the Calorie. A Calorie represents the amount of heat necessary to raise 1000 grams (1 litre) of water one degree Centigrade. One Calorie of heat is obtained from 4 grains of sugar, when this has been completely oxidated.

The bulk foods—carbohydrates, fats and proteins—càn be used by the body to supply energy. Any diet which satisfies hunger probably supplies enough Calories, but we should not thrive if all our Calories were derived from one type of food— —either carbohydrates, or fats, or protein. We need a mixed diet for other reasons already apparent. The number of Calories needed depends on the amount of energy expended in work.

Meals may be divided roughly into those supplying (1) carbohydrates and fats, and (2) proteins, carbohydrates and fats. The bread and butter, toast, jam and cake of tea-time give mainly carbohydrates and fats, while the bacon (lean and fat) and eggs, toast, butter and marmalade of breakfast, or the roast meat, potatoes, vegetables and pudding (mainly starch) of dinner give these with protein added.

The white and yolk of eggs give protein: the yolk gives in addition fat, salts and vitamins; the fat parts of bacon and meat give fat and the lean parts, protein; bread gives some second-class protein in the form of gluten, but it gives mainly starch, that is, carbohydrates; jam and marmalade supply sugar, carbohydrate, fruit juices and water. Meals of one foodstuff lack interest and put a strain on digestion. That is why, to give one illustration, we put butter on bread.

127   5*

Dinner, the most substantial meal of the day, should be at midday for children, but is probably better for adults at night, after mental concentration and stress of work is over. A rest and change of thought before meals, as well as after, conduces to better appetite and digestion. Many institutions rush their people from work to a meal with hardly time to wash hands. A fifteen-minute rest before and thirty minutes after a midday meal may be a real economy.

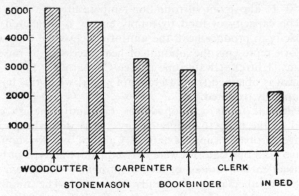

Energy requirements from food (24 hours)

FIG. 72.—*Energy requirements from food* (24 *hours*)

This diagram shows the approximate amount of energy, measured in Calories, required by men of various occupations in twenty-four hours. A Calorie is the amount of heat energy necessary to raise 1000 grams (1 litre) of water 1 degree Centigrade in temperature.

Probably the best plan for most people is to have three good meals a day, supplemented by a light one. The light meal may be taken either at tea or at supper time according to convenience.

Eating between meals is not desirable because such supplements, being often sweets, make for indigestion and obesity. In addition, sugar between meals or early in a meal depresses the flow of gastric juice, taking the edge off appetite. If there is not to be eating between meals, however, children and adolescents must have plenty of appetising, nourishing and varied food at meal times.

On the other hand, however, while what might be called " chain " eating is not good, there may be people who are better suited by, say, six smaller meals a day than by the three larger meals. People with relatively small stomachs need more frequent meals.

Children do not need appetite-stimulating condiments and pickles as adults may to induce interest in food. For all ages carefully cooked food, well served, and not in too large portions should be sufficient to stimulate appetite. Actually, the flavour and serving of food stimulates appetite and the flow of digestive juices more in excitable than in phlegmatic people. Cooking should make food more digestible and interesting ; it also preserves it, killing harmful bacteria.

Meals should be eaten under comfortable, leisurely conditions. Pleasant talk helps digestion, but the talking of " shop " with its calling up of small worries and annoyances is unsound. The sight of a dog can call up anger and fear in a cat, the movements of whose stomach immediately cease, owing largely to the outpourings into the blood of secretions of the adrenal glands (see Chapter XV). Similarly, to quarrel or be angry at meals upsets digestion. Failing pleasant conversation, it is probably better for digestion to read a satisfying book, than to think worrying thoughts, which may cause eating to be unduly hurried.

Children need, bulk for bulk, more food in proportion than adults. Adolescents of fourteen to twenty may well be expected to eat more than adults. They are growing as well as living. There should be no question of limiting children's food in quality or quantity, as far as money will go. To do so affects physique and health throughout life, for their quality, whether of good muscular tone and good health or of poor tone and continued minor ailments, is to a large extent settled, apart from inherited tendencies, during the first twenty years of life.

Everyone must have met, sometime, people who are prone to state with almost passionate emotion that they " never touch that " or that so-and-so is " poison " to them, with an implied assumption that anyone eating these often very harmless foods has low taste, and is in some way personally insulting them in doing so.   They are using their *food fads* to emphasize that they consider themselves different

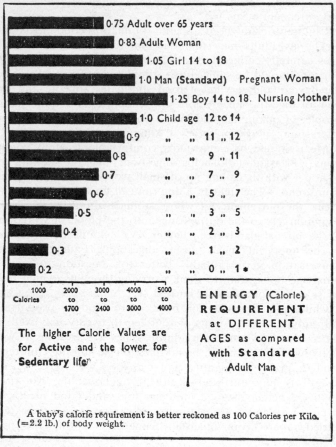

FIG. 73.—(*From Plimmer's " Food Values at a Glance "—Longmans.*)

from the ordinary run of people.   It is quite possible for individuals to know what does not suit them and to avoid it, but other people ought not to be bothered with such diet peculiarities. Actually, many food fads are caught by suggestion. Most foods suit most normal unfussy people. Children unfortunately copy faddy adults. As far as possible they should not hear talk about digestion or, more often, indigestion, and should take food for granted, nor should their healthy appetite be curbed by adults who use, or better abuse, their adult authority to inflict their personal food fads on children under their charge.

Similarly, with patent foods, though some are good, we should guard against being suggestible to what the manufacturer says about his own product. He, after all, wants to sell it. Most of such foods are dear in comparison with their food value.

School Meals

School Dinners have become, under the Education Act, 1944, a recognised part of the school's responsibilities. It has become, in the words of the Act, " the duty " of the Local Education Authority to provide " milk, meals and other refreshments for pupils in attendance at schools and county colleges."

One essential requirement of a school dinner is that it should supply a sufficiency of first class protein. This is expensive and there may be a tendency to try to economise on it. Soups and even stews without variation are not satisfactory. Soup is not a substitute for the meat course. It is valuable chiefly because it stimulates the flow of " appetite juice." It supplies little protein and that of second class quality, such as gelatin dissolved from bones.

School meals should provide social training as well as food. A well-laid table, gay with flowers, with a clean cloth and polished cutlery, adds interest to food and encourages good behaviour. Hands should be washed and hair tidied before meals, and such matters of behaviour as scooping food up roughly, failure to pass food to those needing it, reaching or snatching, failure to take food after fingering it, matters that have to be taught to all children, can be lightly dealt with here.

Senior boys and girls can act as monitors at the heads of tables, and teams of responsible boys and girls serve as waiters to the younger children. Good eating habits thus learnt may help to influence home habits, and knowledge of ordinary conventions may well be of service to children in later life. Eating conventions, of course, vary widely in different countries, but to teach children the normal usage of their own country is not to make them class conscious, but to break down class barriers and make a larger number of people comfortable in a wider range of society.

The *school meal menu* should be arranged so that a lighter meat course is balanced by a more substantial suet pudding, and winter puddings should be more substantial than summer. A regular routine of the same dishes on the same days is to be avoided. It takes away the stimulus of the unexpected to be able to say, " Friday—hot-pot day," or " Monday—cold beef again."

Teachers and education authorities recognise that it is of little use to maintain schools and staffs to teach hungry children, and teachers are obviously the best people to supervise children's school meals. At the same time, it should be recognised that such supervision is an additional strain on the teacher, for whom a full day's work is already planned in actual teaching. It would probably be better to enlarge staffs than to give extra pay for such work.

School feeding schemes are supplemented by the supply of cod or halibut oil and orange juice with satisfactory results in growth and health.

Malnutrition

Malnutrition is partly a problem of the food source from which Calories are supplied. Carbohydrate sources are cheaper but supply less all-round nourishment.

One acre of land planted with cereals produces 4–10 times as many Calories as if the acre were used to feed animals, which would supply milk, flesh and eggs. Peasants with poor land, unmechanised methods of cultivation and little fertiliser, tend to grow cereals to get enough cheap Calories.

They therefore get too little first class protein, calcium and vitamins A, C and D in their diets.

Malnutrition may be said to be of two types : (i) because of lack of food providing animal products—meat, milk—and fresh fruits and vegetables and (ii) because of using debased cereals such as polished rice, white flour and maize. The two types tend to be associated and to be related to ignorance and poverty.

Under-nutrition in child or adult shows as chronic fatigue, loss of interest in work, inability to concentrate, poor spirits and a sense of being over-driven in normally easy work. It is not the efficiency for muscular work so much as the will to do it that is affected. Such under- or mal-nutrition is not due only to food shortage. Food of the wrong kind, as tinned food, is equally likely to contribute to such a condition. In addition, malnutrition may result from a combination of such conditions as bad home surroundings and neglect, lack of sunlight and air, sleeping too many in a room and bed, late hours and insufficient sleep and habitual uncleanliness.

Unhealthy, crowded, ill-ventilated school buildings would help to cause malnutrition, as might employment out of school hours, and, in rural areas, long tiring walks to school combined with poor feeding and damp feet and clothes. Children debilitated from birth readily fall into this condition. Ailments such as adenoids, decayed teeth, rheumatism and the beginnings of tuberculosis would also help to push children into the malnutrition group.

Combinations of these health-destroying circumstances will affect a child adversely. The main causes of malnutrition, however, appear to be poor feeding, defective tonsils and the presence of adenoids, and tuberculosis. Some authorities go so far as to consider all mal-nourished children as pre-tubercular. School feeding can do something, but attendance at an Open-Air School with its specifically healthy conditions and the care it gives to the health of every individual is better still (see Chapter XXXII). Statistics seem to show that there is less malnutrition in the country than in the town. This is probably due to less crowding, greater space, more fresh air and sunlight, and greater chance of fresh foods, such as raw milk, vegetables and fruit.

The Six Fundamental Needs for Health

No consideration of health education is complete without some mention of the vogue for indiscriminate *medicine taking* that probably arose as a result of the Industrial Revolution with its increase of town life, condemning people to eat preserved food, to take little exercise and to work in artificial light, largely cutting them off from the benefits of sunlight. The tendency is for doctors to prescribe few medicines and rather to advise people how to live healthily. Medicines can and do help to alleviate illness and to hasten return to normal health. The constant taking of medicines merely to allay symptoms (as when soothing powders are given to infants whose fractiousness is due to ignorant nurture, or when aspirin is taken continually for headaches or aperients for constipation), probably means that the real cause of the ill-health is not being found and treated.

Sir George Newman, in a recent report, gives the *six fundamental needs for health* as suitable food, fresh air and sunlight, warmth, exercise, rest and cleanliness, and it is at once obvious that these are not to be got out of a bottle of medicine, but depend on a balanced habit of life.

Popular education, which taught people to read without necessarily making them critical of what they read, has made the newspaper advertising of patent medicines commercially valuable, and, as newspapers depend largely on their advertisements to keep themselves solvent, they cannot afford to be very critical of advertisements of patent medicines, of which, though some are useful, many others are both dear and fraudulent.

Taken as a whole, the advertisements and pamphlets of the less reputable patent medicines aim at frightening people, and suggesting to them that they are ill, inducing them to magnify trifling or non-existent ailments, so that they will spend money on the remedy advertised. The antidote lies in the education of public opinion so that people will take a lively interest in being well rather than a morbid interest in being ill.

The Pharmacy and Medicines Act, 1941, prohibits the advertising of remedies for Bright's disease of the kidneys, diabetes, epilepsy and tuberculosis.

Chapter XI

TEETH AND DENTAL HYGIENE

ALL teeth, whether back or front, have the same structural plan. Any tooth is made up of a *crown*, the part that pro-

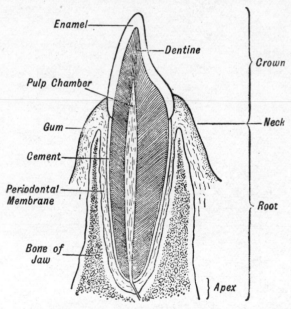

FIG. 74.—Diagram of *side view of a tooth*. The blood-vessels and nerves enter the tooth at the tip of the root, and penetrate to the pulp cavity.

trudes from the jaw, and the root, considerably the larger part, embedded in the jaw. The mass of the tooth is a hard sub-stance, mainly lime, called *dentine*. Over the crown is a thin layer of very hard material, the *enamel*, which ends where the crown joins the root at the *neck*. The root dentine is covered by a thin layer of *cement*, shiny, bone-like and yellowish. Inside the dentine, running up from the tip of the root, is the *pulp cavity*, containing nerves and blood-vessels, which enter at the root tip.

Enamel is harder and more brittle than dentine, which, however, has the greater elasticity. Dentine is continually being worn away and replaced by dentine-forming cells, fed by blood-vessels.

The first signs of teeth occur in the fœtus at about the sixth week of gestation. At birth the set of twenty milk teeth are all in the jaw and are cut between six months and two and a half years of age. They last till about the sixth year, when they begin to be gradually replaced by the permanent teeth, thirty-two eventually, as the jaw and face grow larger. Eruption goes on fairly rapidly from six to ten years, and then more slowly until the wisdom teeth are cut, usually in adult life.

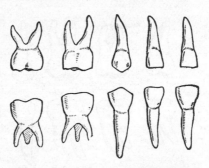

FIG. 75.—Of *the twenty milk teeth*, the first to erupt are the central incisors at 6 months, being lost at about seven years, while the last are the second molars, which erupt at about 18 months. (*After Campbell.*)

The four front teeth for cutting off pieces of food are termed *incisors*. The two *canine* teeth are for tearing food, and are longer and more prominent in animals, such as cats, dogs and tigers, who consume their food thus. The four *premolars* or *bicuspids*, not present in the milk set, are small grinding teeth, and at the back of the jaw are six molar teeth with four pronged roots and rough flattened surfaces for grinding food, so that it can be well mixed with saliva.

Thus in the *milk teeth* there are in each jaw, upper and lower—

4 incisors.
2 canines.
4 molars.

In the *permanent set* there are in each jaw—

4 incisors.
2 canines.
4 premolars or bicuspids.
6 molars.

The permanent teeth exist in the child's jaws, laying down and developing lime salts in their substance, from even before

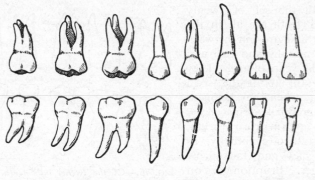

FIG. 76.—Of *the thirty-two permanent teeth*, the first molars and the central incisors erupt at between six and seven years, and, except for the third molars, the " wisdom " teeth, all should be in place by from fourteen to fifteen years. (*After Campbell*.)

birth, and any severe illness during the first six years of life tends to leave a permanent mark on the developing teeth ; less lime is laid down and points where decay is very likely to occur are left. Similarly, severe illness in childhood disturbs bone growth, and leaves marks which can be seen in X-ray films of the children's bones (see Fig. 142, p. 344).

Why Do Teeth Decay ?

Views on the causes of decay of teeth and on how to prevent and arrest decay (caries) have been fundamentally influenced by the work of Dr. King and by the findings of Lady Mellanby and Dr. Helen Conmoulos published in an article

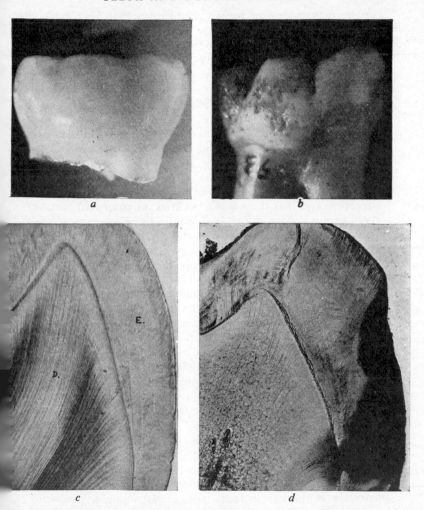

FIG. 77.—Different appearances of children's teeth due to differences in diet. A satisfactory diet produces teeth such as figs. *a* and *c*, with smooth external enamel and dense tooth substance as is shown in long-section. A poor diet results in pitted enamel as in *b* and this also shows in long-section as in *d*. (*From " Nutrition and Disease," by courtesy of Sir Edward Mellanby and Messrs. Oliver and Boyd, Ltd.*)

in the *British Medical Journal*, 19 October 1946, on ' Teeth of Five Year Old School Children.'

The teeth of children of the 5–6 year old group were surveyed in 1929 and again in 1943 and 1945, the same district and as far as possible the same schools in London being used.

In the 1929 group, of the 1,293 children examined, none was completely free of caries ; $4 \cdot 7 \%$ showed only slight caries.

In 1943, the proportion of children showing no or only slight caries was $22 \cdot 4 \%$, and by 1945 this proportion has risen still further to $26 \cdot 5 \%$.

In general terms, the results of these surveys showed that in the 1943 and 1945 groups, the children's teeth were of better structure and that there was less caries, as compared with the 1929 group. Also in the 1945 group, twice as many showed *spontaneous* arrest of caries than did the 1929 group.

These figures can be taken to give a reliable index of the general condition of the teeth of children of all ages at the relevant times, that is in 1929, 1943 and 1945, because both older and younger children would be eating much the same type of food and experiencing the same type of teeth care as would the groups examined. Hence it is safe to conclude that children of all age groups had poorer teeth in 1929 than in 1943 and certainly than in 1945.

The cause of dental caries—that is of decay of teeth—has been ascribed to (i) carbohydrates, (ii) poor dental hygiene and (iii) heredity. Mellanby and Conmoulos state that, " as far as their knowledge goes, there is no sound scientific foundation for any of these contentions."

(i) *The carbohydrate theory* of the cause of caries, is based on the premise that sugars and starches, such as chocolate, sweets, biscuits, bread and cake foods tend to leave a film of sugar or starch over and between the teeth. On this film, bacteria in the mouth feed, particularly at night, producing weak acids. These acids are considered to act on the enamel causing breaks in it, which then allow micro-organisms of decay to enter and to start decay.

To test the carbohydrate theory, King (1946) over a period of 6–24 months gave chocolate-coated biscuits and boiled sweets to a group of young children living in an institution, *after* they had cleaned their teeth last thing at night.

There was no increase of carious activity in these children over this period, and at the end of the test it was noted that previously active caries had been spontaneously arrested. The children had a good calcifying diet supplemented by cod-liver oil.

These findings are also supported by the survey of London school children's teeth 1929–43–45 because though the teeth condition was clearly better in the later groups, there was no evidence that less carbohydrate was eaten in one form or another in 1943 and 1945 than in 1929

(ii) *Dental Hygiene*.—The reduction of caries in the 1943 and 1945 groups as compared to the 1929 group of children cannot be related to better dental hygiene, because in the War years there were progressively fewer dentists to give dental treatment and fewer tooth brushes and less teeth cleaning material in the shops.

(iii) *Heredity*.—If resistance to decay is due to the inheritance of sound teeth, African and American Negroes should keep their good teeth *after* meeting Western civilisation, whereas they do not. Similarly the sound teeth of Eskimos do not withstand contact with Westernised trading stations. It would therefore appear that Westernised diet in some way affects the teeth of these peoples adversely.

Resistance to Decay

It is clear that resistance to decay is related to the structure of the tooth, which depends on (i) fluorides in the drinking water and (ii) right diet.

There is growing evidence that some *sodium fluoride* added to water supplies ($1 \cdot 2$ parts to a million parts) hardens the enamel of teeth and lessens the incidence of decay. This cannot be added by the house-holder in proportions small enough to be safe against mottled teeth and, in large doses, poisoning.

For well-formed teeth, resistant to decay, there must be enough Calcium, Phosphates and Vitamins A, D and C in the diets of (i) the pregnant and (ii) the nursing mother and (iii) the child during growth as well as throughout adult life. If the diet is deficient in these factors, then certain constituents of cereals—for example, oatmeal—may be harmful to the teeth.

Over the last twenty years diets have improved all round. Much more information is available as to the balance of foodstuffs needed and as to the effects of minerals and vitamins on optimum health.

Of recent years, and increasingly during the 1939–45 War, pregnant and nursing mothers as well as infants and children have been encouraged (a) to consume more milk and eggs and so to get from their diet more calcium, phosphates and vitamins A and D ; (b) to take extra vitamins A and D in cod and other fish liver oil and (c) extra vitamin C, as orange juice or black currant or rose hip syrup, which helps teeth development.

In addition, vitamins A and D have been added to margarine, at first voluntarily and since 1940 compulsorily. Since 1945, vitamin D has been added to national dried milk. Similarly, calcium was added to some flours before the War, but since 1943 this has been compulsory.

It must be noted that in spite of definite improvement, there were still in 1945, 73·5 % of the children in the age groups examined by Mellanby and Conmoulos with marked caries, so that there is room for considerable improvement yet.

In addition to correct dietary, other factors operating to prevent decay include the following ;—

(i) *Immune saliva* prevents teeth decay. All dogs, for example, have such saliva, whereas the saliva of monkeys and of man varies with the individual. In man, the possession of immune saliva is most frequent after adolescence and is commoner in men than in women.

(ii) The use of *raw milk* that has not been boiled or pasteurised helps to prevent decay. Also milk sugar lactose, helps calcification, unlike other carbohydrates.

(iii) The eating of *hard foods* that have to be chewed well is of great value. It brings additional blood to the tooth roots and also cleans the surface of the teeth. Such foods are raw fruits, like apples, raw vegetables, specially celery, lettuces, radishes and young carrots, crusts and whole-meal bread.

Typically non-cleansing foods are jams, chocolate, sweets, cakes, biscuits, milk puddings, soft white breads and bananas. If possible meals should end with teeth-cleansing food, such as apple, raw carrot, cauliflower or lettuce.

(iv) At all ages, the *general health* affects tooth soundness. Plenty of sleep, exercise, fresh air day and night, and nose breathing help to keep teeth healthy.

(v) *Teeth Cleaning* is practised for two reasons—(i) appearance and (ii) preservation. Manufacturers of tooth pastes have sponsored a slogan " Clean teeth never decay," but this was recognised to be unsound even before the importance of diet was understood. From the good teeth of Negroes living in un-Westernised conditions and from the research on children's teeth, noted earlier, it does appear that, given the right diet, teeth cleaning for preservation is not essential. As, however, it is difficult if not impossible to be certain that our rather synthetic diet is right in this sense, it is still important that teeth cleaning should be a routine matter both because of appearance and because it may help to ward off decay.

The teeth should be cleaned last thing at night and nothing should be eaten afterwards. Cleaning before meals, as before breakfast, makes the mouth feel fresh, and has a value for appearance. A small brush with good wired-in bristles that are unlikely to come out and be swallowed, a convex rather than a concave surface, and of medium stiffness is the best. Too stiff a brush tears the gums and makes them bleed, which is undesirable.

Brush the teeth up and down so that particles of food wedged between the teeth in biting may be dislodged ; brush also inside and outside and on the surfaces of the back molars. Avoid brushing the teeth horizontally, as it tends to tear the gums round the root neck of the tooth. Tooth-brushes should be kept clean by sterilising at intervals and by being put to drain and dry after use.

Tooth powders mainly aim at removing the film of food from the teeth surfaces by friction, whereas many tooth pastes, by becoming very thin and frothy, are able to penetrate easily, by capillary attraction, into the smallest crevices. The disinfecting quality of such dental pastes is probably so transitory as to be of little real value. They give, however, a clean fresh feeling and make the cleaning a more pleasant process.

Cracking nuts with the teeth, poking the teeth with pins, and eating very hot food should be avoided, as they may

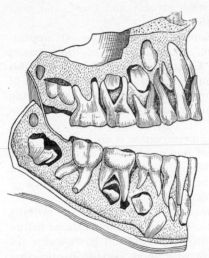

result in cracking of the enamel and thus start decay. The cleaning of teeth should start with the milk teeth, which if allowed to decay infect the permanent teeth below them in the jaw, so that these erupt already decayed.

Dentists

(vi) Every six months there should be a *routine inspection* of the teeth by a dentist, so that any beginnings of cavities can be stopped before much damage or pain results. No tooth should be left to decay so badly that it cannot be stopped and must be

FIG. 78.—The *milk teeth* of a child of 6½, showing the permanent teeth growing in the jaw bones. Their position is such that if the milk teeth decay, the permanent teeth are likely to be affected, even before eruption.

extracted. *Conservative dentistry* is concerned with filling small cavities and preserving teeth sound in the jaw for as many years as possible.

If the mother lacks vitamins A, C and D in her diet during *pregnancy and lactation*, the child's teeth are likely to erupt late and irregularly ; the enamel may be irregularly formed and poorly calcified, the surface being pitted and pigmented instead of smooth and white. The growth of dentine is likely to be irregular, with failure to lay down enough calcium and the membrane round the tooth's root may develop irregularly.

For irregular teeth once erupted, there should be early treatment and judicious extractions of extra teeth, so that the proper teeth can erupt into place evenly. Care must start with the milk teeth and little can be done after the age of ten or twelve. Mouth breathing, by subjecting the enamel to continual currents of cold air, conduces to decay; so does the eating of hot food followed by the drinking of cold water.

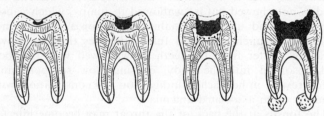

FIG. 79.—*Four stages of dental decay.* In stage 1, the enamel has decayed, while in stage 2 the dentine also has broken down. The dentist can remove the decay, disinfect the cavity, and insert a filling, and there is probably little or no pain. In stage 3 the pulp cavity is affected, and there is pain because of the inflammation in a confined space and of the nerve being involved. In stage 4 abscesses have formed at the tooth's root. Such septic foci, if neglected, may cause defects in other parts of the body, such as the joints or the heart, the poisons being carried by the blood and lymph streams. (*From " Those Teeth of Yours," revised and enlarged second edition, by J. Menzies Campbell, D.D.S., L.D.S., F.R.S.E.—Heinemann [Medical Books] Ltd.*)

In both instances the sudden lowering of temperature causes the enamel to contract too rapidly and produces cracks in it.

Comparative softness of enamel may show itself in pearly-white rather transparent-looking teeth; denser teeth probably have more calcium laid down in them and are more decay-resisting. Vitamin A is associated with healthy enamel (Fig. 77).

If the tooth is filled or stopped while the point of decay is small, there will be no pain and little alteration of the tooth. As the decay penetrates nearer to the pulp cavity, the tooth will become increasingly tender and give pain, both in eating and drinking and in the process of being stopped. Once the pulp cavity is reached more constant toothache is likely.   Furthermore, an opening has been made for bacteria from our mouth to travel down the pulp cavity and cause an abscess at the root of the tooth.

Effects of Carious Teeth

The *effects of decay of teeth* are widespread.   Immediately, decay results in pain, loss of sleep, fretfulness, bad breath, disfigurement and preventable absence from school, entailing educational loss to the child.   If the teeth are painful, the food is not chewed but is swallowed in lumps, which causes indigestion and ultimately malnutrition, for a child cannot absorb such unchewed food fully.   Besides this the brown decaying matter from the teeth is swallowed with the food and absorbed into the body, causing slow self-poisoning, which results in headaches, indigestion and constipation, with which is often associated anæmia.

The tonsils at the back of the throat may become infected from decaying teeth, causing continually recurring septic throats and making conditions for rheumatism to start. Poison from decayed teeth also drains down into the superficial lymphatic glands in the neck, and, if the strain of disposing of the poison is too prolonged, germs from the infected teeth may set up an abscess, a condition known as adentitis.

Pyorrhœa is a dental disease rather of adult life, though it may occur in children.   The teeth become loose and there seems a tendency for good rather than carious teeth to be attacked. The eating of fresh fibrous foods, supplying vitamins A and C, and the cutting down of protein and alcohol in the diet is advised.

School Dentistry

The *aims of school dentistry* are preventive and educational.

As to *prevention*, at present about half the school population can be inspected each year, but only about half of the children needing treatment can have it.   A complete dental service should allow of all children being inspected annually and of treatment being given to those who need it, not less than 70 to 80 per cent. of those inspected probably.

School dentistry, seeking to conserve and not to extract teeth, should not only benefit the child immediately, but also be a safeguard to health into adolescence and adult life. The work of the school dentist can be helped in various ways: by propaganda (the giving away of pamphlets on the care of teeth and suggestions about diet, the showing of films and the displaying of posters), by health education, teaching and tooth-brush drills in school and by the personal interest of the teacher in the particular child. Above everything is the teacher's example and the conviction of the value of the care of the teeth that he or she advocates.

Parents as well as children need to be educated to value the work of the school dentist, so that they always consider trying to preserve a tooth by having it filled rather than insisting on its extraction. This latter attitude is unfortunately strengthened because the early stages of decay are painless and may not show, so that when eventually the tooth comes to be treated, the process of filling is painful, if it can be done at all. In addition, dental treatment is comparatively expensive and may be put off for that reason. It is encouraging that an increasing proportion of children who are recommended for dental treatment actually come for it.

One matter on which ante-natal clinics give advice is about diets to preserve both the mother's and the child's teeth.

CHAPTER XII

THE SKIN AND KIDNEYS

THE body gets rid of solid waste products through the bowels and of liquid and gaseous waste through the lungs, skin and kidneys. The skin and kidneys balance each other in the work of excreting excess water with its dissolved urea and uric acid. That is to say, in cold weather we perspire less and micturate more; whereas in summer, we perspire actively and excrete less urine.

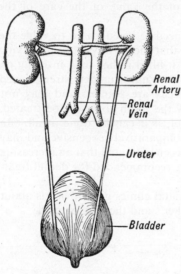

The *kidneys* are two glands lying either side the lumbar or waist region of the spine. The substance of the kidney is made up of coils of small tubes, intertwined with blood capillaries. Urea is extracted from the blood as it is circulated, and the urine drains down the ureter, the tube connecting each kidney to the bladder, at the rate of a drop a second. The bladder is emptied through the urethra, controlled by a sphincter muscle. Six to eight ounces of urine collect in the bladder before the reflex feeling to empty the bladder occurs. Control of this reflex is part of the training of young children.

FIG. 80.—The *kidneys and bladder* viewed from behind. The arteries and veins bring blood to, and take it from, the kidneys. Urine is extracted and drains down the ureters into the muscular-walled bladder, which contracts to expel the contents.

148

Adolescents and adults may, however, do themselves harm by long delay in emptying the bladder. Girls and women, particularly, are able to delay thus, but by doing so they may over-stretch the ligament that holds the uterus in place and cause permanent weakness, which may later lead to displacement of the womb. This ligament can withstand jars but not such continued steady pressure as an over-full bladder exerts. Continued constipation also exercises similar undue and harmful pressure.

Infants in school incited by suggestion are apt to ask to leave the room in order to get a run rather than because of need. It is better for the teacher to be easy than over-strict on this point, the children gradually being trained to go to the offices in recess. Inflammation of the urinary tract may make children need to micturate with what seems like over-frequency. Inflammation of the kidneys, even leading to Bright's disease, may occur as a serious after-effect of scarlet fever. Great care must be taken therefore to avoid the exciting cause, chill, during convalescence.

The Skin

The *skin* is a waterproof elastic protection which is continually wearing away and being renewed. It consists of two layers, the *epidermis*, or outer layer, and the *dermis*, or true skin below. In the epidermis the cells, as they get nearer to the surface, become flattened and dried up and are eventually washed away, or they are worn away as dry scales of skin on clothing. The dermis is well supplied with capillaries. Nerves of feeling end in touch corpuscles there. Sweat glands, opening on to the epidermis surface, are coiled round, and continually take sweat from the capillaries that surround them. Hairs, into the follicles of which open sebaceous or fat-supplying glands, grow from the dermis. In plump people fat accumulates under the skin. Women have more subcutaneous fat than men, and are the more rounded in form and resist cold better. Note the success of plump people, who lose less heat, in long-distance swimming.

Between the dermis and epidermis is the *malpighian layer*

of cells in which is deposited in dark-skinned people the pigment that gives their characteristic colouring.

The work of the skin is (i) to protect the tissues beneath

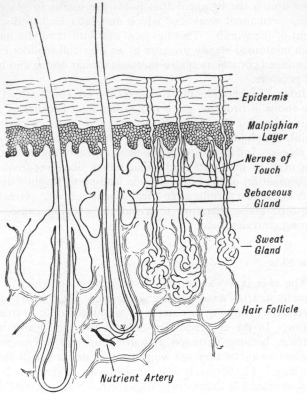

FIG. 81.—The skin.

from bacterial invasion (ii) to excrete sweat (iii) to regulate the body heat, and (iv) to act as an organ of touch.

The Skin and Heat Balance

Loss of perspiration goes on constantly to the extent of from two or three pints daily, but if the body is inactive, sweat does not appear on the skin as visible drops of moisture, as in activity. Sweat is 98 per cent. water, and its solids include common salt as well as urea. There are some two and a half million sweat glands over the whole skin, fewest, 400 to a square inch, on the back, and most on the palm of the hand, the sole and the axilla (the arm pit), where there are from two to three thousand to the square inch.

Five-sixths of the body's heat is lost from the skin by evaporation and by convection currents of air, produced by the heating of the layer of air next to the skin. The surrounding atmosphere is always cooler than the body. If the body is in a hot atmosphere, or if by movement it makes extra heat inside itself, the nerves that control the blood-vessels to the skin allow the muscular walls of each small artery to dilate, so that more blood can flow through the skin capillaries. Thus the skin surface becomes flushed and warmer, and loses heat to the air around it, unless, as in a stuffy room, the air is already over-hot and moist (see Chapter VI).

If, on the other hand, the air is cold, the nerves of the skin arteries contract them so that less blood goes to the skin, which is blanched and possibly cold and dry. In this way the blood is conserved in the deeper parts of the body and heat is retained. However cold the body may feel, the deep body temperature in normal health always remains at $98\cdot4°$ F. *Shivering* is a device by which the muscles, in contracting rapidly, squeeze still more blood out of themselves to the deeper organs, again conserving heat. The involuntary muscle contractions of the shivering also liberate heat.

Skin as a Sense Organ

The skin is not a specialised sense organ such as the eye, which receives sensation of light, and the ear of hearing, but it contains organs of feeling. Distributed in the dermis are end organs of sensory nerves differentiated to feel heat and others to feel cold, others to register the amount of pressure and (most widely distributed of all) end organs to feel pain.

Round the root of each of the small hairs that are distributed all over the skin is a belt of nervous tissue that gives the feeling of being tickled if the hairs are gently stroked and thus pressed

6

against it. In addition to end organs in the dermis, there are sense organs in muscles and round joints that indicate to the brain the position of the limb and the amount of contraction

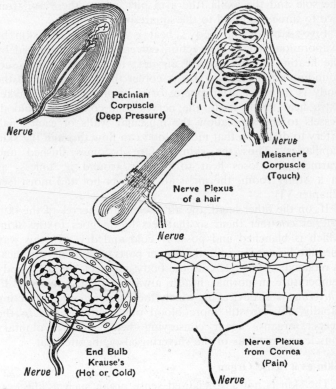

FIG. 82.—Different kinds of *sensory nerve endings in the skin*. The most widely distributed of all are those conveying sensations of pain.
(After Starling.)

of muscle-groups that is being made. This is the kinæsthetic sense.

In judging the solidity of an object, without looking at it, in addition to the skin sense organs, the sense organs in the muscles indicate to the brain the amount of pressure that is necessary or possible for them to exert. It can readily be seen that almost all touch sensations will be made up of the sensations reported by a number of differing nerve endings.

A golf ball, for instance, differs from a tennis ball, if neither is looked at, in being less susceptible to pressure, in having a smooth, hard yet patterned surface against a yielding cloth surface, and in being colder to touch and smaller. In feeling something hot, both heat and pain end organs would report. Damp skin is more sensitive to impressions than dry skin.

The sense of touch is much more acute in some parts of the body, such as the lips, tongue, cheeks, finger-tips, than in other areas, such as the back and thighs. Relative sensitiveness is tested by touching the skin, out of sight of the subject, with the two blunted ends of a divider, the subject saying whether he feels the divider is touching at one or two points. On the back, nerve endings are so sparse that the points have to be set 3 inches apart before the subject can feel two points of pressure. Anything less is felt as one point only. On the cheek anything less than 1 inch is felt as one point touching, but on the finger-tips 1/12 of an inch gives two points, and on the tip of the tongue 1/24 inch. These figures of course vary slightly from person to person, but their relative differences are constant.

How the Skin Protects the Body

The skin protects the tissues below from injury, forming blisters and callosities against undue rubbing. It prevents the ingress of harmful bacteria, which are continually present on the epidermis. If the skin is clean, it appears to have some power of gradually killing micro-organisms on its surface. This power is lost if the skin is dirty.

Hence if the skin is to fulfil its functions satisfactorily it must be kept clean. In ordinary life, it is constantly exuding perspiration and grease and is in contact with air heavily charged with dust particles. Thus it is continually accumulating layers of acid sweat and grease-holding dirt that need regular washing off, apart from the dirt accumulated by special work, such as coal-mining or sweeping a room. This temporary need to wash happens to everyone.

Habitual Dirt

It is *habitual uncleanliness* that matters ; not to-day's dirt but yesterday's or last week's dirt. If the body is not washed regularly, it smells stuffy and acid and people who smell thus suggest fears of disease and are unacceptable socially. The sebaceous glands (not the sweat glands), may become stopped up, and their greasy openings on the skin surface becomes a focus for dirt, forming blackheads. Habitually dirty-skinned people are likely to have parasites, and any cut or abrasion on the skin has the more chance of becoming septic and of healing less rapidly. Habitual dirt also goes with ignorance, a lack of self-respect, and suggests tolerance of squalid living (see Chapter XIV).

Soaps

Water alone is not sufficient to remove greasy dirt. *Soap* is made from boiling fat with an alkali, potash forming soft and soda hard soaps. The free alkali in the soap helps in removing grease, but too much, as in cheap or in household soaps, roughens the skin. Carbolic and disinfectant soaps cannot have enough disinfectant incorporated in them to kill germs. Their effect is mainly psychological, their smell being reassuring. Ordinary yellow soap would do just as well, however. Used for toilet purposes carbolic soap is definitely harmful, because it roughens the skin and is thus more likely than most other soaps to cause openings for the ingress of the bacteria it is supposed to kill.

It is a mistake to think that the face does not need washing with soap. Use as good a soap as can be afforded and wash in warm water, using a face-cloth to apply the soap, particularly into the crevices. Such washing will do much to remove and prevent blackheads and make the skin fresh and attractive. A cold sponge afterwards tones up the skin and closes the pores, again helping to prevent blackheads.

Powders, habitually used, tend to enlarge the pores so that they show too much. If powder is used, finish the day with a nourishing greasy cream to prevent the skin from getting prematurely dried and wrinkled.

Not everyone can have a bath in a tub every day, but, given a quart of warm water a day, it should be possible to wash all over in from five to ten minutes. Washing to the waist only is not enough. Cold baths in the morning have a useful tonic effect for people who feel warm after them. They are not cleansing. A warm bath, the temperature about 110° F., may be enervating if continued over long.

Of the *common skin affections* that recur in school, it is important to differentiate clearly between those originally caused by dirt and the non-dirt diseases, though, of course, clean people may catch dirt-encouraged diseases too.

Ringworm

Of the *non-dirt diseases*, *Ringworm* stands out, because of the amount of school absence it has caused. It is actually due to a vegetable fungus, and may occur in the form of body or head ringworm.

Body Ringworm occurs at any age, and begins with a pink, smooth, irregular patch, which heals in the centre and spreads out round the edge. Infected children should be excluded from school, and in order to prevent the disease spreading, other persons should not use their bedding and towels. Regular application of sulphur and white precipitate ointment should cure body ring-worm in three to four weeks. It is not usually irritable.

Head Ringworm shows itself in bald, scurfy patches on the scalp, not necessarily in ring form. The hair breaks off short. Teachers should learn to recognise early possible symptoms and refer children for examination by the school nurse or doctor, thus getting cases treated promptly and minimising fresh infections. Talks to mothers at welfare centres also help. All brushes, combs and pillows should be kept for the personal use of the patient, and clothes, taken off over the head, boiled at frequent intervals.

Ringworm is very catching, and is carried from child to child by caps and hats. Infected children should be excluded from school. At one time it used to take as long as four or five years to cure, thus entailing educational loss for the child and loss of grants to the local education authority, because every child on the register and absent used to mean about $3\frac{1}{2}d$. loss in grant per session. Over a period of months, and for a number of children, this loss became a serious one for the local rates.

Thus when it was found that X-ray treatment for ringworm meant comparatively speedy cure, it became both of

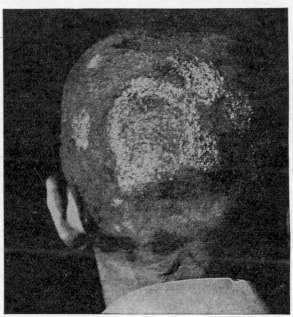

FIG. 83.—*Head ringworm*, a scurfy patch (not a ring) with stumps of broken hairs. (*From Adamson's " Skin Affections in Childhood "*—*Oxford Medical Publications*.)

educational advantage to the child and of grant-earning value to the authority to set up this fairly expensive apparatus for giving treatment. Only skilled operators should apply such X-ray treatment, during which the infected hair falls out and a new growth of hair occurs. Cure should be effected in about three months, and no child should return to school till microscopic examination has demonstrated freedom from spores. School nurses and health visitors co-operate in examining home contacts and in giving advice about preventing spread of infection.

Ringworm occurs rather more frequently in boys than in girls, possibly because of the shorter hair, and quite as much in middle-class as in poverty-line children.

Alopecia is a non-infectious condition in which bald, shiny patches appear on the scalp, which may become normal again over a period of months or the effects may be permanent. The condition is sometimes confused with ringworm. It is thought now to be due to disturbance of the nerves, whose nerve endings serve the area affected. Artificial sunlight treatment, local and general, has effected cures, and open-air school life may be advised.

Acne, the appearance of little pus-forming spots, often occurs in adolescence on the face. Pus-forming staphylococci (Fig. 6) probably lie quiescent in the mouth of sebaceous glands and, particularly in greasy skins, are apt to form small suppurating heads. A diet with ample vitamin content is of value. Constipation should be avoided ; chocolates and sweets should be eaten sparingly ; the spots should not be scratched, for this causes re-infection. Pus heads should be fomented with hot, wet cotton wool. Regular washing with a good soap helps to prevent acne.

Warts are caused by a virus and are infectious.

Impetigo

Of *skin diseases associated with dirt*, one of the more common forms is *Impetigo* or *Scald Head*. It shows as little blisters first, at the corners of the mouth and round the nose, possibly spreading to the body and head. The blisters, caused by bacterial infection, break to form a yellow amber crust. There is some itching. Impetigo is very contagious and is spread easily by dirty hands and finger-nails. It is associated with grime and neglect, dirty heads and body lice. Children of school age may be persistently re-infected after treatments from a pre-school child at home. Scratches on knees and hands may be self-infected. There is a rise in the number of children with impetigo after holidays, a fact which shows the value of the teacher's and school nurse's care.

Treatment is preferably by the closed (Elastoplast) method. Quicker and more effective healing occurs than in the older " open " treatment by bathing and the application of ointment, and the children need not be excluded from school. Dressings of sulphonamide are effective. In using this, the plaster should be applied generously because small pieces fall off. Malt and cod-liver oil, Parrish's food, and aperients may be prescribed. Persistent cases should be considered for extra feeding and for admission to an open-air school.

The disease is not considered as it once was to be solely confined to unclean children. It occurs fairly frequently among debilitated children, who are inclined to have colds. Though not dangerous, it causes considerable discomfort to the child and vexation to the parents, takes up much clinic time and interferes with school work.

To curtail and prevent it the school nurse should survey classes from which cases have come to detect early further infections ; leaflets may well be distributed to parents on treatment and prevention ; school towels and drinking vessels must not be used indiscriminately, for infection may pass from one child to another. An infected child should, if possible, sleep alone, and the finger-nails be kept cut short to minimise scratching, and old gloves be worn at night. The health visitor should follow up cases and give advice in the home.

Scabies

Scabies or Itch is a dirt-associated infection due to a parasite, just visible, which burrows under the skin, especially in the creases of joints and between the fingers, and lays eggs, making a little vesicle at the burrow opening. The usual incubation period is a fortnight to three weeks, but it may be as much as two months. At night, when the skin is warm, the young parasites crawl out of the burrows and the itching is intense, causing the scratching of sores and scars. Scabies is spread by intimate contacts such as sleeping in the same bed, rather than by clothing or bedding, but towels in restaurants for the use of all comers are specially to be avoided.

Treatment : a lotion of benzyl benzoate 25 per cent., soft soap 25 per cent., with methylated spirit up to 100 per cent. and a little boric acid. The lotion is painted all over the body.

One application only is usually sufficient. If there are sores, the lotion is made up without soft soap. Re-infection is prevented by changing and boiling or stoving all clothes and bedding. Treatment centres may be necessary, since baths and complete changes may be difficult to arrange in some homes. Frequently the house and the people in it are sources of infection. The sanitary authority may therefore, undertake wholesale disinfection of clothes and bedding while the family is removed to a treatment centre. Although clean people may be infected, continual family re-infection is an index of social inefficiency.

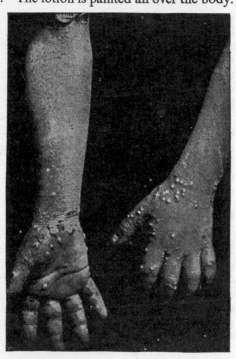

FIG. 84.—Scabies or Itch, a dirt disease. (*From Drummond's " School Hygiene "— Edward Arnold & Co.*)

The continued presence of body lice, fleas, bed-bugs and pediculosis is an indication of the acceptance of dirty and squalid living conditions. Cleanliness and freedom from parasites, however, are difficult for families that live

6*

in one room, especially in crowded slum conditions where lice are possibly swarming on the walls.

Great improvement in housing has been made in the last twenty years. Dirt conditions must be combated in the long run, not by penal methods but by educating people so that they *want* to be clean. Under the Children's Act (1907) the local education authority is empowered to require parents to cleanse a child and, failing this, may arrange for such cleansing at cleansing stations. Parents may be fined for the non-attendance at school of a child excluded for uncleanliness, whom they have failed to cleanse. Publicity for prosecutions is a useful deterrent.

All slum clearance schemes help to provide conditions making for cleanliness, but the urge to be clean must be in the people themselves. Dirty people may still be dirty even in a garden city. The schools are doing progressively more to make children understand what being clean means, that is, to have a standard.

Head Lice

Head lice are more common among girls than among boys, Dr. Kenneth Mellanby in 1944 found that there was a higher degree of infestation in industrial cities than in country districts and that the highest rate was among pre-school children, girls of three reaching a proportion of $51 \cdot 6$ per cent. with ' dirty heads ' and there was little decrease in rate until fourteen. For boys, the highest percentage of infestation—40 per cent.—occurred at four years of age. Permanent waves that are not combed out and brushed regularly, lead to infestation in young adult women. In some drafts of the women's services during the 1939–45 War, 50 per cent. of the intake were infested.

The head louse is a colourless, inert, blood-sucking insect. The female lays up to a hundred eggs in her three to four weeks of life. The eggs, called nits, are cemented obliquely on the hair near to the scalp, pointing downwards, rather under the surface of the hair. The nit hatches in about six days, the egg case remaining cemented to the hair. The louse in biting injects a poison which increases the irritation. In prolonged cases, the occipital lymphatic glands at the back of the neck become enlarged and even tubercular. Nits can often be seen in the hairs behind the ears.

Treatment : (i) For the Lice, rubbing in of " Lethane 384 " special hair oil is effective and does not itself smell noticeably It does not remove nits but kills those it wets.[1]

Nits must be cut out or can be dissolved off by soaking in vinegar for about 30 minutes. No head is clean until it is free from nits.

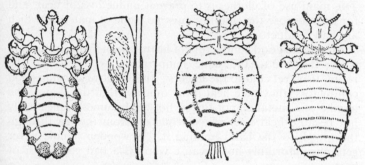

FIG. 85.—Different kinds of lice, and a nit or egg cemented to a hair, the point of growth of which is from below in this diagram, hence the impossibility of brushing or combing nits from the hair. (*After Hewer.*)

(ii) Benzyl benzoate emulsion destroys the lice and also dissolves the cement by which the nits adhere to the hair. It is relatively expensive.

Any tooth-combing of the hair must be done with a good quality steel comb.

The powder " D.D.T." has given a new power of exterminating insect but is harmless to other life. One dusting with " D.D.T." destroys, for example, fleas, head and body lice, bugs or flies, all of which in different ways are responsible for spreading infections.

Use of " D.D.T." must be accompanied by routine cleansing to destroy eggs and dirt conditions favouring breeding.

[1] *Gammexane*, which needs to be diluted just before use with four parts of water, is now used alternatively with " Lethane." " Gammexane " is easy to apply, does not irritate child or nurse and, unlike " Lethane," has some effect in discouraging lice, even after washing the hair. It does not, however, kill nits. D.D.T. lotions are also used when " Lethane " is not procurable.

Chapter XIII

CLOTHING

The main use of clothes is to prevent undue loss of heat, and for this purpose the clothing must be made of materials which are bad conductors of heat.

Metals are good conductors of heat. Even in a warm room, where they are at the same temperature as the air in the room, they feel cold to the fingers; this is because, being good conductors, they take heat away quickly from the skin. The handle of a metal teapot full of hot tea becomes unpleasantly hot because heat is conducted quickly from the tea through the metal, to the hand holding it. A wooden handle never gets uncomfortably hot because wood is a bad conductor of heat.

Any substance, like cloth, carpet or asbestos, that does not strike cold to the touch, is a bad conductor of heat. Though some objects in a room feel colder than others, they may all actually be at the same temperature,[1] that of the room, say, about 60° F. The differences are due to differences in the rates at which heat is conducted away from the body, the temperature of which (98·4° F.) is always higher than that of things in the room.

Wool *v*. Cotton

Air is a bad conductor of heat, so that rough materials that hold air in their interstices, such as woollen tweeds, knitted stockings, woven underwear and furs, are the best to wear in cold weather, when heat needs conserving; smooth materials, such as cotton, linens and artificial silks, which allow the body to lose heat, are preferable in warm weather. Wool fibres

[1] Except, of course, things like hot radiators and any living people, mammals or birds.

162

have a natural curly bend or camp in them that, when woven, holds air in the material. Cotton fibres can be worked up to simulate wool in this respect. Materials of this sort containing cotton, however, tend to be heavy, whereas wool materials are relatively light.

Wool also retains some natural oil of the fleece, and this makes it able to absorb moisture slowly and to dry slowly, whereas cotton absorbs moisture quickly and dries quickly. Contrast the effect of being caught in a rain shower in a woollen tweed coat, in which the rain-drops stand on the material's surface and can be shaken off, and in a cotton or linen dress, in which each rain-spot shows as a circular wet patch and the soaked material is soon clinging damply to the skin. This hydroscopic quality of wool ensures that when the skin perspires and the body tends, on a cold day, to lose heat over-quickly, the wool next

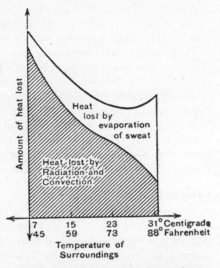

FIG. 86.—Heat lost by radiation and conduction warms the air around the body. This is greater at lower temperatures when the difference between the body temperature $98 \cdot 4°$ and the air temperature $45°$ is greater. The higher the air temperature the less heat is lost thus, and the body's excess heat is then adjusted by quicker loss of heat in sweating.

to the skin absorbs the perspiration *slowly* and dries *slowly*. This prevents noticeably rapid loss of heat and the chilled feeling that means that the body resistance is lowered, and that, given a dose of cold germs, a cold may be caught.

A cotton vest soaked with perspiration after exercise feels cold and damp against the skin. Heat is being lost over-rapidly. We should not be conscious of this cooling down, and this is the time to put on an extra coat, so that heat may be lost more slowly.

Analogously, sitting on damp grass, sleeping in a damp bed, or putting on unaired clothing, chills the body, because the body heat is used to dry up the damp. This makes for special susceptibility to an active attack of rheumatism.

A school of thought exists that doubts the value of wool next to the skin. It is argued that by keeping the skin over-warm and by absorbing moisture and drying slowly, wool may tend to keep the skin in a continued state of dampness, and so over-ready to lose heat rapidly and be chilled, whereas cool air passing over a dry skin has comparatively little power to chill. Similarly, tightly fitting clothes, such as woven vests round the body, and armholes closing in the axilla, are considered to lead to habitual moistness of skin from perspiration. The aim is for the skin never to be so hot, either from clothes or from over-heating of air, as to be perspiring visibly, except during and after strenuous physical exertion.

Cellular Cotton

Aertex cellular cotton material is an alternative to wool for wearing next to the skin. It holds air in its cellular structure and so is a bad conductor of heat as is wool. Hence it feels warm. It absorbs moisture slowly and does not feel cold against the skin when saturated with perspiration as does ordinary cotton. It is relatively cheap, non-inflammable, and it washes well and does not shrink.

Continual warm dampness of the skin from wearing wool next to the skin is considered to cause increased susceptibility to " head " colds, rheumatism and tuberculosis. In this connection, it is perhaps significant that rheumatism occurs less frequently in the hardy gipsy and the middle-class child than in the still over-clothed and coddled child of the artisan.

Children need to be brought up to be hardy and not to be afraid of cold. This does not mean that they should be made to suffer from cold, as in having cold baths or sitting in an unheated room on the annoying and uneconomical plea that it is " good for them." The hardening process can be gradual and unnoticed. A good average power of resisting cold and heat, hunger and thirst, injuries and disease is a useful emergency asset throughout life.

Whether wool is worn next to the skin or not, excessive clothing, especially when it is too tight, makes one less able to stand adverse health conditions. It is of interest, perhaps, to note that the average total weight of a man's clothes is 15 lb., whereas a woman's is about 4 lb.

The temperature indoors, as in classrooms, should be such that children do not need, and are not encouraged, to wear top-coats and scarves while there. If outdoor clothes are worn indoors, there will tend to be relatively too much blood in the skin (causing the skin to perspire and lose heat) and too little in the brain ; and when outdoors the child will be hot-skinned and enervated and inclined to catch cold, instead of being braced and stimulated mentally and physically. Outdoor clothes with open-air classrooms are, of course, better still.

It should be remembered also, that wool shrinks and loses its natural oil unless it is washed carefully. Cotton washes and wears well, can be boiled, and is relatively cheaper than wool. Wool, however, unlike cotton, does not catch fire easily. Cotton wool and flannelette are entirely cotton and are very inflammable. Flannelette can be bought impregnated with chemicals to counteract this, but washing removes this safeguard.

Silk is a bad conductor of heat, but is relatively expensive and not hard wearing. Linen, though hard wearing, is more expensive than cotton. Like cotton it is a good conductor of heat.

Values of Loose Clothing

Clothing, as noted earlier, should be loose and light, and the weight should hang from the shoulders. *Tight boots and gloves* hinder the circulation of blood, causing cold feet and hands, and possibly chilblains. *Tight garters and knicker elastics*, that make a mark on the leg, also hinder the circulation and they conduce to varicose veins in later life. Tight knicker elastics and belts round the waist compress the abdominal organs and tend in the long run to induce a deposit of fat along the line of constriction. *Tight corsets* are, fortunately, now unfashionable. Those worn in former days used to constrict the lower part of the lungs, preventing adequate breathing as well as displacing the liver and stomach by downward pressure.

Records kept among College women from 1891 onwards show a decrease in " green sickness " (a form of anæmia), in digestive disturbances, in tendency to faint and in menstrual disability. An increase was observed in average height and all-round fitness and joy of life, which kept pace in an interesting way with the enlarging of the average waist measurement and with the shortening and lessened voluminousness of the skirt (*Mosher*). Brassières should be carefully chosen so that they give support, especially forward and inward, to the breasts without pressing them out of place.

Boys suffer from tight collars more than girls. *Tight, stiff collars* press on veins on either side of the neck that take the blood from the head back to the heart, causing relative congestion in the head and so less oxygen in the brain. Such collars, by over-clothing the neck, also increase susceptibility to cold. An open-necked shirt with a pull-over is neat and free. Collars also impede muscle development at the base of the neck. Contrast sailors' necks with those of a regular collar wearer. *Tight hats*, among other things, probably conduce, among other influences, to baldness by constricting the scalp circulation and by pressure on scalp nerves.

Loose clothes are always warmer than tight ones, and two loose thin layers than one thick layer, because of the air that can be held in the interstices and between the looser garments. The air held in the clothes of children sitting continuously in a hot, moist atmosphere gets over hot and stagnant, and one advantage of a quick break in the open air is the bracing moving and changing of this enveloping " garment " of warm air.

On the other hand, a cold, damp east wind blows through the interstices of clothes, so that the body has a continually changing cold layer of air next to it, which it tries in vain to warm. Skin and fur coats and closely woven materials resist this kind of wind, but loosely knitted jerseys do not. Rubber mackintoshes, because they keep in moisture which condenses on the inside rubber surface, are unhealthy for regular use, as are rubber gymnastic shoes, particularly for people whose feet perspire markedly.

Dark clothes absorb heat more than light ones, as was shown by the following experiment cited by Dr. Argyll Campbell. A piece of black material put on the surface of snow in the sun sank in deeply, while a piece of white material of similar size and shape scarcely sank in at all, in the same time ; the snow under the black material had received more heat and had melted more. For protection against heat, colour counts more than material, white being coolest, then yellow, pink, blue, and black last.

Underclothing worn during the day should never be worn at night. In garments worn next to the skin, bacteria increase rapidly ; after one day's wearing 400,000 bacteria to the square inch were found, and they increased after six days' wearing to nearly ten million per square inch. Such bacteria probably increase stuffy smells. Frequent washing and sun drying lessen them.

Dark woollen knickers need to have washable linings to wear with them, and a vest and cotton knickers are preferable to combinations to wear next to the skin, because knickers can easily be washed and so changed more frequently.

Clothing should be of about equal thickness all over the body. Children who wear socks and very short skirts or knickers in winter may tend to lose too much heat. In summer, girls as well as boys should play games and do physical training stockingless and, if possible, in bathing costume, thus getting out of doors the benefit of the ultra-violet rays from the sunlight. Both boys' and girls' clothing should fasten in front, where fastenings are necessary, so that the children can dress and undress themselves.

Shoes

For *footgear*, shoes are preferable to boots for normal people, because boots tend to take the place of the muscles in supporting the foot and leg at the ankle and make for weaker joints, just as the old type of corset weakened the abdominal muscles.

Shoes should fit firmly round the heel and over the instep, and give room in the front of the shoe for the toes to spread out uncramped. In the natural foot the inner side is straight, with no inward bend of the big toe at that joint. Shoes then should be similarly straight on the inner side, so that they do not press the big toe inwards out of place, as over-pointed shoes do ; in order to avoid deforming the foot, the point of the shoe should come in front of the big toe and not of the third toe as it often does (Fig. 20, *a*).

On the inner side the shoe should fit smoothly to the hollow of the instep, without any wrinkles. When laced up there should be a space between the two laced sides. If these touch the shoe is too big round the instep and will not fit firmly on the foot. A blocked-up toe leaves the toes uncompressed. In buying new shoes there should be half an inch between the big toe and the end of the shoe, when standing up.

Bunions and Corns

Short shoes cause *bunions*. Pressure on the end of the big toe causes " give " in the big toe joint, and inflammation of its synovial bursa, called synovitis. The first symptoms are pain and redness ; if the joint is painted with a counter-irritant, such as iodine, and the shoes discarded at once, there should be no more trouble. Wearing out such short shoes, in a mistaken sense of economy, results possibly in a lifetime of foot pain from a bunion and in unsightly foot shape.

Corns come from the continual rubbing on the same spot of an ill-fitting shoe. Careful choice of shoes and the keeping, possibly, of several pairs of shoes in wear in rotation, never the same pair two days running, does something to prevent corns from coming. Corns should not be allowed to get very painful before they are dealt with. Regular daily washing and care of the feet are essential.

High Heels

High heels shorten the normal stride in walking and give a jerky " clack clack " tread, because the body weight is changed over-abruptly at each step from the heel to the ball of the foot. A medium heel makes for foot comfort and economy of output in walking. People who say they need high-heeled shoes for support probably need instep arch supports for flat-foot. High heels also put undue strain on the muscles and ligaments of the ankle joint, so that the heel " goes over," that is, wears down markedly on the inner or outer side (see Chapter II). Certainly children should wear low-heeled shoes over the muscle-straining period of growth.

Chilblains

Tight shoes, and those with very thin soles, cause continual cold feet, because damp readily permeates the shoe. This causes loss of heat and leads again to chilblains, colds and rheumatism. *Chilblains* are excited by too rapid warming of cold feet and hands by the fire or on hot-water pipes. The value of warm, snugly fitting shoes may be diminished by the wearing of over thin or tight stockings, so that too much heat is lost or the circulation impeded. Warm stockings or spats or gaiters, and warm underclothing are useful in cold weather. Important factors in treatment appear to be comfort and good food, especially butter and eggs. Ultra-violet light is also valuable.

Apart from the effect of cold, proneness to chilblains seems to depend on individual metabolism, for some people get them very readily. The regular taking of cod-liver oil and of calcium *before* the cold weather sets in is sometimes advised. Painting with iodine relieves the irritation to some extent. Vigorous exercise, such as long walks, helps to get rid of chilblains, by increasing the circulation locally. This increase of circulation is also the object of the rubbing which is often advised.

Prolonged cold feet conduces to congestion of the nasal mucous membrane, thus reducing resistance to colds. Constant wearing of bedroom slippers causes an habitual slovenly walk and a relaxing of foot tone of muscles and joints. Stockings should be changed after exercise, both because continued soaking of perspiration spoils the stocking foot and because a change freshens and braces the feet. Teachers should impress on their classes that the feet should be as clean as the hands and that there is no danger in daily feet washing, as is still thought in some areas.   Physical training done barefoot emphasises this.

Nails

Nails on hands and feet should be kept clipped short and clean and the quick be kept pressed evenly down, to prevent hang-nails developing.   A stiff nail-brush, hot water and soap are better than a sharp instrument poked under the nail to clean away dirt.   *Ingrowing toe-nails* on the feet can be prevented by cutting the nail straight across with a slight concave shape in the middle, the opposite way to finger-nails, which grow and are cut to a convex shape.   A slight filing of the nail surface down its middle line also helps.   This concave cutting makes the nail tend to grow towards the middle line of the nail, and so away from the sides, where there is the possible tendency to grow in painfully.   Tight shoes conduce to ingrowing toe-nails.

Verruca are a form of wart that occurs on the plantar (under) surface of the foot.   They are infectious and are caught by walking barefoot, for example, round swimming-baths. Medical treatment is necessary.

Chapter XIV

THE PRACTICE OF HEALTH

It is one of the school's duties to train children to assume all-round cleanliness as part of their average standard of living, not as a matter of what might be called "party manners," for it is what is *assumed* rather than what is asserted that shows people's real views. For example, it is normal after dressing in the morning to leave a bed stripped to air ; getting up late might preclude this, but in proportion to the strength of the habit, there would be a sense of disgrace in having failed to reach a standard. In a different case is the person who does not know that such bed-stripping is usual—who does not even assume it.

Cleanliness training is concerned with more than just cleanliness of the skin. Cleanliness and trimness of clothes—buttons on, shoes cleaned ; freshness and tidiness of rooms, house, gardens and particularly back premises ; the putting away of used articles ; fresh and airy beds and bedrooms ; the leaving of baths and lavatory pans clean and the keeping of streets and town litterless—all these come among the aspects of cleanliness training with which the school must deal.

Conditions in towns tend to cause relative overcrowding so that dirt of person and of habits in using public conveniences or in leaving refuse about rapidly bring harmful results, and not to the offender only. Adults will have a pleasanter and healthier time individually and be less expense and annoyance to the community if, as children, they have been systematically trained to *prefer* cleanliness. Infants and juniors have no instinctive preference for it.

171

Stages in Health Training

In *the practice of health* three stages can be distinguished :—

(i) *The "drill" stage.* This is the stage in which the young child carries out health practices regularly without question because he is expected to do so by an adult. He uses his handkerchief, cleans his teeth, washes, because no other course occurs to him. It has always been assumed. This stage merges into the next—

(ii) *The stage of social approval.* At this stage the child

    (*a*) in the infant school carries out health practices to win the approval of parent or teacher or of other adults.

    (*b*) Later in the Junior School he carries out health practices to be acceptable in the gang to which he belongs. He follows the child leader of the gang, and practice is largely due to imitation and so to indirect suggestion. The Cub and Brownie stage of the Scout and Guide movements have this incentive.

    (*c*) Later still, in Secondary and Modern Schools, the adolescent carries out health practices because the adults or older pupils do so. His motive for doing so is to save attracting unwelcome attention and comment or reproof. His standard is set not by what he believes himself but by the standards of the people around him. Adults who orient their behaviour by what the neighbours think, or, as most of us do, follow fashion in dress or pattern of living, are still partly at this stage.

(iii) *The stage of self-respect* is reached when adolescents and adults carry out health practices in order not to fall short of their own ideals, regardless of what others think or do or feel in the matter.

At the "drill" stage, children should learn, by constant repetition, a number of specific habits, which are built up and reinforced by living in an atmosphere in which, for example, regularity of bedtime and eating without personal fuss are taken for granted. Such habits hold their influence in some degree throughout life.

As the stage of social approval is reached people admired are imitated, blindly perhaps, but insistence on cleanliness tends to make the child proud of being clean. Being clean, too, brings small privileges and being dirty deprivations. There is, however, no real understanding of the reasons for cleanliness. Continual griminess, in infants and junior children, is a reflection on the home and school and on the way the child is supervised, rather than on the child himself.

In the infant and lower junior school, rewards, that is, concrete symbols of approval, can be used to stimulate children's interest in forming health habits. " Buttons " for children reaching a high standard, labels for clean books, charts on the class-room wall noting clean hands, brushed teeth, incite interest and effort, but they must not be over-stressed, so producing smug self-satisfaction in those gaining them and defiant despair in the unsuccessful. Emphasis should be laid on the value of and pleasure in reaching the standard rather than on the failure of those not doing so. It all depends on the tact of the teacher. She must stand away and not allow herself to be emotionally involved in the matter.

To the teacher and home the establishment of good habits in the child means less effort and strain in discipline, and so more energy available to be applied elsewhere. For example, wash basins are left clean after use, and there is no need to recall a child to clean up a basin left dirty.

Knowledge and Feeling

Practice needs to be based on knowledge and feeling. Some teachers think it is sufficient to see that children carry out certain routine activities with regard to health matters. They rely upon mechanical repetition alone.

Repetition is necessary to the formation of good habits but it must be purposive, effortful repetition. The learner must *know* why, to what end, with what result in view the action is performed. He must also *feel* that the action is worth carrying out and must make some effort about it.

Health practice must not therefore continue to be just a matter of blind obedience, for then the pupil would probably give up the practice on leaving school. The knowledge behind the practices must be taught to the children. Specific health teaching is necessary. It will arise in an almost incidental way in conversation with the youngest children. It will find a somewhat larger place in the projects and general activities of the junior school and it will need a fuller and more organised treatment with older children of the secondary school age range.

Sentiment Towards Health

As is well-known, we only pay attention to and master completely that knowledge or skill which we feel is worth while. If, therefore, this teaching and practice of health is to be of lasting value, children must be led to feel that it matters to them, that it is something of importance, of value and worth.

This attitude or *sentiment towards health* is not a matter of direct training, but is largely caught from the teachers and the school community. Analogously it is said that morals should be caught, not taught.

Once, for example, a real feeling for cleanliness (a sentiment for or love of cleanliness in the terms of the psychologist) has been aroused in a child, that individual is likely to carry this attitude towards health into the bigger adult world. He is likely to see the desirability of cleanliness not only in those directions in which he first learnt it but cleanliness and health of all kinds and in all its aspects.

We speak then of the practice of health but we must acknowledge and provide for the three sides of health education—

(a) knowledge of health facts,
(b) feelings and attitudes towards health,
(c) action with regard to health.

The third stage of health practice—self-respecting practice—will only be reached by those individuals who know, feel and act aright with regard to health.

Child's Attitude to Health

So far the question of Health Practice has been analysed and reviewed from the teacher's angle. It is not suggested that health is something elusive, to be pursued and captured only at great cost by the children. The teacher realises that the child's health and attitude towards health affairs is largely her responsibility and as such a weighty matter.

To the child, however, it should be no such weighty matter, it should cause him no anxiety, he should assume that it is a natural state of affairs. He assumes that the plants in his garden will grow and flower and fruit. He nevertheless takes it as a matter of course that he must tend them, water, weed and safeguard them.

In short, the child adopts the practice view of health and accepts teaching on the ways of maintaining sound health and does not think in terms of cures. Health teaching should be positive and hopeful.

Mental and Emotional Health

Teachers need also to bear in mind that health is not merely a physical matter. The mental health of a child is at least as important as his physical well-being. In fact, each reacts on the other. If the child is unhappy or frightened or, for example, finds that his different respected authorities do not agree, this may react adversely on his health. It is important that the teacher should not antagonise the parent, and so destroy the child's confidence in his parents.

Apart from the material advantages of cleanliness in a community, older children and adults can recognise the value of personal cleanliness in ensuring good health, and, more altruistically, they can see that dirt is dangerous to the community and aim at being clean as a personal duty owed to other people and expected of them in return. This relates hygiene to civics teaching.

In an adolescent or adult cleanliness may be an indication of character. If an adolescent girl comes to school with a dirty neck it is not unfair to assume that other of her personal habits are defective.

The school then must aim at influencing and training children by reinforcing good home teaching or by attempting to supply some substitute for home influence, if it is defective.

The Teacher's Example

First in importance is the *teacher's own example*, based on a sincere belief in the value of cleanliness. A teacher whose own skin and nails are grimy, or who lacks trimness, is valueless as a teacher of cleanliness. Children are quick to see through shams, but, on the other hand, an attractive freshness of person in a teacher will set a standard and be imitated.

Constant personal interest in cleanliness by the head teacher and staff is essential and helps to form a good school tone. A high standard should be assumed, surprise being expressed when a child fails to live up to it. Individual comments in public should be avoided, but a personal word in private about some point that might be improved, followed up by recognition that effort has been made, may well be useful.

Any attitude of contempt or self-righteousness is to be avoided. It is worse than useless, for it may well produce a defiant reaction. Everyone has had to learn recognised behaviour conventions, and the teacher will rather seek, by general suggestions to the class first, and later by individual advice, to give the children the chance of doing the right thing, without making them feel in the wrong and inferior. The method of appeal varies, as has been noted earlier, at different ages.

A problem that must continually recur in this connection is how far punishments can and should be used to enforce cleanliness. While no absolute ruling can be given, it is preferable, as being of wider and more positive scope, to work up such a school tone that children *feel wrong* if they do not reach what is the ordinary school standard. To make a dirty child wash publicly in front of his class will injure his self-respect, and may incite him to resort to a display of defiance before equals to balance up his inward shame. There may also be trouble with an affronted parent, who sides with the child against the school, a position very bad for the child's views on authority.

The school can offer *training in health habits* in many practical ways. The possession of a handkerchief or rag and a pocket in which to keep it, the daily inspection of hands, and arrangement of tooth-brush drill (possibly with imaginary brush and water), the routine opening of windows and tidying of rooms by child monitors, all help. In many schools of the older type there are, unfortunately, too few lavatory basins, only one roller towel and no hot water. Individual or paper towels are preferable to a common towel, which may spread scabies and infectious eye conditions. If there must be roller towels, they should be changed daily.

There should be nail-brushes, and either liquid soap, which the child tips out drop by drop on to the hand from a fixed container, or powdered soap into which a finger only can be dipped. A more homely expedient is to put the soap powder in a tin with holes bored in the top. For satisfactory washing warm water is essential. It is important that children should have the opportunity and should be taught to wash after going to the toilet.

Children should be trained to let out the water and rinse out the basin after use, and not to leave dirty water standing in the basin, and also to wash off the dirt from hands into the water, not to wipe it off on the towel. Basins or troughs with a continual flow of water obviate this piece of supervision for the staff, but give less training for the child.

School offices should be inspected regularly by the head teacher, both as to how the children are using them and how the caretaker is keeping them. Thus, even if the child unfortunately encounters malodorous conditions and lack of care at home, the school will offer a standard of fresh cleanness and decency. School conditions should certainly not be less satisfactory than home in this matter. It has been said that the real value that a family places on cleanliness can be judged by the way in which closets, water or earth, are kept (see also Chapter XXXIII).

School baths include shower-baths for cleansing and swimming-baths for recreation. The possession of shower-baths identifies the school closely with personal cleanliness training. The economic problem of providing them has to be considered, and they must be planned to use as little heat, water and space as possible. Their value lies in their practical training for the children, the easing of the problem of providing baths in bathless homes, and the fresher atmosphere in the classroom both for teacher and children. It also indirectly results in an improvement in the home care (mending and washing) of underclothing.

At least two showers a week should be the aim, one the minimum. The shower or douche kind use least water. If girls use overhead showers they need bathing caps to keep their hair dry. Showers that spray from the wall at about four feet up are a possible substitute for girls. Older girls may prefer cubicles, but the bulk of the children are better dealt with in an open douche room, some twenty to a room, and there should be a set of dressing-rooms at either end so that one batch of children can be dressing while the next batch is undressing and douching. The newest plans for girls' showers supply no separate cubicles at any age.

The best time for use is after Physical Training lessons. The children should be under the shower for five minutes, and the whole dressing need not take more than twenty minutes. This allows one minute to soap, and one to douche with the shower at 95° F. Then the water is gradually cooled to 65° F. and stopped. The school should provide liquid soap and towels. Showers allow no long soaking of the skin, which is injurious to some children. Tub baths get a fatty line of deposit round them that has to be cleaned off, and they use more water and heat and are thus more expensive in upkeep than showers.

Hygiene of the Swimming Bath

The chance to use *swimming-baths* influences cleanliness, though indirectly, because swimmers using public baths conform to a recognised standard of body cleanliness and clothes care, and they get used to and like the opportunity to discard clothes and feel the tonic effect of cold water on the skin. Swimming is also excellent all-round exercise, and ability to swim helps to give courage, self-confidence and poise. It is a sport that can be carried on in after-life, unlike team games for the playing of which a club and accessible ground are necessary. It might also lead to the saving of life. The school aim should be to make every child a swimmer.

The swimming-bath should preferably belong to the school or be attached to a group of schools, as in Bradford. If public baths are used they should be reserved at certain times for the children. The bath should be white tiled, both for cleanliness and to avoid accidents, as of a child sinking unseen in opaque water. It is important that some form of filtering should be used or that the pool should be disinfected by the addition, for example, of chloride of lime ; it should be emptied frequently.

In some baths all bathers take a warm soap shower-bath before entering the pool, their sterilised costume being hung over the top of the cubicle during the shower, so that the attendant can check that the shower has been taken. At the least, lacking such facilities, all children should, as a matter of routine, use the foot-bath. This obviates the need for invidious picking out of children with dirty feet for a foot-bath by the teacher.

Cold water often stimulates the bladder reflex, and all children should empty the bladder before entering the water. Bath attendants complain that there is wholesale fouling of the water if this is not done.

People with cuts, skin diseases, colds or infectious eye or ear diseases should not be allowed to enter the water, both for their own good and that of other bathers. It is probable that a large proportion of the colds bathers suppose they have caught from being in a bathing costume too long are really due to bacteria of colds from uncared-for pool water. Caps should be worn, some authorities suggest, by all bathers ; others suggest that they are necessary only for girls with long hair. Damp hair needs drying carefully.

Children with short-sight and children with a past history of middle ear inflammation should not be allowed to dive. Not more than thirty beginners should be taken in a class at a time, and there should be at least two adults present, the teacher and the bath attendant. Every care should be taken to see that children arrive home properly dried, with clothes fastened and with their full complement of clothes. Tactful and enthusiastic teachers can do much to obviate the withdrawal of children from swimming by doubting parents, who, if hostile, will be ready to attribute any cold or ailment the child contracts to the swimming-baths.

The school cleanliness aim, then, is to train children to *prefer* to be clean, and to *feel wrong* if they are not. This will be effected not by punitive methods but by the teacher's own example and interest, by the carrying through of practical drills and duties, making the children responsible for and proud of results, and, by giving children the chance to use shower- and swimming-baths. All through one should work on the assumption that " it is better to keep clean than to make clean," and that good habits formed at school age will promote health and social acceptance throughout life.

CHAPTER XV

ENDOCRINE OR DUCTLESS GLANDS

GLANDS are classed as being of internal and of external secretion. Those of external secretion, such as the kidneys, liver, sweat and parotid glands, manufacture in their tissue a specific substance which is collected and carried away by a duct. Glands of internal secretion, also known as ductless or endocrine glands, supply the body with substances that give signals, and influence growth, emotion and metabolism. Blood flows through the gland tissue and picks up on its way the specific hormone or chemical messenger that, while it means nothing to the majority of the tissues, is the signal for some specific part of the body to act in a particular way, as when the secretion from the intestine wall, *secretin*, signals to the pancreatic juice to flow.

The endocrine organs include the thyroid and para-thyroids, the islet tissue of the pancreas, the interstitial tissues of the gonads, the adrenals, the pituitary and the thymus and pineal bodies.

Thyroid Gland

The bilobed *thyroid gland* is situated in front of the trachea. It secretes into the blood thyroxin, which contains iodine. It is active in infancy, childhood and puberty and becomes less active in adult life. Its normal function is to increase metabolism, that is, the rate at which the body processes go on. Its effect is thus analogous to the holding of a paper in front of a dull fire to increase the draught and draw up the fire.

In children thyroid deficiency produces a stunted, over-fat, coarse-haired and -skinned dwarf who has defective speech and low mentality. Such children are termed *cretins*. Treatment by sheep's thyroid or by synthesised thyroxin gives good results. If the condition is recognised within the first six months of life, mental as well as physical improvement to normality is possible. If treatment is delayed till the second year or later, while the physical development can be made to

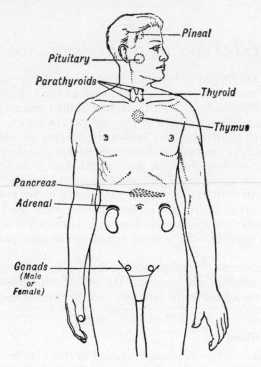

FIG. 87.—The position of the chief Endocrine Glands.

proceed normally, some degree of mental retardation—ultimately three to four years—is likely.

In adults, thyroid deficiency is associated with *goitre*. Lack of iodine in the diet precipitates goitre, the tendency to which appears to be initiated by too much fat, calcium or cabbage in the diet, too little vitamin A, and by water-borne infective agencies.

Goitrous districts, where iodine is known to be lacking, include Switzerland, the Middle West of U.S.A., China, Argentine and Hungary. People living within three miles of the sea get air-borne iodine. In districts lacking in iodine, iodised table salt—1 part to 100,000, can be used.

Marked deficiency in adults shows as Myxoedema. In this condition metabolism slows down, the hair falls, the subject becomes lethargic and slow of speech. Continued small doses of thyroid extract counteract this.

An over-active thyroid produces a nervous, excitable, over-active and rather worrying, irritable type. Such children and adolescents should not be allowed to over-exert themselves (as they are apt to do) particularly if the pulse is abnormally quick. Exophthalmic goitre, in which the eyeballs become over-prominent, is due to marked over-activity of the thyroid. It is rare in children.

While there are obviously types of thyroid excess and deficiency so marked as to be pathological, there are also in the range of normal people, on the one hand, fat, heavy, lethargic types who take life perhaps over-easily, but are good-tempered and easy-going, and, on the other, excitable, worrying people who, if interfering, will at least worry and care enough to get things done. It is probable that these and many other differences in emotion and urge are due partly, at any rate, to differences in balance of ductless gland secretions, not just of the thyroid, but of others as well.

There is a slight normal enlargement of the thyroid gland at the menstrual period. Exposure of the skin to a reasonably low temperature stimulates the gland. Thus cold baths and showers, playing games out of doors in the winter, brisk walks and winter sports all make for greater energy and for slimness.

Para-thyroid Glands

The four small *Para-thyroid glands* are embedded in the thyroid, but they are not connected with it functionally. Their work is to conserve and to help in the acquisition of Calcium (lime), which is needed for the bones and teeth, to maintain the tone of the blood vessels and nervous system in a state of

7

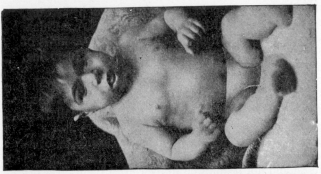
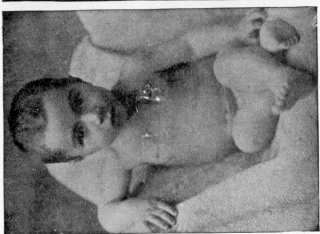
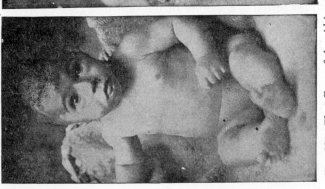

FIG. 88.—*The effects of thyroid insufficiency.* On the left, a child showing marked deficiency of thyroid, producing physical deformities and mental deficiency. Centre—the same child after some months of treatment with sheep's thyroid. Right—the same child a year later, showing the return of symptoms after its parents had refused to continue the treatment. (*Reproduced by permission from the "Journal of Heredity."*)

optimal irritability. Shortage of calcium tends to make people irritable, touchy, lacking in serenity and easily provoked to anger. Deficiency of the para-thyroids causes muscle cramps and tremors which are relieved by the injection of calcium.

Adrenal Glands

The paired *Adrenal or Supra-renal glands* lie just above each kidney, with which they are unconnected functionally. They are made up of two kinds of tissue, the cortex and the medulla. When any emergency arises causing anxiety, fear, rage, cold or fever, the sympathetic nervous system (see Chapter XVI) excites the secretion of adrenalin into the blood from the medulla, and the animal is immediately mobilised for a maximum effort, whether of fight or flight.

Digestion is stopped and the extra blood is ready for use in the skeletal muscles ; the liver rapidly turns the animal starch stored in it into sugar for use in the muscles ; the hair stands on end and the pupils dilate, giving the animal a terrifying appearance ; if the body is wounded the blood clots more easily to stop bleeding ; fatigue of muscles is staved off longer than normal, and the muscles are keyed up to make contractions much beyond their normal willed power.

Pursued by a bull, a man will jump a hedge quite beyond his capacity in cold blood. Adrenalin makes the hair of an angry cat or dog stand up along its back. Probably in a smaller way, every time we key ourselves up to cross a busy street, there is a similar but lesser output of adrenalin into the blood.

All this helps the body's capacity to meet emergency, enabling a maximum effort to be made and so increasing the animal's chances of survival. It is probably because of this upsetting of metabolism and emotions for the battle that, having lost our tempers, we find ourselves afterwards suffering from indigestion, headache and a feeling of being unsettled. Once launched it becomes progressively more difficult to control rage. Adrenalin is making us different, and it is more difficult for us to be reasonable or to see reason.

Some people are more, others less, inclined to be overcome by such unreasonable rage. Probably their adrenal balance is respectively above or below normal. Over-activity of these glands causes high blood-pressure and excessive restless energy. Adrenalin is used in dentistry to check bleeding. The adrenal tissues are rich in vitamin C.

Cortisone, a hormone of the adrenal cortex, produces striking and prompt relief of rheumatoid arthritis.

Thymus and Pineal

The *Thymus* lies behind the sternum. It is largest during childhood and atrophy begins at puberty. It is thought to hold back sexual growth until the skeleton is relatively mature so that the young animal is robust before its reproductive phase starts.

The *Pineal* is situated in the mid-brain. In the lamprey it appears as a third eye and is sensitive to light. It is thought to hurry the onset of puberty in opposition to the effect of the Thymus.

Pancreas and Insulin

The *Pancreas* secretes its digestive juice into the intestine, but, in addition, as the blood flows through the gland tissue, a hormone, *insulin*, is secreted. Insulin helps to regulate the storage and use of carbohydrates so that the store is gradually made available to the body. It also prevents protein being used up as a fuel.

If too little insulin is secreted, *diabetes* results. The body, then, cannot make use of the carbohydrates eaten, the liver is unable to store glycogen (animal starch) and sugar is excreted in the urine because, although the body needs sugar, it cannot use it without insulin. The normal amount of sugar in the blood is about $0 \cdot 1$ per cent.

Insulin injected under the skin corrects the diabetic condition. The treatment is combined with careful dietary so that the carbohydrates and insulin intake are balanced. The effect of each insulin injection is transitory and the treatment must be continued throughout life. If too much insulin is given and the blood sugar sinks to about $0 \cdot 07$ per cent., convulsions and unconsciousness supervene. Glucose, given by the mouth, quickly allays these symptoms.[1]

[1] See footnote, p. 189.

The Gonads

The *Testes* and *Ovaries*, apart from producing male and female gametes, supply hormones which initiate the development of the secondary sex characteristics and the sexual rhythms. The development of the beard and the breaking of

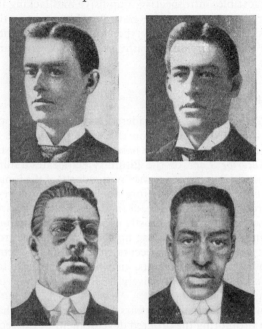

FIG. 89.—Shows the progressive effects of Acromegaly at 29, 37 and 42, on the facial bones of a man, normal at 24 years of age. (*From Schafer's " Endocrine Organs."*)

the voice in the boy and the development of the breasts, body hair and menstruation in the girl, are controlled thus.

Hoskins suggests that races that mature early sexually tend to be relatively short in height because with sexual maturity the growing points of the long bones close, whereas in races that mature sexually relatively late, the growing points will remain open and allow of longer continued growth in height. He contrasts the African pigmy with the tall Northern European type.

The *hypo-gonadal type*, in whom adolescence is delayed, is thin and tall, with extremities always cold, a " velvet " mat complexion with a tendency to acne and a childish manner ; he is suggestible, introspective, impulsive and lacking in drive. Consider the phrase " gentle giant." Castration in the male produces the allied eunuch type, tall, beardless, with wide feminine hips. Timidity, apathy and lack of drive are characteristic of eunuchs.

The Pituitary

The *Pituitary gland* is considered last because it appears to exercise a controlling effect on the whole endrocrine system. It lies in a bony hollow at the base of the brain and is bilobed.

The *Anterior Lobe* of the Pituitary elaborates a number of hormones which control growth, particularly of the long bones. Over-activity, if it occurs before adolescence, produces giantism. Growth may continue until thirty and heights of over 8 feet have been recorded, mostly in boys. The growing points of the long bones fail to close normally and allow growth to continue. If over-activity occurs in an adult, the condition known as Acromegaly results, in which the hands, feet and facial bones enlarge progressively. Under-activity in children results in dwarfism (Fig. 89).

The anterior lobe also appears to act with the gonad hormones in promoting the ordered development of the secondary sex characteristics. It controls lactation and also possibly broodiness in hens and maternal behaviour in mammals, including responses relating to the care and feeding of offspring.

One of the activities of the *Posterior Lobe* of the Pituitary is to increase the blood sugar antagonistically to the effect of insulin. It helps to regulate the output of water from the kidneys, preventing too great a loss. It is also connected with the control of fat metabolism. Under-activity produces a fat, sleepy type of person, with small hands and feet and retarded sex development—the " Fat Boy " in *Pickwick Papers.*

The Endocrine Gland Pattern

Finally, it must be recognised that while few people are deficient in these gland secretions sufficiently to be ill and definitely abnormal, the emotional and physical balance that we call normal does almost certainly depend on the balance and inter-relationship of these secretions. Such balance is spoken of as the individual's *endocrine* or *ductless gland pattern*. Mental cases are now judged as to treatment partly in relation to their possible lack of endocrine balance.

Racial differences, such as differences in height (compare the Scots and the Japanese), in amount of hair growth (compare the white races and the Chinese), or in type of temperament (compare the phlegmatic Norseman and the volatile Mediterranean), are probably partly due to inherited differences of racial endocrine pattern.

The waste product of activity, CO_2, is utilised in the body as a chemical messenger, though not gland produced. When the concentration of CO_2 in the blood rises as the result of muscular activity, the centre in the brain that hastens breathing rate is stimulated by the increased amount of CO_2 that comes to it in the blood and lymph. The breathing accelerates and the panting gets rid of excess CO_2. This explains why CO_2 is administered to re-start respiration in cases of suffocation.

The effects of endocrine organ secretions can be summarised as (i) transitory like the effects of secretin, insulin and adrenalin, or (ii) permanent like the effects of the thyroid, and the pituitary on growth or the production of secondary sex characteristics by the secretions of the gonads.

Note to p. 186.

Hostels for Diabetic Children

[1] In this country one child in 62,000 between the ages of 4–15 is diabetic, and under the 1944 Education Act special Hostels are now provided, though home supervision is always preferable, if satisfactory.

Each Hostel is run by specially trained nurses and the children are taught to give their own injections of insulin and to test their urine for sugar. They attend the ordinary schools of the district and are encouraged to take part in all social activities and in swimming and games, and to live as normal a life as possible.

CHAPTER XVI

THE BRAIN AND NERVOUS SYSTEM

THE brain and nervous system tend to ensure the smooth working together of all the other systems of the body, the circulation, breathing, digestion, movement. They co-ordinate sense impressions, the mind initiates action in relation to these impulses and the brain stimulates the appropriate response by muscles and glands. Where past experience is of value, as in remembering things that are dangerous or pleasant, the nervous system works in conjunction with the mind, that is, consciously, whereas, where consciousness of past experience is not necessary, it works automatically without consciousness.

The heart-beat and the tone of the artery walls, the constant peristaltic movement of the alimentary canal, the perspiring of the skin when heated, are only some of the many automatic processes, the rate and regularity of which are continually kept going by orders initiated by the nervous system. If we had to keep on remembering these processes we should probably continually be held up because we had forgotten to will them to go on, and we should have very little time for work or play, for trying new ideas or seeing fresh things and storing up and sorting impressions.

One benefit of having a great many of the body's processes ordered automatically so that we have both time and energy for learning and resorting experience, that is, for thinking. Further, while we are asleep, and not consciously thinking, the automatic regulation of the heart, breathing, digestion never stops.

Similarly, the body automatically withdraws itself from sudden dangers, the eyelids blink when anything flicks across the eyes, at the touch of something over-hot the hand is rapidly withdrawn. Such automatic responses, called *reflex actions*, are a protection to the body. The original development of a nervous system in lower forms of life—worm, shell-fish, jelly-fish—resulted only in the inheritance of set patterns of behaviour called *tropisms*, for protection, food-getting and reproduction which are carried out blindly whether they lead to the destruction of the animal or not.

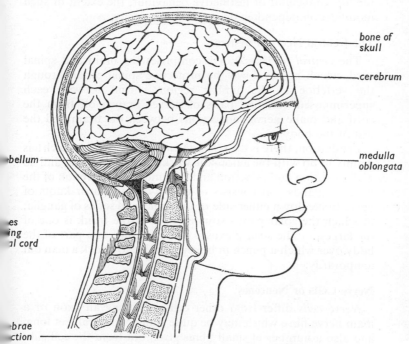

FIG. 90.—*The brain*, showing relative positions of different parts.
(*After Huxley*.)

In higher forms of life, in addition to the inborn automatic invariable reflex reactions, are to be found other inborn reactions known as *instincts*. Here the response is less automatic and is accompanied by definite feelings or emotions, which are absent in the case of reflexes. For example, the animal's impulse either to run for shelter or to lie hidden at the sight or sound of something strange is instinctive, and the emotion which accompanies the action is fear.

7*

Instinct has been called "congenital behaviour," which can be contrasted with what may be called "intelligent or learned behaviour," which depends on individual experience and involves such brain and mind activities as remembering and thinking. An intelligent animal can then obviously modify congenital or instinctive behaviour, the extent of such modification depending on its mental capacity.

The Central Nervous System

The *central nervous system* comprises the brain and spinal cord, which passes down the protective spinal canal through the vertebræ to the lumbar region. From between each superimposed vertebra, pairs of nerves branch off from the cord and make nerve connections between the brain and the rest of the body.

In addition, there is the *sympathetic nervous system,* which has mainly to do with the automatic working of the viscera, and so with digestion and excretion and the amount of secretion of the ductless glands. It consists of chains of ganglia or knots of nerve tissue down either side of the spine, and series of ganglia, of which the solar plexus situated deep in the trunk is one of the largest. The solar plexus is chiefly known as a part of the body over which a punch in boxing is liable to knock a man out temporarily.

Nerve Cells or Neurones

Nerve cells differ from other cells in having an axon or a main nerve fibre which may be quite short or several feet long, and also a number of small fibres given out from the cell substance, called dendrites. The *axon* is a nerve fibre covered in an insulating envelope of white fat. An ordinary nerve looks white because it is a bundle of many such axons, each insulated from the others and carrying its own message. The longest axons run from the nerve cells in the lumbar spine to the toes, where, as in other places, each one spreads into special receiving or message-giving end organs.

The *dendrites* interlace themselves with dendrites of neighbouring nerve cells rather as it is possible to link the fingers of the two hands, so that though they are almost touching, there is no real continuity. Nerve impulses are able to flash along such dendrite connections from one nerve cell to another, the impulses having, as it were, to jump the connection points as the electric current jumps across the points of a sparking plug in a motor-car engine.

The point of jumping is called the *synaptic junction* or the *synapse*. When a person is tired, impulses jump less

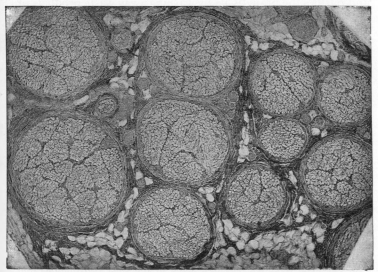

FIG. 91.—Section of *sciatic nerve of man*, showing a number of bundles of nerve fibres. The little rings are the sheaths of the nerve fibres. Nerve impulses travel at the rate of about 400 ft. per second. (*By permission of Sir E. Sharpey-Schafer.*)

readily, and it is at these synaptic junctions as well as in end organs in muscles that any nerve fatigue shows itself first. Nerve tissue consists of grey and white matter, of which the grey is always the cells and the white the nerve fibres or axons.

The Brain

The *brain* is made up of three main parts, the cerebrum, the cerebellum and the medulla oblongata, which continues down the spinal canal as the spinal cord.

Inside the skull the brain is enveloped in three membranes, the stoutly protective *dura mater* outside, a vascular, delicate *arachnoid membrane* inside, and innermost, the *pia mater*, which also are continuous down the cord. The brain is surrounded by and permeated with watery *cerebro-spinal fluid*, which, being between the dura and pia mater membranes helps to minimise jars from knocks on the head. The fluid cleanses and purifies the brain tissue by washing away waste products of

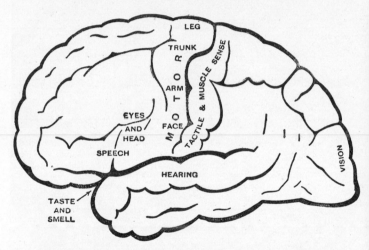

FIG. 92.—The *cerebrum*, showing some of the chief convolutions and areas associated with particular functions. The vision centres are at the back of the cerebrum.

brain activity. In the thin walls of the vessels that conduct the fluid all over the brain are moored phagocytic bodies, which swing out and engulf harmful matter and remove it in a way analogous to the work of white corpuscles in the blood.

The *cerebrum*, the largest part of the brain, fills up the skull roughly above the eyebrow level. From an evolutionary view point it is the latest developed part of the nervous system. Here take place those brain changes that accompany changes in consciousness, such as willed activity, abstract thinking, remembering and forgetting, changing emotions, likings and dislikings. It is divided into two longitudinally from back to front, the halves being connected by a wide band of white nerve fibre tissue (Fig. 93).

The outside surface is very much wrinkled (which enlarges the surface area that is packed into the space), and is grey because the nerve cells are in its outer layers, *the cortex,* whereas the inside bulk is white, consisting of fibres joining innumerable nerve cells or neurones to each other. In lower animals the outer layer of the cerebrum known as the cortex is comparatively smooth, whereas in man it is considerably convoluted ; the greater the complication of the convolution the more intelligent is the animal. The right half of the cerebrum controls the left side of the body and vice versa. The cerebral cortex consists of some seven layers of neurones with their inter-connecting network of axons and dendrites, the different layers doing different work.

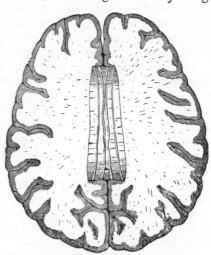

FIG. 93.—Horizontal section through the cerebral hemispheres, showing the white and grey matter. The longitudinal division of the cerebrum into two parts is shown.

The *cerebellum* lies below the cerebrum at the back of the skull. In it the grey matter or nerve cells are outside and the white matter inside. Its work is continually to adjust the balance of the body. Thus to try to sit a doll on a fence so that it balances in a sitting position is difficult, whereas any child or adult could balance there immediately. It is the cerebellum that thus co-ordinates the easy adjustment of muscle-groups so that some contract and others relax smoothly.

Every time a movement is made the rest of the body has to

be adjusted, and it is done without any sense of effort.   In this the cerebellum is helped by the semi-circular canals of the ear which register the position of the body in space and in relation to gravity.

In locomotia ataxia, in which the cerebellum is injured, the patient has to think continually about the balance, instead of assuming it unconsciously.   Thus a patient leaving the clinic, where she had been re-learning to walk, was seen to clutch on to the railing before she could tell a casual enquirer the time, because she could not think simultaneously both about standing and about telling the time.

The *medulla oblongata* lies below the cerebrum, and in formation it is an enlargement inside the skull of the spinal cord, which is continuous from the medulla down the spinal canal. It is connected with the cerebrum above it and with the cerebellum behind it.   In it and in the spinal cord the grey matter or cells are inside and the white matter or nerve axons outside. Cut across horizontally the grey matter is in the form of an H with the horns pointing forward and backward (see Fig. 95).

The medulla is, from an evolutionary view-point, the part of the brain that evolved earliest.   From it are controlled such vital processes as the heart-beat, breathing, digesting, perspiring.   All the nerve centres to and from all parts of the body pass through the medulla.

A dog in which the cerebrum has been removed loses initiative and ability to recognise people and things for what they are.   He is inert, but he continues to breathe.   If he is lifted and placed on his legs, he will stand up, and though he will not recognise or seek out food, if it is put by his nose so that the smell reaches the olfactory nerve endings, or if food is put in his mouth, he will eat it.   All this is done unconsciously by reflex action.

Sensory and Motor Nerves

The nervous system has been likened to a telephone system. Actually, however, nerves carry impulses only in one direction. *Sensory nerves* collect impressions such as of heat, cold, roughness, smoothness, pain, from the skin ; impressions of light images from the eyes ; of sound from the ears and of taste and smell from the mouth and nose. These impressions the nerves communicate to the spinal cord and the brain. Other nerves, called *motor nerves*, convey impulses from the brain and the spinal cord to muscles mainly, but some to glands.

Thus a fire is seen to be getting low, and as the result of im-

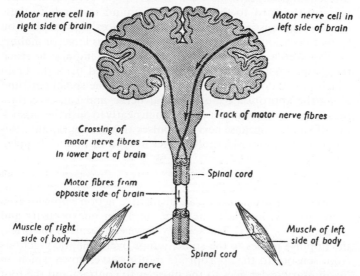

FIG. 94.—Diagram of the front aspect of the brain and spinal cord, showing how a *motor impulse* from a neurone on the left side of the cerebrum passes to a muscle on the right side of the body. Follow the small arrows running parallel with the nerve fibres. The cord is shown in sections only ; it is really continuous. (*From Campbell's* " *Readable Physiology and Hygiene* "—*G. Bell & Sons, Ltd.*)

pulses from the brain along certain motor nerves the appropriate series of movements to put on coal is made.

The thirty-one pairs of nerves that leave the spinal cord are mixed nerves containing both sensory and motor fibres. However, in the cord the sensory nerve centres and fibres are at the back of the grey matter H, and the motor in the front. Each spinal nerve has one root from the sensory area at the back and another from the motor area in the front, which join up in front of a ganglion or knot of nerve cells and then pass each to different parts of the body, giving off sensory and motor branches in the course of each.

In any *willed or voluntary action*, such as feeling a hassock with the toe and pushing it away, sensory nerve endings feel the hassock's pressure on their end organs, the impulses pass up the sensory nerve to the back of the spinal cord, and thence pass up the cord to the brain. The mind responds to these impulses because of past mental experiences gained when on former occasions impressions of the hassock as large, or shabby, or displaced again, had caused such sensory impulse to reach the brain. As a result, an impulse is initiated from the brain which passes down the front motor part of the spinal cord and along the appropriate motor spinal nerve and causes certain muscle-groups to contract just enough neatly to push the hassock out of sight. Because nerve impulses travel very rapidly, this sequence takes considerably longer to read of than to happen.

Reflex Action

Either a *reflex action* or an instinctive action happens even more quickly, as when one steps on a pin unexpectedly and withdraws the foot. The sensory nerve ends register the prick, the impulse passes to the spine, jumps over synaptic junctions from sensory to the appropriate motor nerve, down which an involuntary order goes to the muscles to contract and the foot is withdrawn. Possibly also there is an instinctive springing away, calling out and even weeping.

A reflex arc of action is, therefore, a sensory stimulus, a jumping of this impulse across synapses to the motor nerve and a muscle or gland response. Actually the border line between a pure reflex and a pure instinctive reaction is not clear cut, the mechanism being of the same nature, but an instinct embodies more than a reflex, and may be a series of reflexes.

Protective reflexes such as blinking, and instinctive actions such as the inclination to turn the head on hearing a sudden noise, are inborn, not learnt. Another example of an inborn reflex is the *knee jerk* in which, when a person is sitting down with crossed legs, and the tendon below the knee-cap is hit

sharply, the extensor muscles of the thigh contract and the
foot flies up.

Sneezing, coughing, blushing are similar reflexes, as is the

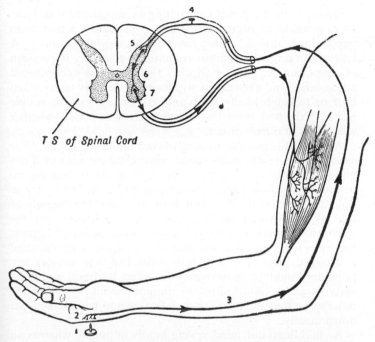

FIG. 95.—Course of a spinal reflex arc of action. The pin (1) excites the
sensory nerve endings of pain (2), and an impulse passes up the sensory nerve (3) to the back of the grey matter of the spinal cord. It
jumps the synaptic junctions (5 and 7) and passes down the appropriate motor nerve (8) so that muscles contract to jerk the hand away.
When such a reflex is inhibited, as it can be by a controlled person,
the impulse also travels up the cord to the brain, there is a conscious
mind process of deciding not to jerk the hand away, and a motor
impulse prevents the quick reflex muscle reaction.

tendency to much weak, mirthless, instinctive, giggling and
uncontrolled social behaviour. Certain reflexes set up a
chain of reflex responses, each one setting light, as it were, to
the next, as when a cat is held by its legs and dropped, the

sensation of falling awakes a chain of reflexes so that it turns over and alights on all-fours.

Inhibited Action

Owing to man's power of profiting by experience it is, however, possible to prevent a reflex or instinctive action from happening; this is termed *inhibition* or *inhibited action*. A reflex is an immediate motor response to a sensory impression of, for example, pain or shock. Children and uncontrolled adolescents, and even adults will tend instinctively to cry when hurt or to laugh loudly when amused, or say, as such people put it, " the first thing that comes into their head," whether wounding to others or not.

Actually it is possible to control such inborn reactions. For example, where an uncontrolled person, taking hold of a hot plate, would drop it instinctively, a more controlled person would have a first impulse to drop it and a second to try to hold it because of the mess and disturbance and the discredit of looking foolish that the dropping of it would entail. In the uncontrolled person, with the sensory impression of hotness there is a reflex arc of action leading to relaxing of muscles and a dropped plate. In the more controlled, the sensory impression would be immediately followed by brain and mind activity, and a modified motor impulse would be sent to the muscles so that the plate, though hot, would be held and put down quietly.

A child does not mind crying loudly in public, whereas an adult with a similar feeling would be self-critical and feel aware of the risk of looking foolish. Knowing that such an exhibition of uncontrolled emotion is considered childish, he would suppress it as far as possible.

A good deal of educational training in good manners and other forms of social behaviour involves training in such inhibiting of reflex and instinctive reactions. Some one enters in an unusual hat, and you all but open your mouth to remark on it, even to laugh and then by a rapid but separate process, decide to say nothing and drop into some banal remark perhaps to fill up the conversational gap. The sensory impression from your eyes prompted a motor impulse to the muscles of speech to speak, but the inhibiting impulse to the conscious part of the brain and so to the mind makes for remembrance that the person will be emotionally distressed by laughter, so that the original impulse is inhibited and the muscles keep their usual tone, and do not contract in laughing, and the speech muscles do not move.

A child who takes the nearest cake on the plate offered to him instead of the largest, as is his first instinctive inclination, is exercising inhibition.

If a puppy is tickled on the back he will kick reflexly with his back leg, probably into the air and with no direct relation to the tickled spot, but if the tickling continues, he, after a set time, ceases to be irritated by it and to kick. This particular synaptic junction in his spinal cord is now temporarily blocked. With an electric instrument called the " mechanical flea " it is possible to tickle a puppy thus, so that the reflex is tired, but if the " flea " is moved so that it tickles only half an inch away, a fresh reflex arc is tapped, and the kicking begins all over again, until this reflex arc too is blocked. If the dog is responding reflexly by scratching with its left hind leg and the " flea " makes irritation causing the reflex call on the right leg to scratch, the dog does not fall over, for the first reflex is inhibited automatically by the response to the second.

It is probable that it is a general, gradual blocking of synaptic junctions by chemical fatigue products that helps to induce sleep.

Habit Formation

While reflexes, such as blinking or sneezing, are inborn, any sequence of actions repeated in a series many times is likely in time to be done in exactly the same way and order, that is, reflexly. The particular nerve paths become worn, and the movement, that had to be thought about at first, becomes easier to execute and more and more nearly automatic ; thus a *habit* is formed.

Most people, for instance, dress and undress in a certain unvarying order, which they are surprised possibly to find is not everyone's natural order, and this quite elaborate sequence of movements comes to be carried on with less than full attention, the wave of attention rising, as a decision has to be made about a hole in a sock or a mislaid collar stud, but mainly being carried out as a series of " learnt reflexes." People, for instance, have been known to forget when changing during the day, and to have undressed completely and got into bed.

Professor Pavlov's name is associated with the long and careful series of experiments he made in training dogs to acquire what he termed *conditioned reflexes*. In these, the action is not called forth by the natural stimulus but by a substituted stimulus.

A small operation is performed on the dog to make one salivary gland open on to the cheek instead of into the mouth, so that the saliva can be collected and checked as to amount and time of flow. When men or dogs see or smell food, the salivary glands are stimulated reflexly to pour saliva into the mouth, and the amount of flow is an index of the degree of emotion aroused.

Among many experiments Pavlov found that if the dog saw food and at the same time heard the bell ring, the dog very soon began to connect the bell with the food, and the ringing of the bell, the substituted stimulus, would cause a reflex flow of saliva without food being seen at all. Also, later, if the bell were regularly rung and the food produced in ten minutes' time, the dog would not have the flow of saliva until ten minutes after the bell had been rung, the reflex flow of saliva being prevented or inhibited until then. This ten minutes' period of inhibition was found in some dogs to take the form of a general inhibition, so that the dog went to sleep, but woke up promptly at the end of the ten minutes. This suggests a further possible line of research as to what sleep actually is.

A further line of experiment of Professor Pavlov's was to train dogs to connect a white circle of light with food, giving a salivary response, and to connect an elliptical patch of light with an unpleasant electric shock. When the two responses were quite clearly defined for any dog, Pavlov began to vary the ellipse until it approximated to a circle. The dog continued to distinguish and to react accordingly, until the distinction between the ellipse and circle was very fine. At last, being unable to distinguish by habit, the dog became excited and began to howl and struggle, showing symptoms suggestive of hysterical and neurotic states in human beings.

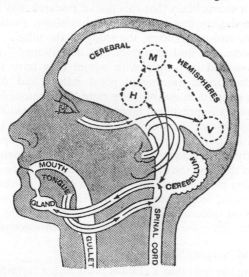

FIG. 96.—Diagram to show *the difference between inborn and conditioned reflexes*. If food is put in the mouth, impulses flash up to the brain along a nerve from the taste organs on the tongue. In the brain, owing to an inborn nervous connection, they travel to the centre controlling the salivary glands and so out, along another nerve, to the glands themselves. Thus the mouth waters and the food is lubricated for swallowing.

That is an unconditioned, that is a natural, reflex.

When we learn things, similar nerve connections (shown dotted) are formed in the cerebral hemispheres. The man shown has learnt that a particular cooked dish is good to eat. When he sees the dish, impulses travel from the eye to the visual centre (V) in his cortex. As he has formed a connection (dotted arrow) between this centre and the motor centre (M) controlling his salivary glands, the impulses follow that route and his mouth waters. Similarly, when he learns that a particular gong heralds dinner he forms a connection between the hearing centre (H) and the motor centres concerned. Compare Fig. 58. (*From Wells, Huxley and Wells' " The Science of Life "—Cassell & Co., Ltd.*)

Similar experiments with training of responses to pleasant food and to disagreeable acids give like results. It seems possible that the human nervous breakdowns may be similarly connected with such contradictory stimuli. Pavlov's work over thirty years is of great importance, among other reasons because it seems likely that this line of research may ultimately elucidate the connection between physiology, particularly of the brain, and psychology, the study of the mind.

Everyone can find examples of " conditioned " reflexes in themselves and in people with whom they have to do, and much educational training in good habits and community manners consists in establishing right " conditioned reflexes."

All sensory impressions, however, are not immediately translated into physical action. We may, for example, see a book on the floor but not direct our muscles to pick it up. We are constantly experiencing fresh sensations and storing up impressions through the cerebrum and the mind to be correlated with others and recalled and acted on later. Books are read, pictures seen, lectures and music listened to and worked on, information pieced together, definite conclusions reached ; this and much more is found to modify future activities.

Growth of Nervous System

It is usually held that a child is born with a certain supply of neurones or nerve cells which cannot be added to in growth. What it is supposed can be added to, however, is the dendrite and axon connections between neurone and neurone by *association fibres.*

Thus a baby discriminates nothing that it sees or hears. Then, early on, it distinguishes the sound, " dad, dad " from other sounds in its auditory centre, and repeats the sound by the stimulus of its motor speech centre. Gradually it comes to connect the sound " dad, dad " with a seen impression of a characteristically dressed trousered person, and with a heard impression of a deeper voice.

These centres in the brain have been connected up by association fibre paths between them, so that if the child sees any man, the chemical upset in its seeing centre, together with some mental interpretation, will cause an impulse to pass along the already worn path to the speech centre, and the child calls " dad, dad ! "

Later, again, " dad " will be differentiated from other men,

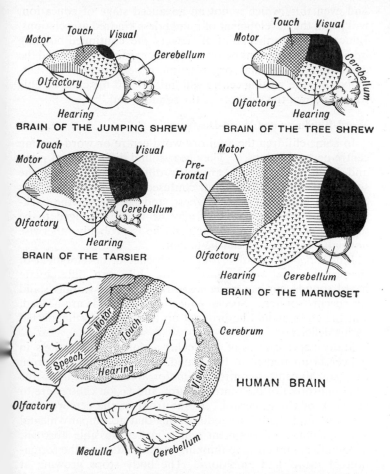

FIG. 97.—*Four stages of evolution of the mammalian brain and the human brain.* The *jumping shrew* is a small night animal with a long nose, and mainly depending on sense of smell. The *tree shrew* is a more agile, arboreal animal, needing clearer sight and better controlled movement. Note the corresponding differences in areas. The *tarsier*, between the lemur and monkey, and the *marmoset*, a primitive monkey type, show progressively less " smell " areas and more for general senses. (*Adapted from the " Evolution of Man," by permission of Prof. G. Elliott Smith and the Oxford University Press.*)

and even this, which is not an advanced stage of education, will mean the development of numberless kindred associations. Education, from this point of view, is the continued building up of such associations between already existing centres and the corresponding mental organisation of experiences. Eventually, too, the writing centre will link up and the child be able to write down the symbols of the sound " dad."

Word-Blindness and Word-Deafness

In some children the auditory word centre or word-hearing centre never develops. They hear sound differences of pitch and loudness but they can never differentiate between the sounds of words ; talk is all confused noise to them. This condition is termed *word-deafness*, and because of the backwardness it entails the child may be wrongly judged to be mentally deficient, whereas actually he is probably otherwise normal. Lip reading can be taught.

Word blindness results from the absence of development of the usual visual word centre. The child can differentiate heard sounds but can never learn that certain symbols stand for specific sounds. Special educational methods are needed, and the child should be brought up to some work unaffected by his deficiency.

Many nerve centres of particular action or impressions in the cerebrum remain to be located, but, as can be seen from Fig. 92, the centres controlling motor areas lie mainly in the neighbourhood of the central fissure, and vision centres are to the back of the cerebrum. In the front of the cerebrum we probably find the brain modifications that accompany mental development, a development which makes possible abstract, imaginative, and creative thinking of all kinds, and the formation of ideals and ambitions. The body stops growing at about twenty-five, but the brain, if used, can go on growing and improving till at least sixty, and possibly longer. Unused, however, it soon loses this latent capacity.

Cerebral Palsy

Paralysis in school children is roughly of two kinds (i) *flaccid* in which, as in infantile paralysis, little contraction of the muscle occurs and (ii) *spastic* where the damage is in the brain and muscle contractions occur but cannot be fully controlled or co-ordinated. In the spastic individual, the movements of the affected limb are stiff, awkward and jerky. Such a child might make a voluntary effort to pick up a book but be baulked by a series of involuntary movements which he cannot control.

Brain damage may be hereditary or may arise before or during birth and occasionally from an illness such as meningitis during childhood. Different forms of spastic paralysis occur according to the centres in the brain tissue which are damaged.

Spastics need special education and the earlier it is begun the better. It should include (i) massage and exercises for the specific physical handicap; (ii) speech training (Spastics are often " late developers " and probably because of this are educationally retarded.); (iii) treatment of emotional difficulties resulting from their physical handicap; (iv) attention to actual speech disabilities and writing difficulties, both of which are frequent.

Until recently treatment has been by surgical interference in the hope of obtaining maximum use of the limbs. Massage, exercises and occupational therapy are now increasingly utilised. Some of these children go to Open-Air schools or to schools for the sub-normal, but schools run *only* for children with cerebral palsy are preferable.

Chapter XVII

ECONOMY OF WORK—FATIGUE—REST
AND SLEEP

A view of work that has come down from the Victorians is that work is synonymous with toil, always wearisome and boring, and only to be done as a disagreeable duty by the exercise of " will power." This view is assumed in many of the older hymns, which appear to have been written by old people, who might perhaps physiologically be expected to feel in this way about work.

Now some work is like this to everyone ; immediate drudgery but possibly with an ultimate aim. Newer psychology, however, demonstrates that congenial work suited to the worker is stimulating and a source of satisfaction, both immediately and possibly as an expression of ideals. It gives a sense of power in achievement, and is done all the better for the interest that the worker brings to it. Congenial work, in fact, is rarely too hard.

The worker, however, must fit the work. It is useless to make a boy who wants strongly to be a sailor into a clerk, or vice versa, and expect satisfactory work. Neither must the worker be over- or under-intelligent for the job. The over-intelligent child is bored and may think of intelligent but illegitimate ways of amusing himself, while the under-intelligent child will get worried and feel a failure. Sound training, too, gives a stimulus of confidence (see " Vocational Guidance," Chapter XIX).

Then, too, environment must be reasonably unobtrusive. To work continually in a stuffy room, or, for some kinds of work, in noise, or in an irritating, awkward, dark environment that increases difficulties results in loss of rhythm and poorer work. The Institute of Industrial Psychology at one time gave disinterested advice to firms on these and other matters.

There were in a large restaurant breakages of crockery running into hundreds of pounds a year, and the Institute was asked to advise on this. Coffee cups in the rush hour suffered greatly, and it was noticed that the girl at the coffee urn had to take each cup, fill it and pass it on to the waitress, and that she was being hurried and made irritable both by the girl who took the full cup from her and by the next girl, impatient for hers to be filled.

It was suggested that each girl should be given something to do, the girl who brought her cup was to push it along a groove under the urn tap, the filler simply turned the tap on and off and the next girl took the full cup away. This resulted in considerable saving of emotional energy for the whole staff, and of large sums of money formerly spent yearly in replacing broken coffee cups. It is one example only of the use of intelligence in planning work.

Another point that industrial firms have recognised is that a healthy worker is more contented and does better work than the less healthy. Welfare schemes, with proper rest rooms, provision of inexpensive meals, opportunities for games and physical training are not based only on sentiment and humanitarian principles. They pay the manufacturer because better work is done, and the distributor because customers are more likely to buy from healthy, cheerful, interested assistants than from grumbling, depressed ones.

When the Factory Acts were first considered in the last century, children were working physically for fourteen, or even more hours a day, and manufacturers cried out that if hours were shortened all profits would go. Actually, however, a reduction in hours improved the quality and ultimately even increased the quantity of work done. Different types of work can be carried on efficiently for varying lengths of time, the more skilled for shorter times. Watchmakers cannot go on for more than four hours a day, because of the fine adjustments involved. There comes, of course, a point in shortening hours at which a decrease in output results.

Rest Pauses

Intervals during work are found to improve the quality of work and to reduce the amount of spoilt work. They are of similar value in school, particularly if children can get out of doors and be active. The maximum of efficiency in work is

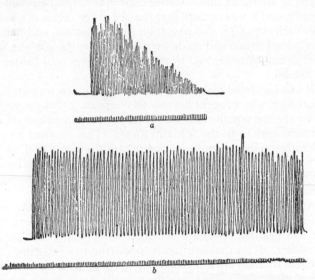

FIG. 98.—The pace and fatigue. These two ergograph records were made by the same student on the same day. *a* was made by pulling as rapidly as possible, and shows rapid accumulation of fatigue ; *b* was made by a slow, steady pull every two seconds, and although the time was twice as long as in *a*, and the work performed about four times as much, there is no appreciable evidence of fatigue. (*From Gruenberg's " Elementary Biology "—Ginn & Co., Ltd.*)

not reached immediately after a rest, so that too long a rest might not justify itself, because the workers would take too long to warm up again to their best work, the time taken to warm up being partly dependent upon the length of rest. For a similar reason, Tuesday is a better day for results than Monday, just after the week-end, and the second period in any morning than the first, because by that time the child has adapted himself to work.

Supervisors of all kinds, foremen and forewomen, head teachers and managers, can facilitate their workers' economy of work by their wisdom in exercising supervision. Some workers need keeping up to scratch by encouragement, others are irritated by continual unnecessary fussing. A supervisor should be calm and unflurried, and should beware of exerting pressure to show off authority. His shop, or school, or class will reflect his attitude all too faithfully. He should take every opportunity of mixing with equals who will be able to criticise with that frankness that he cannot so well get from subordinates.

It is economical then for work to fit the worker, but whatever the work, some understanding of how to get the best output from mind and body is of value to all workers, just as a man who buys a car aims at learning how to get the most economical results from the particular engine. Comparatively little is yet known about the incidence and exact causes of mental fatigue, and experiments are continually being devised and conducted to investigate this question further.

Mental Fatigue

The mind, like the body, works better the more regularly it is exercised, but, like the body, it needs consideration as to rhythms of work and rest. Pushed to extremes of fatigue the mind gives progressively less work and less reliable work for progressively greater output of effort, an uneconomical method.

While to concentrate on work, mental or physical, may need effort of will, determination alone cannot ensure a high standard of work, say, at the end of a hard day. There are definite conditions governing maximum mental efficiency, but everyone should find out his or her own best personal rhythms and try to arrange work in relation to these. This is not saving the machine from hard work, but aiming at getting the best results from it, by intelligent foresight.

To turn more definitely to an educational view-point, the development of mental life is a transition from the impulsive actions of babyhood to the increasingly considered behaviour of adults. One fairly obvious difference between children and adults is the latter's power of *deliberate volitional attention*, as in listening to a lesson or lecture. *Spontaneous attention*, on the other hand, is of the kind shown when a child or adult cannot be torn away from a new toy, a camera, or a car.

The border-line between the two is difficult to define, because, for instance, a stimulating teacher may turn deliberate into spontaneous attention. Forty-five minutes is probably the longest economical time that an adult can give attention to work involving much deliberate effort. He can, of course, listen longer, but there will have to be an increasing effort of will to concentrate with decreasing ability to do so fully.

Adolescents from 12 to 14 years can give such concentrated attention for from thirty-five to forty minutes, children aged 9 to 12 from twenty-five to thirty minutes, and those from 6 to 9 from fifteen to twenty minutes. Infants below 6 need shorter periods still.

It is best, if possible, to have classrooms that are sufficiently spacious, and classes small enough in numbers to allow children to get up and move about the classroom in frequent intervals between short spells of oral and written work. With these conditions lessons can, in any one subject, be rather longer, but in the average crowded classroom, though such freedom is difficult to arrange, periods at least can be short, so that the child gets frequent changes of aim and so of interest. Relief drills (between desks) are also useful, as a help to the teacher against the child's fidgeting that comes from sitting still too long.

Deliberate attention of this kind is easier to maintain earlier in the day, when the children are physically fresh. It is therefore better to put subjects with less intrinsic interest and more need for concentration, such as arithmetic, in the morning, and to leave story work, which has more natural interest for children, to the afternoon, when it is more difficult to hold their attention. By ten years of age a child should be able by habit and training to sustain attention, for a short period, even when interest and pleasure of novelty is waning.

Power to attend depends partly on *environment*. A hot, stuffy or too cold room, cramping desks, undue crowding together of children, poor lighting, backless seats, and noise of traffic, all hinder concentration, making the teacher's work and discipline more difficult. Teachers should be alert, in

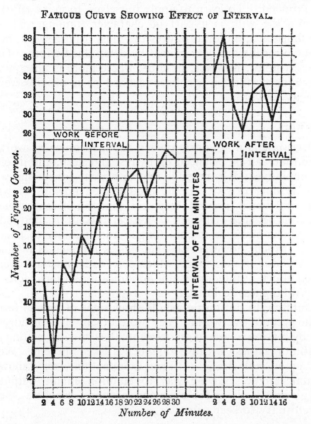

FATIGUE CURVE SHOWING EFFECT OF INTERVAL.

FIG. 99.—The graph shows the value of a rest pause in on the quality and amount of work done. The work done here was a laboratory test—the multiplying of columns of figures—but the principle is applied to industry with success. After the pause there is an immediate and marked improvement in the "number of figures correct." (*From "Valentine's Experimental Psychology"—University Tutorial Press.*)

their own interests, to sum up signs of incipient restlessness and inattention, and deal with the cause before loss of control has become obvious.

In considering *mental and physical fatigue*, it is important to recognise that, at times, we must all play and work when we feel fatigued. To learn to apply ourselves, to make effort, to exercise the will, is a part of character training. Though spontaneous attention produces the most fruitful work, many valuable results are only gained by determined effort. There comes a point, however, in effort where more is uneconomic and, indeed, fatigue has been defined as a progressive incapacity to work.

Overwork

Overwork is not working when tired, so much as working more than can be balanced up by rest and sleep, and its effect is cumulative. It is possible that incapacity for mental work may be due, in part, to the accumulated poisons of waste products which prevent impulses jumping across synaptic junctions between neurones. Physical discomforts that induce restlessness show as mental fatigue and inability to concentrate. Much, however, of what passes for mental fatigue is *boredom* due to monotony, which everybody must get over by willed effort. Boredom is not an indication of incapacity but of unwillingness to work.

Children do not on the whole show signs of mental fatigue to the point of overwork. They protect themselves by fidgeting and by ceasing to attend on occasion, thus possibly getting into a habit of laziness, because too much is asked of them. Worry and emotional stress, as from examinations, may show as mental fatigue. Giving way to emotion entails output of energy and is tiring for everyone around; teachers should therefore try to keep calm.

Rest

A *rest* may take the form of a change of activity or a complete cessation of work, the former being the more interesting and natural for normally healthy people. Thus a sedentary worker, such as a clerk, might rest by gardening or playing tennis in his spare time, while for a physical worker reading or playing bridge gives the necessary change. Children need to be guided to a certain number of interests such as stamp collecting, reading, or using building blocks or Meccano that give them rests from continuous physical activity.

A rest is more than a safeguard against overwork, for during rest periods mental processes of assimilation continue unconsciously. In doing a piece of work, such as writing an essay, it is often advantageous to collect and think over all relevant facts available, and then to leave that work and think no more about it for a matter of hours or days. Often there will be an almost sudden recognition of facts suitably fitted together. This unconscious co-ordination shows also in physical activities where a skilled activity, attempted clumsily on the first day, can often be done in three or four days' time, with no intervening practice, relatively easily and in tolerably correct form. Judicious allowance of time for such consolidation makes for economy of work.

For infants, a *midday rest*, which becomes probably a sleep, after dinner, is of value both for digestion of the fairly heavy midday meal and for mental relaxation, and because growth in height and weight almost certainly takes place actively during such passive rest and sleep. A midday rest, preferably out of doors, and in an open-air shed if wet, forms part of the routine of open-air and nursery schools, and might well be more widely adopted in all infant schools.

Hammocks on inverted tables, or frames or cane beds, some 6 inches from the ground, are cheap, light to handle and quickly adjusted and put away. Lying on mats put out for the purpose on the floor is a possible solution, but floors are generally draughty. Sleeping in a sitting position, huddled over a desk, cramps the chest and heart and digestive organs and gives little general bodily rest (see Fig. 156).

For rest during the day or for sleep, a horizontal position for the body is preferable, because the muscles that continually contract to maintain sitting and standing posture can then relax, and because the heart rests as the pulse rate slows down.

Conditions for Healthy Sleep

The exact physiological cause of *sleep* is not understood, though Professor Pavlov's experiments suggest that it is a

8

state of general inhibition. As noted earlier, it appears to be connected with the circulation of fatigue products which gradually block the passage of impulses at the synaptic junctions. The difficulty of making oneself remember some trifling point when sleepy and of holding in one's thoughts several ideas and evaluating them, seems to show this.

It also seems likely that the nerve centre in the medulla that automatically controls the constricting of blood-vessels all over the body becomes affected by fatigue products and constricts rather less. Thus more blood will get into the body blood-vessels, and so less into the brain, promoting sleep. For concentrated thinking there must be proportionately much blood in the brain. Note the difficulty of such effort immediately after a heavy meal, when extra blood is needed to facilitate digestion in the stomach walls.

Absence of stimuli such as noise and light also promotes sleep. Worrying about a problem, reading an exciting book or doing absorbing work till just before bedtime—such activities stimulate thought and so bring blood to the brain, thus tending to prevent sleep. Reading an unexciting book or playing patience are soporific for most people.

No one can go to sleep with cold feet, and it is better to have a hot-water bottle or bed-socks than to waste time staying awake. If the feet are warm, there is then proportionately more blood in them and less in the brain. Similarly, a hot drink may help to induce sleep by attracting blood to the stomach. A heavy meal, however, would be of less value, because it might rather bring indigestion and wakefulness.

A hot bath, because it draws the blood to the skin's surface and so from the brain, conduces to sleep. By increasing circulation it is also helpful in getting rid of muscular fatigue after strenuous exercise, such as a long day's walking. However, all these are matters that are dependent on personal idiosyncrasy.

It is important always to *sleep with open windows*, and, if possible, with a current of air through the room to the chimney, which should never be blocked up. The habitual breathing of fresh cool air throughout the night makes for better growth, resistance to disease and all-round good health. There is nothing the matter with night air. Indeed, it is possibly purer than day air, because it will contain less dust from traffic and less factory smoke. Tuberculosis has been called a " bedroom disease." Open windows at night help to prevent the contracting of such chest complaints.

The Healthy Bedroom

Students who are about twenty have spent nearly seven years of their life asleep in bed. It is important, therefore, to make *bedrooms* healthy places. They should be airy and not full of ornaments and upholstered furniture and hangings to catch and retain dust and germs. Light furniture that can be moved readily for cleaning is desirable. Rugs, that can easily be taken up, are preferable to a carpet which is likely to become dust-impregnated between infrequent cleanings. A vacuum cleaner partially obviates this.

Washable, fadeless hangings are best. Beds should have no valances, so that dust underneath can be seen and removed. Single beds are healthier than double ones. Coverings should be as light as is compatible with sufficient warmth. Wool is better than cotton, which is heavy and not as warm. The room temperature should not be much over 60° F. Bed coverings and room temperature should be so adjusted that the sleeper does not wake up perspiring heavily.

A fixed bedtime is best for children and for adults. The body then gets a conditioned reflex for sleeping at that time. Children should not be sent to bed for peccadilloes, for this will lead them to associate bed with punishment. They should not be allowed to get into habits of demanding to be rocked or sung to sleep. Sleeping in the dark is best, though a nightlight, put out later, may help to obviate fear of the dark. Adults should never ridicule a child about such fears.

Children from 4 to 8 need at least twelve hours' sleep ; from 8 to 12, eleven hours ; from 12 to 14, ten hours ; and from 14 to 20, nine hours. Adults' needs vary, seven to eight hours being the average. There is no substitute for sleep, and curtailing of sleep very soon results in premature wrinkles and the loss of good looks, as well as of lessened efficiency.

Sleeplessness

Children's sleep should never be curtailed for study. *Sleeplessness* in children points to overwork in school (and the work should be immediately cut down), or to unwise feeding, or to too little chance of exercise and play out of doors. Sleeping draughts for adults or children should never be resorted to save on specific medical advice. It is well to be philosophic about occasional loss of sleep. To lie quietly in the dark and horizontally gives considerable rest, and it is best to try to think about happy unstimulating things, rather than to worry about how tired one will be next day. To take half a dozen deep breaths of fresh air, thus dosing the blood with oxygen, sometimes induces sleepiness. Continued loss of sleep retards children mentally.

It is a good thing to have one's sleep out and to wake naturally. Sleep has been deeper and of more value if the sleeper, when roused, wakes unwillingly and slowly. People who are fully awake at once probably need longer hours of sleep than slower wakers. *Night terrors* may be due to neurotic temperament in a child, but treatment of adenoids, or of a tendency to rheumatism or constipation may help to eliminate them.

CHAPTER XVIII

ATTITUDE TO HEALTH—HYSTERIA—TIC—
STAMMERERS

PERSONALITY is made up of physical, intellectual and emotional
factors, and it is impossible to have a healthful personality
without a balance of function on all these sides.   Disturbances
of any of these factors upset the whole.   It is hard to concentrate mentally if one has toothache ; bad temper, worry or
pleasurable excitement upsets digestion and appetite.

Personality is recognised to be partly conditioned from the
outset by the ductless gland pattern, which shows, for example,
in body shape, tallness or shortness, fatness or thinness, and
in the vehemence or feebleness of emotional response to given
situations.   By training and education, physical and emotional
tendencies can be intelligently controlled.   Thus each individual can learn how to get the most out of his mixture of
qualities, to attain reasonable success and happiness.   The
teacher can largely help in this by understanding the child's
mental and physical development and by influencing him to
form good mental habits.

The child is not just an adult in little, with adult values and
feelings.   Every year, every day even, the body is developing
and changing.   The child's reactions to difficulties, to success
and failure, though not less poignant than an adult's, are yet
different, and every age needs intelligent understanding from
the teacher.

The potentiality of the developing neurones, as of the rest of
the organism, depends on heredity, but whether they will
develop to their full powers is settled by education and the
chances given by environment, physical and mental.   Heredity
creates, but as far as knowledge now goes education can
create nothing, though lack of right education may leave
powers only partially developed (see Chapter XXV).

219

It is now recognised that on the mental side many abnormalities, kinks and even breakdowns have their origin in childhood, and could possibly have been prevented or at least minimised by a more understanding upbringing. Just as important as physical health habits, such as sleeping with open windows or teeth cleaning, is the fostering of sound intellectual and emotional habits. A healthy balanced outlook on life is of value both to the growing child and to those who have to work with and for him.

Perhaps the teacher's chief difficulty in fostering mental habits arises from the fact that, until the approach of puberty, children are capable only of simple reasoning on concrete issues and not of abstract thought. Asked what health is, they will say it is " drinking milk " or " cleaning your teeth." A certain amount of direct teaching and encouragement will be given, but very largely the training makes use of the child's natural imitative impulses and his suggestibility, that is, his willingness to accept as correct facts, views and methods advanced on trust, without adequate or any reasons.

Suggestion and Persuasion

Everybody is suggestible to some extent, but lack of knowledge of the subject being discussed, combined with the authority and impressive manner in which the *suggestion* is put, are important factors in successful suggestion. An impressively worded advertisement, or the pointing finger of a dignified eye-piercing man on a placard, or the sunny brightness of a seaside poster on a dull day in town influences us by suggestion.

The difference between persuasion and suggestion is that in using persuasion, reasons are given and people know they are being persuaded, whereas suggestion has largely failed if its use is suspected by those receiving it. The more educated people are the less suggestible do they tend to be.

Up to the junior school age free use is made of suggestion, both in mental and physical things. If the school and home environment are good, then the child has a high standard by which he unconsciously judges other environments later. This is the reason why the nursery school ought to be a bright, clean, attractive building, with well-groomed courteous teachers, careful service and a high standard of table manners at school dinners, open windows and wholesome offices. All these things go to make the child assume these and similar conditions as a standard. The child also assumes the rightness of doing things for himself.

Children imitate expressions and attitudes. They are very suggestible to an atmosphere of vigorous work and of honest effort, while the process of obtaining mastery over material is of natural interest to them. Boys and girls, too, admire a person who can do practical things they can understand, and in consequence they will accept unquestioningly and with enthusiasm what such a hero says and does.

If, too, children are treated courteously and reasonably, they are likely to act similarly themselves. They learn, by example rather than precept, to judge other people generously and not to try to seek to increase their own importance by depreciating all success in others. They will be willing to admit mistakes, and they cannot come to the conclusion too early that everyone, themselves included, is fairly average, with special abilities and disabilities ; that everyone has a superior somewhere.

On the other hand, school and home should take children and their interests seriously, and not ridicule or shame them or be too heavily disapproving of those mistakes due to ignorance, which all of us have made at some stage. Maybe the one who laughs does so in order to increase his own feeling of self-importance.

All children should have frequent chances of achieving small successes. When these achievements are praised he realises that the praise has been justly earned. Such experiences make a cheerful and reasonably self-confident child, who, while not too self-assertive, will not continually need, when adult, to be reassured and urged on at every undertaking.

Postive Health Teaching

Health teaching must be positive and optimistic, and not play on fears. Similarly, care should be taken not to suggest vague but worrying fears of ghosts, death, the dark, bogies, policemen, doctors and dentists, nor should children be dubbed, in moments of exasperation perhaps, " stupid " or " stubborn," or " little spitfires " or " always late." They tend to see themselves thus and to act accordingly ; they give up all effort to alter, and excuse their conduct as being after all what adults seem to expect of them. A sense of inferiority, too, may result. The effect is similar when parents say, " You will never be any good at arithmetic—I never was." The child ought to be encouraged and to be better taught and so have more chance of learning.

Health education, too, must avoid making a child introspective. From an American school syllabus comes the advice," Early to bed, and a long night's sleep will rest my mind and body and keep me from being nervous." Such items can easily make children self-centred and morbidly introspective. Emphasis should be laid on the possession not on the lack of health. To be healthy is mainly to be unaware of the body's workings.

Practice of health habits should be natural and a matter-of-fact part of the child's daily routine, while, later, at adolescence, some simple physiology will be of intense interest, along with all the other interest of this age in how things work. Also everyone's duty to the community, as in not spreading infections, will be appreciated at this age. Knowledge should replace ignorance and superstition, and the individual be trained not just to want to be self-centredly fit, but to be " fit for something."

Adolescents

As children reach early *adolescence*, they should be trained to be able to resist suggestion, to appreciate reasons for a course of action, to think out reasons for themselves, and to reach unprejudiced conclusions. The more knowledge possessed on a given topic the less suggestible should one be, and adolescents should be trained, by being critical about matters on which they have evidence, to be cautious about accepting statements about which they realise they necessarily lack knowledge. This view-point would prevent the constant ready expression of confidently stated but worthless opinion by ignorant people, who have prejudices rather than reasons.

Honest teachers will be on their guard not to abuse this power of influencing children by suggestion that their authority affords them. Children catch prejudice as readily as reasoned opinions, perhaps more so. The teacher should beware of offering ready-made opinions on matters which the children should be thinking out for themselves. Over-emphatic suggestion, too, defeats its own end by being annoying and results in contra-suggestibility.

Attitude to Authority

The home environment will settle largely the child's view of *authority*, and will condition his response to it possibly throughout life, but the school can help. If the child finds authority in the person of the teacher and parents definite, reasonable, just and kindly, he is likely to react comfortably to it, to co-operate willingly, to expect courteous treatment.

If the grown-up is uncertain in moods, sometimes lax, sometimes strict, or tries to make up for mistakes by bullying or ridicule, or if he is pushed into displays of temper or is over-repressive, then the child may well carry into its adult life a permanent bias and prejudice against those holding authority. Such adults are always likely to be " agin the government " ; they are difficult to employ and unwilling often to accept criticism and readily inclined to think themselves wronged, and they are equally unreasonable as masters.

If a teacher has goodwill and exercises authority reasonably, the children will have courage to state their difficulties rather than weakly to grumble among themselves, wasting energy and emotion. The ability to state an opposition view with dignity, unemotionally and without giving offence, is sure to be of value in life, for everyone is certain to need it sometime.

Development of Independence

Children crave sympathy and affection and to have notice taken of them. This is only natural and right when they start out in a world full of new things and experiences, and for the

8*

first four or five years they are chiefly interested in themselves as individuals.   They should, however, gradually grow out of this to relative independence and self-sufficiency.   A mother or teacher who over-mothers a child, doing too much for him, is satisfying her own urge to have someone dependent on her. She is possibly sacrificing the child's ultimate happiness, for no one likes a spoilt child.   He is too apt to over-value himself and to assume that others, adults and children, should yield to his whims.   His awakening among contemporaries is often rude and cruel.

Illness may aggravate the situation, for a child becomes the centre of too obviously anxious care.   Grown-ups who make a good deal of their ailments and their coughs and insomnia, are still trying to get an interest taken in them by the methods they used successfully as children.

Children, then, need to grow up intellectually and emotion-ally, and not to remain dependent on parents or teachers, but, on the other hand, growing up should not be presented to them as so threatening a process that they become old men and women before their time.   It is the teacher's business to strive to get this well-balanced outlook.

A normal healthy child is then at least up to the average for his age in height and weight, he eats and sleeps well, is energetic, optimistic and self-confident, full of curiosity, and takes pleasure in play and activities.   He also has a good resistance to childish ailments, and shows evidence of satisfactory mental development.

The " Highly Strung " Child

All teachers will come across, among adults as well as among children, that constitutionally nervous type of person who is spoken of as " highly strung," " nervy," " all on edge," " jumpy."   Children of this type may be capable of great achievements ;   they are potentially the creative artists and thinkers, but they inherit, in differing degrees, an unstable emotional balance.   If treated wisely, however, during child-hood, they will develop into normal, useful, happy adults, but wrongly nurtured they may become the neurotics of adult life.

These unstable children are often precocious and rarely still. To press them unduly is to risk dullness later. The child who, according to popular tradition, wins prizes at school and does nothing outstanding in later life is possibly one of these. They need to have liberal, careful feeding, to have plenty of sleep and to be shielded from emotional strains. All this should be given unostentatiously, so that they do not realise that they are the object of special concern. These, and all children, should be treated with special care after returning to school convalescent from some infection. Children then may be fretful and pettish, and may easily be over-pressed by a full normal routine of activities.

" Nervousness " in adults often expresses itself as an inordinate response to a relatively small stimulus. Such people are easily startled or provoked to unrestrained screaming, laughter, gesticulation, or even crying. A good deal of it can be controlled, with advantage to everyone, by appropriate training and education. The tone of a good home and school, the playing of well-coached games, demanding as they do coolness in emotional crisis, control of temper and the need to work for the team, not for self, are of value here.

It is to be noted that people who proclaim themselves as " highly strung," " nervous," and " so sensitive " are often, unconsciously perhaps, using this supposed special susceptibility to allow themselves the luxury of not controlling their emotions, thus impressing themselves unduly on those around them. Finely sensitive people do not say they are. They do not want to be hurt, and so aim at keeping their sensitiveness mainly to themselves ; they do not talk about it.

Hysteria

Hysteria, like neurosis, is a functional nervous disorder in so far that, though there are well-marked and characteristic symptoms, there is no change apparent in the nerve or other tissue, as there is, for instance, in the formation of an abscess at the root of a tooth. Organic nervous disorders are those showing definite lesion, as in infantile paralysis. Crichton Miller defines the hysteric as " one who uses dramatic means to influence her environment in order to escape from some form of humiliation."

In extreme cases of hysteria there may be apparent paralysis, loss of speech, hyper- or in-sensitiveness to pain, and vomiting, but the teacher is mainly likely to come across hysteria in the form of uncontrolled laughter and crying, apparent fainting, or exaggeration of some relatively slight injury. The hysteric aims unconsciously at making herself noticed and interesting. She is too absorbed by her own emotions to see herself as she appears to others. For example, hysterics are careful to fall so that they do not hurt themselves, and, having " fainted," have a good normal colour, whereas a true faint brings paleness.

The immediate treatment is to be brisk and not particularly sympathetic, to send away sympathisers, and not to take too much detailed notice of symptoms, which will probably be produced in a sympathy-compelling way, " such a *dreadful* headache." There is no need, however, to be callous, though one must be judiciously detached, for the hysteric needs help of a robust kind. A sense of humour, that implies an ability to laugh at oneself, is useful.

It is said that people doing hard manual work are rarely hysterical. For the adolescent, work and gradually increasing responsibility will be a useful antidote. There should be few chances of being introspective, and religion, that expresses itself in doing work for other people, is preferable to too much meditation. Living out of doors, plenty of sleep and regular habits all help too. Pronounced hysterics often show a history of unstable nervous inheritance, and maybe of undue coddling in upbringing. Unbalance of endocrine gland secretions may also contribute to the emotional instability.

Neurosis

Neurosis is a functional nervous condition. Undue worrying and depression, lack of sleep, indecision, suspicion of slights, indigestion and irritability, undue susceptibility to noise, are some symptoms. Teachers are perhaps particularly liable to this form of illness. Unlike those who deal only with small numbers of people, they have to work in a team with the rest of the staff, and to deal with large classes ; they have the constant low-grade strain of dealing with human instead of inanimate, inert material (contrast the work of a librarian), and they have often to teach over and over again facts that may well have lost their stimulating freshness. They should, therefore, take all opportunities of mental change and holidays away from their usual surroundings, and train themselves to leave school worries behind them.

Cutting down of meals, getting too little fresh air and exercise, cause loss of health standards. A teacher who begins to be afraid of change, in work or in recreation, should beware. There is a possibility that neurasthenia is associated with insufficient activity of the supra-renal glands. It is to be noted that the hysteric tends to be of rather lower intelligence than the neurasthenic, who is the more self-critical.

Habit Spasm or Tic

Habit Spasm or *Tic* is the term used for nervous recurrent compulsion habits, such as nail biting, blinking, twitching of the face, or drumming, or the jerky moving of body or hands. Trying not to make the movement produces an intolerable urge. Tics are most common between five and ten years of age. Often such habits start from some minor exciting cause, such as clothes that are too tight. A case is recorded of a boy whose incipient facial twitch was found to be due to an over-bright, unshaded light just over his head in a classroom. The recurrent retreat from this glare started the series of movements.

Once a nerve path is worn, complete cure is difficult. The tic becomes worse if the child is unduly strained. Parents and teachers can best help by preventing the establishment of such nervous habits. Once such a tic is established, angry emotional comment is useless, and merely adds to the strain. The co-operation of the child must be obtained, and the personal fight can then be helped by judicious adult encouragement to persevere. The general health should be built up. Contrary to common belief, habit spasms are rarely copied by schoolfellows.

Stammering

Stammering is a functional nervous disorder, that is, there is nothing the matter with the child's speech mechanism ; it is the nervous control that is disturbed. The stammerer lacks confidence and it is at moments of strain that the speech defect is most marked. Stammering in boys and girls is in the proportion of three to one.

Many Local Authorities now supply special treatment. The school sends the names of children with speech defects to the school medical officer. The eyes are first tested as the correction of astigmatism is found to benefit speech defect. The teeth are put in order and malnutrition and any cause of undue fatigue dealt with.

The Centre for the *Speech Therapy Class* must be quiet and away from traffic or a noisy playground. The teacher, who is specially trained, visits the home to discuss and explain the treatment, especially with the father. Lack of home sympathy prevents cure. The stammerer feels insecure and needs encouragement. He is taught (i) to *think* before speaking, (ii) to breathe in before speaking, (iii) to speak slowly and (iv) to keep calm. Children attending the special class need to be at least ten years of age, because they must be able to co-operate intelligently.

Class teachers can help greatly. The stammerer should be spoken to quietly and given ample time to reply. Quick questions and answers should be taboo. The stammerer should not be made to feel different from the other children. For example, he should have his turn at reading aloud. Ridicule from other children should be prevented. Anything to give confidence will help.

After the treatment classes are over, children should be " followed up " to see if further help is necessary, and to collect statistics of the permanence of results. Stammering or tic may be due to an emotional upset in the child's or even in the parents' life.

Allergy—Hay Fever—Asthma—Headache

Allergy is a state of exaggerated sensitivity to some protein which is harmless to the normal person. Examples of states caused in this way are hay fever, asthma, certain rashes, digestive disturbances and migraine.

In *Hay Fever* the individual is especially sensitive to the protein of wind-borne pollens—not to all pollens, but to those of particular plants—grasses or conifers, for example. An allergic condition so caused would be seasonal. The symptoms are sneezing, nasal discharge and running eyes.

Asthma occurs in boys more than in girls. The attacks of breathlessness and wheezing often occur at night. The cause may be proteins taken in food—egg, milk, fish, wheat, or meat, or the inhaling of proteins in dust from feathers or horse-hair or even from the coats of animals.

Many people have idiosyncrasies in connection with certain foods which cause rashes or other disturbances. Rhubarb, oysters, strawberries, cinnamon, mackerel, are examples.

Heredity is of considerable importance in the incidence of allergies ; asthma tends to occur in highly strung, nervous children. The conditions are not diseases and are not usually dangerous to life.

Headache is usually a symptom only of disturbance elsewhere in the body,[1] and the cause should be found and treated as early as possible. Poisoning from the toxins of inflammation, or from decayed teeth or anæmia, feverish conditions, too much alcohol, concussion, sunstroke, neurotic states, and working or sleeping in a stuffy room are some causes of headaches. Eye defects may show themselves, not as failure of sight, but in recurring headaches. Fatigue in fast-growing children, rheumatism and adenoids may also be causes.

Chorea, or St. Vitus' Dance, though often classed as a functional nervous disorder, is probably due to the toxin of rheumatism (see Chapter XXX).

Infantile Paralysis, though its after-effects show as a disability of the nerves, is an infectious disease (see Chapter XXVIII).

---

[1] A persistent cough is similarly a symptom, the reason for which should be sought.

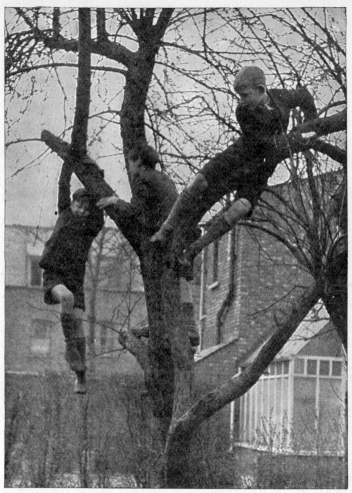

Fig. 100.—Play Therapy in the garden of a Child Guidance Clinic. These boys are satisfying their emotional difficulties and feeling power in the adventurousness of tree climbing. (*From Craig's " Child and Adolescent Life in Health and Disease "—E. & S. Livingstone, Ltd.*).

Child Guidance

The *Child Guidance Clinics* are for the treatment of behaviour problems in nervous, unstable and difficult children. They are not primarily for the treatment of the innately dull child. Just as the work of the School Medical Service is to treat early and slight ailments to prevent minor from becoming major defects, so the Child Guidance Clinic aims at preventing adult neurosis by attention to mental hygiene.

Cases are referred to the clinics by school medical officers, teachers, parents, children's courts and care committees. The difficulties are mainly those of nervousness, backwardness at school and lack of adjustment to home or school which, if left, might end in delinquent behaviour. Tics, bed wetting, excitability, tempers, stammering, theft, truancy, sex difficulties, night terrors and fears are some of the causes of reference among London children.

The basic staff of a Child Guidance Clinic consists of a psychiatrist, an educational psychologist and a trained social worker. Of these, the *psychiatrist* has a medical qualification and carries out the physical and general mental examination. The *educational psychologist* contributes knowledge of the attainments and development of normal and abnormal children at different age levels. Intelligence testing is carried out and the educational psychologist can judge, for example, whether a child is emotionally upset from being asked to cover too much or too little work at school, or to do unsuitable work. The *social worker* investigates the home environment. Home visits are made, before and after treatment, and it is frequently possible to persuade the parents to make some adjustment in the child's regime which helps to solve the behaviour difficulty.

Play Therapy

Play Therapy. It is generally agreed that children express and resolve their emotional difficulties through their play. The child, for instance, plays at being a soldier because the soldier seems strong and important in contrast to the relative weakness and dependence of the child. In the Clinic playroom, children are supplied with a variety of toys—large sand trays, running water, ample blackboard space, a doll's house, model figures, animals, trains and motors—and they are left to do what they like with these toys, short of actual injury. Meanwhile skilled observers make records of what the children do, without themselves being seen, thus avoiding the danger of making the children self-conscious. It is found that for children of a repressed, shy type, this play therapy is a helpful form of treatment.

It has been said that these Clinics should rather be called "Parent" than "Child" Guidance Clinics because almost invariably it is the parent or responsible adult who can, with understanding, alter the child's environment for the better. As the result of the Clinic's investigations, advice may be given as to more consistent treatment in the home, or less stern and repressive discipline, or a change of school may be indicated or medical treatment needed.

Preventive Aspects of Child Guidance

Child Guidance work started in this country in 1926 and Clinics were recognised for Ministry of Education grants in 1935. The early tendency was to deal with marked emotional upsets and to aim at *cure*. Now, in addition, the tendency increasingly is to aim at prevention as at a Child Guidance Centre (*not* Clinic). Here a doctor who specialises in the illnesses of children—a pædiatrician—rather than a psychiatrist, meets parents, teachers and social workers to consider behaviour problems before these have become acute. Parent-teacher associations are of value in this connection.

Hostels for Maladjusted Children

Some L.E.A.'s run Hostels for Maladjusted Children and good adjustment has been achieved in this way. Such Hostels are not suitable for (i) very dull or educationally sub-normal children (who tend to improve in special residential schools for educationally sub-normal children), or (ii) for really delinquent children because the discipline for maladjusted children needs to be firm and kindly but not strict enough for a constitutionally psychopathic child.

CHAPTER XIX

INTELLIGENCE TESTS AND VOCATIONAL GUIDANCE

EVERYONE tacitly, by acceptance of standards in general use, if not actively and consciously, admits the convenience and value of having ratings of abilities and of potential abilities on which to base judgments and decisions respecting individuals. Chronological age is always a factor in such ratings. A boxer is old at thirty, a judge young at fifty. A child of seven or eight should be able to take his place in the junior school, but it is clear, too, that all children of one age have not reached exactly the same stage of growth either physically or mentally.

In addition to the ordinary school examinations there are now a large number of standardised attainments tests which are used to measure a child's achievement and progress in such branches of school work as reading, composition and arithmetic. While they are a guide to the child's level of performance, they do not indicate his real potentialities since the results are partly dependent upon opportunities for learning. For example, a child of not more than average ability may do better in an attainments test than a child of much higher ability, if the former has had the opportunity of better teaching, or the latter been hampered through illness or poverty or home anxieties.

In order, therefore, to measure a child's ability to learn, in contrast to merely finding how much he knows in some particular direction, Intelligence tests are used.

General Intelligence

" General Intelligence " is sometimes defined as innate capacity to make adequate adjustments to environment ; the degree of intelligence of each individual is thus held to be inborn. Standardised tests of intelligence, graded so that a

233

child of normal intelligence should be able to do the tests allocated to his age-group, have been devised and used. The score obtained in these tests determines the child's Mental Age.

The *intelligence quotient* (or mental ratio) is a statement in which the child's mental age is expressed as a percentage of his chronological age. Thus a child of eight who could pass all the tests up to and including those for eight year olds, but no more, would have an intelligence quotient (I.Q.) of 100. If he could pass the tests for nine or a proportion of the ten-year-old and later tests, his I.Q. would be more than 110.

If, on the other hand, the child of eight cannot answer the tests for age seven or six, he is considered *dull* ; his I.Q. would be below 100, probably below 80. In so far as the tests are reliable, we can assume that the child will never outgrow this innate dullness.

The meanings attached to the various values of Intelligence Quotients, as suggested in the *Primary School Report*, are :—

120 upward . .	Very superior intelligence.
110 to 120 . .	Superior intelligence.
90 to 110 . .	Normal intelligence.
80 to 90 . .	Normal but dull, should be able to work in the ordinary school.
70 to 80 . .	Less retarded children, incapable of great intelligence, but can be taught to earn a living. They should be taught in a specially organised small class in the ordinary school.
50 to 70 . .	More retarded children. They need Special School education.
Below 50 . .	Ineducable imbeciles and idiots.

Intelligence tests of the present school type are of little use for adults, whose wider experience allows greater use of judgment. The degree of intelligence is not considered to increase after sixteen years of age, though, the mental content of the individual does and should do so.

Intelligence Tests

MM. Binet and Simon devised the first useful set of tests, for children from three to fourteen. Burt, Terman and Spearman are outstanding names among the many psychologists who have and are still experimenting on such work. Any specific information about the content of tests given here must be considered illustrative and only as an example of the many lines of thought and investigation continually being pursued.

Examples of tests for a child of three are :—

(1) Points to own nose, eyes, mouth, when asked.

(2) Knows own sex.

(3) Names a key, penny, knife.

(4) Gives own name and surname.

(5) Matches colours—three colours of each of the four primary colours.

(6) Repeats two digits, one of three tries to be correct ; as 3, 7 ; 6, 4 ; 9, 5.

At age six an average child would be able to—

(1) Repeat five digits, one of three trials to be correct ; 52937 ; 68532.

(2) Distinguish right and left : (a) right hand ; (b) left eye ; (c) right ear—all correct.

(3) Know days of the week.

(4) Know number of fingers on each and on both hands without counting.

(5) Count 13 pence (not all in a row).

(6) Copy a diamond—three trials—two to be recognisable.

(7) Name four coins—$1s.$, $6d.$, $1d.$, $\frac{1}{2}d.$, shown separately, all to be correct.

At age eleven an average child should, among other tests, be able to—

(1) Detect absurdities in three out of five sentences :—

　　(a) The cyclist who was killed may not get better.

　　(b) I have three brothers, Jack, Bob and myself.

　　(c) The railway accident was not serious ; there were forty-seven killed.

　　(d) The girl was found cut into eighteen pieces, and it was thought that she had killed herself.

　　(e) I shall not kill myself on Friday because Friday is an unlucky day for me.

(2) Give sixty words spontaneously in three minutes.

(3) Repeat sentences of twenty to twenty-three syllables.

(4) Repeat five digits backwards.

These examples of tests are quoted from Herd's " Diagnosis of Mental Deficiency."

Performance and Non-Verbal Tests

It is realised that in order to eliminate as far as possible the influences of education, tests which demand the minimum of

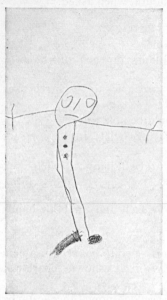

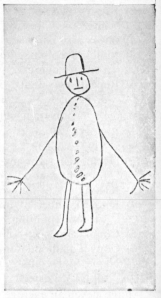

FIG. 101.—Typical drawing of a man by child aged 5. The drawing is full-face, and there is little observance of detail, the arms growing from the head, and the wrong number of fingers. The limbs are shown by single lines, but the feet and buttons have been noticed. (*From Burt's " Mental and Scholastic Tests" —P. S. King & Son, Ltd.*)

FIG. 102.—Typical drawing of a man by child aged 6. More detail has been noticed here, such as the legs shown with double lines, the attempt at showing five fingers, the hat. The body is oval-shaped, and not yet the shape of clothes. Though buttons are included, there are too many. Most children, however, do not look at the object to be drawn at all, at this age. A few take one look. (*From Burt's " Mental and Scholastic Tests" —P. S. King & Son, Ltd.*)

acquired knowledge or use of special aptitudes need to be constructed. For example, differences in vocabulary and in language ability tend to modify results and so where such modification is likely, Performance and other non-verbal tests are used.

In *Performance tests* the child is required to manipulate

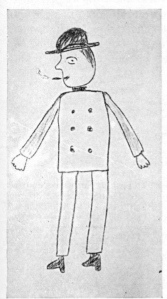

Fig. 103.—Typical drawing of a man by child aged 8. There is considerably more interest in detail here, as in the cigarette, neck, clothes shape for the body, heels to the boots and the more natural shape of the hand. The face is drawn side-face. Note that the line of the head shows through the hat. (*From Burt's " Mental and Scholastic Tests "—P. S. King & Son, Ltd.*)

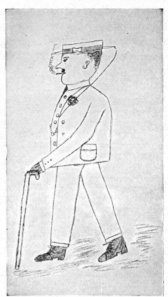

Fig. 104.—Typical drawing of a man by child aged 11. Many more details have interested the child here, such as the ear, hat and guard, moustache, watch-chain, pocket, boot-laces, buttons on sleeve and coat and the shirt cuff. There is also ground on which the figure stands, and the whole figure now faces sideways. (*From Burt's " Mental and Scholastic Tests "—P. S. King & Son, Ltd.*)

concrete material such as blocks, cubes and dominoes or form boards with their incomplete pictures or patterns. The Porteus mazes and drawings of men shown in the figures are other kinds of performance tests.

There is, in addition, a growing use of tests that not only do not require linguistic ability but also make no demand on manipulative skill. Frequent items in sets of Intelligence tests are *Classification Tests*. In these the child is presented with five words, four of which are alike in some respect and the other is different; for example, *shoe, glove, boot, sandal, slipper* or *penny, franc, shilling, farthing, sixpence*, or *some, all, often, most, none*. The child crosses out the " different " word.

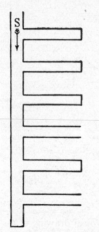

FIG. 105.—*Porteus Maze Test for Fifth Year.* In any of these tests, if the child makes a mistake he is directed to re-start, and not to retrace his course. In this, the openings are demonstrated before the child begins, and, for full credit, he should pass out by the upper opening. A second trial is allowed. (*From Burt's " Mental and Scholastic Tests "—P. S. King & Son, Ltd.*)

In the non-verbal form of such tests, the words " *shoe, glove, boot, sandal, slipper* " are replaced by pictures or diagrams. This substitution of pictures for the written words makes it possible to test in cases when the person has little linguistic ability or speaks in a foreign tongue.

Analogies tests (e.g. *Cup* is to *saucer* as *knife* is to *what?*) can be produced in picture as well as in verbal form in some instances. " *The day before yesterday* is to *the day after to-morrow* as *Saturday* is to *Sunday?, Monday?, Wednesday?, Friday?* " is an example of such a test that can only be given in word form.

The similar *synonyms* and *antonyms* tests can only be presented in word form.

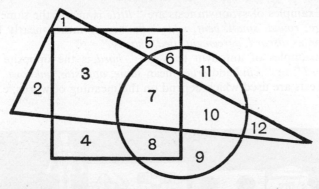

FIG. 106.—This partly *Visual Test* was used in the Mental Survey of Scottish Children, when the complete age-group $10\frac{1}{2}$ to $11\frac{1}{2}$ were given the same set of tests (87,498 children). " Scatter " or range of intelligence was found to be greater than had been hitherto assumed. *Questions* on this test are : (1) What number is in the triangle and square but not in the circle ? (2) What is the sum of the two numbers which are in the circle only ? (3) Subtract the number which is in the circle and triangle but not in the square from the sum of all the numbers which are in the square but outside the circle. (*Diagram and questions reproduced by the courtesy of the University of London Press from " The Intelligence of Scottish Children."*)

FIG. 107. — *Porteus Maze Test for Fourteenth Year*. Starting from the centre S, the child traces the way out without crossing any line, or turning up any of the blocked paths. Up to a fourth trial is allowed. (*From Burt's " Mental and Scholastic Tests "— P. S. King & Son, Ltd.*)

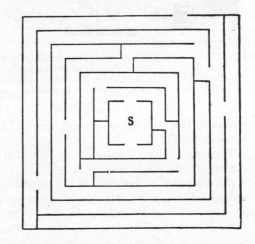

Examples of synonym tests are " *little* is nearly the same as *large, round, small, bent, wide* " or " *unity* means nearly the same as *discord, agreement, tied, charity.*"

Examples of antonym tests are " *hard* is the opposite of . . . ? " or " *kind* and *cruel* mean *same, opposite, unknown.*"

Tests are used which depend on the meaning of words, e.g.,

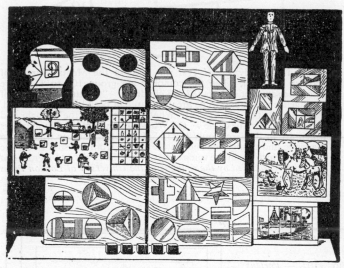

FIG. 108.—*A collection of Inset Performance Tests.*—It is generally held that there is a greater element of chance in the results of Performance Tests than in those of Language Tests. (*Reproduced by permission of Prof. Cyril Burt and the British Broadcasting Corporation.*)

" *Honey, jam, saccharine, treacle,* are all (*liquid, sweet, sticky, manufactured*) ? "

The explaining of *absurdities*, of which the following are examples, is a possible form of test.

(*a*) One day a man fell off his bicycle on to his head and was killed instantly. He was taken to hospital and they fear he may never get better.

(*b*) I have three brothers, George, Albert and myself.

Reasoning Tests

Tests of reasoning are difficult to standardise, but they are considered the best tests for " General Intelligence." Terman, in one test for the " Superior Adult," asks how to measure out exactly seven pints of water, using only a 3-pint and a 5-pint vessel. Burt has found that at seven a child should be able to elucidate, for example—

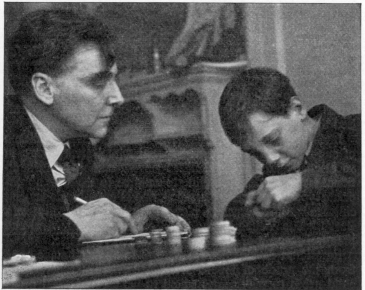

FIG. 109.—Boy doing a performance test of intelligence. He is absorbed and quite oblivious to anyone looking on. (*From Craig's* " *Child and Adolescent Life in Health and Disease* "—*E. & S. Livingstone, Ltd.*)

Kate is cleverer than May.
May is cleverer than Jane.
Who is the cleverest, Jane, Kate or May ?

Or at eight—

" I don't like sea voyages and I don't like the seaside. I must spend Easter either in France or among the Scottish Hills or on the South Coast. Which shall it be ? "

Or at nine—

" Three boys are sitting in a row. Harry is left of Willie, George is to the left of Harry. Which boy is in the middle ? "

The child reads the problem to himself and is told to try to give the answer at the end of it. When the results of a series of intelligence tests suggest that a child has a low mental ratio, it is advisable that further investigation should be made.

Values of Tests

Intelligence tests are useful because they give a basis for considering, comparing and contrasting the intelligence of a group of people in an unbiased and unprejudiced way, which is impossible with examinations of the informational and essay types. The best Intelligence Tests have been so well standardised that the results are independent of the examiner.

Intelligence tests are widely used now in assessing children of sub-normal intelligence for special school attendance ; in vocational guidance for children leaving school, as an additional test for helping to allocate children to the most appropriate type of secondary education, and in assessing delinquent children who, for example, play truant, or commit petty theft. Burt's " The Young Delinquent " gives a detailed, vivid and practical account of the value of such methods in use.

Emotional development progresses to an adult stage apart from the grade of inborn intelligence. Thus the retarded child needs to play games suited to his chronological rather than to his mental age, and to be given text- and story-books of increasingly adult appeal. It is for this reason that the Hadow Report recommended a break at eleven, using chronological age and not mental age as the basis of change.

Tests of Special Ability

While no child of low I.Q. can be really successful in work that involves much thinking, general intelligence alone is not a guarantee of success. This depends on other factors as well, including *Special Abilities, Special Interests* and *Temperamental Qualities*. There is wide variation between individuals in all these directions, and, in consequence, psychologists have investigated methods of measuring these qualities and abilities.

There are a number of tests for measuring special capacities, such as tests for linguistic, arithmetical, manual and musical ability. These tests are constructed to test aptitude and ability, not attainment, in particular directions. There is no suggestion that ability in one direction, say mathematics, is more desirable than ability in another, say music. Two children of the same mental and the same chronological age may rank very differently in the same test of special ability.

Special disabilities also need to be taken into account. A child is sometimes hampered, for example, by " word blindness " or " word deafness " and appears to be less intelligent than he really is. Non-verbal tests are needed.

Testing Temperament

Most people have some special interests but these are not always accompanied by special ability in those directions. Differences of Temperament and Disposition can be seen in the way children attack their work. One child is excited and dashes at it, while another goes slowly and cautiously. Nevertheless, it is difficult to assess how far an individual's emotional make-up, how far his disposition and his temperament help or hinder his progress. It is difficult to estimate the value of such traits as concentration, initiative, industry, persistence, cheerfulness and assertiveness. There are comparatively few reliable standardised tests of temperament, well known ones are those devised by Downey. In the main it is found that, up to the present, the best method of assessing temperamental qualities and the resulting character is the personal interview carried out according to a definite technique agreed upon by representative psychologists.

Vocational Guidance

Bodies such as the National Institute of Industrial Psychology give advice to children on work for which they are best suited. This advice and guidance needs to be given by those who know the demands of the various occupations and also those who understand individual differences. Two children with the same

I.Q. would not necessarily be equally suitable for a particular job. One may lack the special interest or the special ability required for the work. Or again, one may have a temperament quite unsuited for the kind of task in question.

In order, therefore, to insure that the boy is recommended to the type of work in which he is most likely to gain success and satisfaction, educational tests and reports are considered, intelligence tests and special aptitude tests are given, and he is also interviewed. It is, further, necessary to take into account the boy's general health and physical condition, including his sensory and muscular equipment.

A sample case may be quoted. A strongly built boy, with a gruff social manner, asserted that he wanted to become a commercial traveller. On enquiry, it was found that what he liked about the life was the travelling about, but his manner would probably have made him unsuccessful as a salesman. He was recommended to go to sea, and did well.

The vocational guidance psychologist, knowing in detail the work to be done in different vocations and the qualities necessary for success, can direct the boy's choice as no parent can. To put a child to a particular form of work for life, as is often done, because the parent is employed in it and wants help there, or because of immediate financial return, or because of supposed social status, is not the way to make contented, successful citizens.

CHAPTER XX

DULL, BACKWARD AND RETARDED CHILDREN. EPILEPTICS

CHILDREN who are not making satisfactory progress at school can be put into three categories :—

(1) *Dull children*. These are children who are of low intelligence. The dullness is inborn and such children will never reach the standard of attainment of the majority of children of their own age.

(2) *Backward children*. These are children who for some reason have not reached the educational level of the average children of their age.

(3) *Retarded children*. These are the children who have not reached the level of attainment which corresponds to their intellectual ability. They may have reached or even surpassed the level of attainment of normal children of their own age.

The two latter cases are first considered. The teacher of both the backward and the retarded child must investigate the causes of the child's unsatisfactory progress and help to remove these.

Physical Causes of Backwardness

Physical causes of backwardness. Deafness or defective sight may make a normal child appear to be stupid. Rickets causes definite mental retardation until about eight years of age. Adenoids, causing deafness and defective breathing, lead to backwardness. Continued lack of sleep shows in a lowered mental ratio, and lack of adequate food and fresh air, and general malnutrition augment this. Prolonged absence from school due to infectious or other disease, may result in a child falling behind in his work, and unless he has special treatment he may never catch up.

Professor Cyril Burt tells of a boy whose clever thefts at twelve were largely traceable to his having missed learning to read at six: as a result, he was wrongly classed as defective mentally and in consequence he developed no useful interests. Nomadic life—of barge and theatrical children—may lead to backwardness through lack of systematic training.

Teachers should be alert to suspect physical causes for

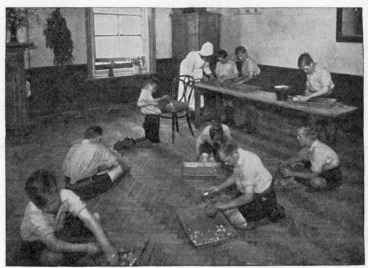

FIG. 110.—Backward Boys making " worlds " in their sand trays. It is found that children tend to express and resolve their own emotional difficulties in the kind of " world " they choose to make. (*From Craig's " Child and Adolescent Life in Health and Disease "—E. &. S. Livingstone, Ltd.*)

backwardness, and, both for their own ease of class control and for the child's good, recommend such suspects for consideration of treatment for adenoids, deafness or provision of glasses. Children backward owing to malnutrition or illness may benefit by the regime of an Open-Air School and have a chance there to catch up educationally.

In the case of *the retarded child* the cause of retardation may be physical, but it is more likely to be the child's maladjustment to his environment at home or at school. It may, for instance, be dislike of the teacher or of school customs, or lack of interest in a subject or the method of presenting it, or it may be due to excessive day-dreaming, pampering by parents or a wrong home atmosphere.

The Dull Child

The aim of the teacher of *the dull child* is to see that he uses effectively and rightly what intelligence he has, so that he may become a happy, fearless individual and a self-respecting citizen.

Congenitally dull children are characterised by *late development*. Most normal children speak at ten and walk at twelve months, while a dull child might well not talk till two or two and a half years or walk till two years or even later. Bowel control, too, develops late. On the other hand, it is not good for any child to be pushed on by over-stimulating adults to precocious development ; steady, unhurried growth all round is healthiest. Some of the most brilliant adults develop late.

The family history of congenitally dull children is likely to include relatives showing unstable tendencies, mental defect, hysteria, epilepsy, syphilis or alcoholism. The incidence of mental defect is much greater in Whitechapel than in Hampstead, for example, because people with defects in the family are likely to be unsuccessful in life, and consequently to drift to slum areas.

Some mentally defective children have a clumsy walk, slack posture and a vacant, unalert expression or a continual mirthless grin. Physical stigmata, such as small head of unsymmetrical shape, malformation of the outer ear, cleft palate and hair lip, may be present. This in no way means that all people showing such physical stigmata are mentally retarded. Other children of marked mental defect have bright alert expressions and show no outward signs of defect. Eruption of teeth and the onset of puberty may be late in dull children. Speech defects are commoner among dull than among normal children, and they persist longer. Personal habits may be dirty and careless and need special emphasis in the education of such children.

The dull child is readily suggestible, but cannot maintain

9

attention long or think abstractly. He lacks sustained purpose. He may be readily excitable or of dull apathetic disposition. Reasoning power is poor. A boy who was told to water his garden, was found doing it in the rain. Some dull children are vicious and mischievously destructive, but lack of anger is to some extent a characteristic of weaklings. Sex impulses may be lacking or over-strong. Dull children are often affectionate and inclined to show off. There tend to be more dull boys than dull girls in the sub-normal schools' population.

While the majority of dull children conform to no special physical type, it is possible to differentiate from among other classes those with markedly small skulls, the *microcephalics*. The spaces between the cranial bones may have joined up too early and prevented the normal growth of the brain. A cranium circumference of less than 17 inches has been taken as a standard below which normal adult development should not fall, but this is somewhat arbitrary. Microcephalics are difficult to train because they tend to be spiteful, dirty and destructive as they grow up.

Macrocephalics, those with heads larger in circumference than normal, may be normal mentally but the condition may go with mental defect. This is not to be confused with the characteristic square and usually bossed skull, due to rickets.

The *Mongol type* of mentally defective has a Chinese cast of face, with high cheek bones and eyes slanting obliquely upward ; so that, though unrelated, all Mongols seem to have a family resemblance. They may be apathetic but are usually cheerful, lively and affectionate, and with a sense of fun. The tongue is often large, the ears small and rounded and the cheeks flushed. Mongols are loose-jointed ; they are liable to congenital heart disease, chest ailments and chilblains. They cannot be educated much, though their pleasant brightness may promise well. More boys than girls are Mongols. The cause is unknown.

Cretins are defective through lack of the thyroid gland secretion (see Chapter XV). They are, as a rule, placid, unemotional, and easy to manage. Puberty is late and sterility possible. Unlike dull children they are educable in so far as they respond to thyroid treatment.

The *after-effects of acute encephalitis* (" sleepy sickness ") are more serious in children than in adults. It seems likely that the virus attacks the basal ganglia of the brain not yet fully developed. The younger the patient the greater the possibility of permanent damage. There is in such children, therefore, a gradual deterioration that shows itself in decreasing intelligence (as shown by intelligence tests) and in inability to concentrate and attend. Moral defects and emotional instability, not present before, may develop, so that a previously satisfactory child lies, steals, falls into violent rages or is wantonly destructive or cruel. Removal to a quiet, ordered environment gives the best chance of recovery, such as it is.

A certain number of people exist who are classed as *moral imbeciles*, that is, they lack moral sense, and they are incapable of recognising that thieving, lying or the infliction of cruelty, physical or mental, is wrong. Apart from having no feelings of pity or remorse, they cannot understand that such lack of morals is anti-social and that a community must protect itself against such menaces to its peace. These children, especially if they suffer also from mental defect, may come under the purview of the school medical service. Some, however, make their way in life ruthlessly. Everyone must have come across the person who is incapable of understanding moral limitations in judgment. This category, of course, should not be taken to include people who make moral judgments different from our own.

The Education of the Dull Child

Formerly, if a child was to attend a special school for mental defectives, the practice was for him to be recommended for examination by his school authorities, and the school medical officer had to certify him as a mental defective, after which he had to attend the special school until sixteen. This procedure is modified by the Education Act, 1944. The medical officer does not now issue a certificate unless required to do so by the parent or unless it is necessary to secure the attendance of the child at a special school.

Normally, the medical officer gives advice to the parent and the local education authority, and this should be sufficient to secure attendance at an appropriate school. The former procedure, to a certain extent, cast a social slur on the child and on his parents, who may be unwilling for him to attend the special school. There, however, he gets much more useful teaching suited to his capacities, than in the ordinary school; he will feel more competent in the less competitive atmosphere of the special school. Furthermore, the ordinary school class can be run more economically if all the children in it are of nearly the same level of intelligence.

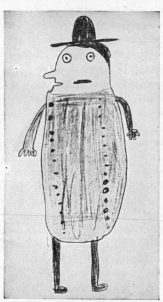

FIG. 111.—Drawing of a man by a backward girl (aged 7, 10/12), showing "mixed profile." "The contour of the head, particularly of the nose and hair, are in profile; the two eyes, two arms, two legs, two rows of buttons, show a front view; while the nose turns to the left, the feet turn to the right; and there are two mouths and no ears." (From Burt's "Mental and Scholastic Tests"—P. S. King & Son, Ltd.)

The Report of the Commission on Mental Deficiency (1929) suggested that there should be three kinds of provision for sub-normal children, special classes in the elementary school (as it was then called), special day schools and special residential schools.

For the *special classes in the ordinary primary or secondary school*, it would be economical to employ a teacher with special training in teaching children of low mental ratio: the dull children would be attending an ordinary school, and there would be no social stigma attached: the children and the teacher would benefit by being in touch with normal children and with the organisation and staff of a normal school. Such special classes provide for the least dull children. This kind of class is cheaper for small local education authorities to establish, for a special school of economic size is impossible unless the total school population of an area is at least 8,000.

The Special School

The aim of the *Special School for Sub-normal Children*, whether a day or a residential school, is to make the child an efficient citizen, self-respecting and self-supporting as far as may be and of socially acceptable habits.

The education given should be practical, concrete and vocational. The children learn by initiation what to do, but it is useless to give them reasons. Children below a mental ratio of 70 cannot usefully, says Kerr, be taught to read or probably to write much. Every case must be judged on its merits, but it is waste of effort and of the child's time to teach reading and writing to such children except the little necessary for present-day life, such as to read direction notices and warnings of the " safety first " type. The child sees the value of this practical work, and so makes some progress, if taught on " Direct " methods. Similarly, arithmetic, which is a very difficult subject for mental defectives, should be concerned mainly with teaching the children to handle money, so that they shall be cheated the less in after-life.

Clear speech will be of advantage to the child, so considerable training should be given in enunciation. It is to be noted that mechanical skill in reading may be much ahead of understanding. A child may be able to read a book suitable for ten-year-olds, but to understand only the ideas and contents of a book for seven-year-olds.

The less dull children may reach ten-year-old level educationally by the time they leave at sixteen, but many never do this. All children in special schools are medically examined yearly and any change in physical and emotional condition and educational progress noted. The classification is rather by attainment than age at first, but in later school years the child should have vocational training suited to his years.

Up to half the time-table period is given to hand-work, which will merge into vocational work for boys, gardening, carpentry, boot-making, book-binding, rug-making, tailoring; and for girls, domestic work, laundry, cooking, needlework and darning.

Training in habits by doing is essential. Thus, all cleaning polishing and attending to domestic duties that can be done by the children should be divided out among them, so that they can feel a sense of responsibility and satisfaction in each bit of work done and approved by the teacher. Each child also should have his own towel, tooth-brush and washing materials, and be supervised in their use, and the elder children should wash out the towels daily.

The sub-normal child should have opportunity of taking part in well-taught games, sports and physical training, swimming and dancing, that accord with emotional development, not with mental ratio. Scouting and girl guide activities are useful. All these activities make for physical development and pride in posture, and they put the child in the position of having to meet practical social and emotional issues, such as keeping temper, and playing fairly, which can be a training for such issues in life.

The education of a sub-normal child costs the community more than that of a normal child, and yet the reports of *After-Care Committees* on the later history of defective children are not very encouraging. About a third of special school children are employable. The defective adolescent is always changing his job. He may have worked well under school supervision and direction, but he is incapable of directing his own life purposefully and is probably over-lavish and easily cheated about money.

Defectives, too, are often sexually uncontrolled, lacking as they do the imagination to evaluate the social results of lack of control.

With the improved infant care in the last thirty years, the proportion of weaklings, physical and mental, that survive to adult life is increased. The proportion of mentally defective people to the total population is steadily increasing, a serious social problem for all normal citizens.

The Colony for Adult Defectives

Thus, for many reasons it seems better, both for the defective and for the normal people of the community (who must support these defectives in prisons, workhouses or hospitals by payment of rates and taxes), that mentally defectives should be segregated into colonies. Here the defective himself is kept happy and protected : his work is supervised and, as far as possible, the colony is made self-supporting by the work done : the defective is guarded from sex contacts, and so from having unwanted defective children that he himself could never support ; and the community is protected from sex assaults and possible crimes.

Sub-normal adolescents, who are employable, can be helped by the supervision and interest of the Care Committee workers, in work and home conditions. Old scholars associations, too, do good work in focusing the interest of the defective adolescent. Religious influences may be useful. In big towns it is possible for the After-Care Committee to set up " *industrial centres* " and some handicraft classes for older boys and girls of both high and low grade, where work can continue to be supervised and directed.

For lower grade notified children, the *Occupation Centre* aims only at fitting the child for the strictly limited environment of his own home, where he may lead a life of happiness for himself and, sometimes, of usefulness to others, but in any case a life in which he ceases to be an intolerable burden to others, and to have his own place in the family circle (Mental Deficiency Report, 1929). All this work, though useful to the community, must be looked upon only as palliative.

Epilepsy

Epilepsy is included here because it is an inherited condition that tends to hamper the living of a full adult life. It is a disease of youth, the onset of 75 per cent. of cases occurring before twenty. There is a strong tendency for the condition to be inherited, so that epileptics ought not to have children. The first fit may follow an accident or shock or an acute illness, or the fits may date from infancy.

There are two forms of epilepsy, major and minor. In the *major form* the epileptic turns pale, gives a cry and falls down unconscious. There is a tonic contraction of the muscles, the face becomes dusky with congestion, and there is foam at the mouth. Convulsions last for a minute or two, gradually subsiding. The patient will generally sleep for some hours afterwards and often wakes with a headache. The tongue is likely to be bitten, so that immediately an attack starts, any hard substance, a tooth-brush or pencil-box lid should be thrust between the teeth to prevent this. Any hard furniture, too, should be moved away from the patient, who may injure himself severely in falling or during the convulsions.

Some fits may be slight and lack the characteristic symptoms. That the unconsciousness is epileptic in origin and not a faint or hysteria can be suspected when the person is found in a pool of urine, for relaxing of the sphincters of the bladder and anus is characteristic. Such a point should be reported to the doctor.

Many epileptics have, a little before the fit comes on, specific sensations, differing in individuals, called aura, which vary from tickling at the wrist, or vague abdominal disturbance, to hallucinations. The aura may enable the patient to get to a place of safety before the fit occurs.

In *minor epilepsy* (*petit mal*) there is a wave of unconsciousness that makes only a temporary interruption in occupation ; for example, a child who is writing becomes pale, stops and is blank, and goes on again after the pause as though it had not occurred. There is no convulsion. If the child were riding a bicycle he would fall off. It is very characteristic that whatever was being done before the fit is continued when consciousness is regained. The eyes may roll senselessly. At the end of the fit the child may, without cause, attack his next door neighbour. Though less disturbing than the major type the likelihood of recovery is no better.

The cause of epilepsy is not known, but *fits can be excited* by indigestion, constipation or undue emotional disturbance or alcohol. They occur in families showing nervous instability, and a family history of syphilis and alcoholism may include epilepsy as well.

Fits may occur at wide intervals of perhaps a year or at lesser intervals down to several in a day. The epileptic is not necessarily mentally deficient. Napoleon and Julius Cæsar are well-known examples of epileptics. Fits, however, may tend to recur at increasingly frequent intervals and, when they do, there is generally a progressive mental deterioration.

Both because of the disturbance of ordinary school classes, and because the epileptic can get more useful specific treatment elsewhere, epileptics should not be educated in ordinary schools. It is the legal duty of the local education authority to find out epileptic children in their district and to arrange for their education and care, if need be.

Epileptics are best segregated in special residential colonies or schools where they can have quiet, regular routine and continual care and supervision. Quietening medicines such as bromides and a diet with little meat are used. Such a regime may reduce the frequency of fits and prevent them from becoming chronic. Many epileptics are intractable, and of uneven temper, falling into senseless rages on occasion. A facile smile is frequently seen.

After-care for less severe cases is important. Suitable occupations are gardening and fruit-growing. Epileptics should undertake no work that involves the use of machinery or fire, entails going up ladders, or standing on scaffolding. They are not suitable for work, for example, on board ship or on railways, where the lives of other people depend upon their actions. For their own comfort, happiness and usefulness, if the fits occur at all frequently, the best plan is for them to live in colonies permanently. Epilepsy cannot be diagnosed in infants, and convulsions in babies are not the same as epilepsy.

Under the Pharmacy and Medicines Act, 1941, epilepsy is one of the conditions for which advertisement of remedies is prohibited.

9*

Chapter XXI

THE SENSES—TASTE, SMELL AND SIGHT

As living became progressively more competitive, animal forms survived better if they developed organs to help them to interpret what was happening around them, to perceive food and enemies by sight and sound and smell and touch. Smell remained perhaps the best developed sense until tree-living animals found sight equally useful, a line of development that has progressed in man. The chief ways in which the body collects impressions of its environment are by sight, hearing, smell, taste, touch and muscular sense. In the first four cases, the sense-organs connect directly with the brain, while impressions gained from touch and muscular sense-organs reach the brain mainly via the spinal cord.

Smell and taste are closely allied. The sensations of smell follow the alighting of minute particles of the matter smelt on olfactory nerve endings, a patch of yellow tissue high up at the back of the nose. In quiet breathing air is not brought into contact with this patch ; to smell anything purposefully, air is sniffed sharply. In man the olfactory patches are about a quarter of a square inch in area, whereas in a dog the area is nearer 10 square inches. A dog's world is thus much more one of smells than a man's (see Fig. 97).

Taste impressions are collected by nerve endings of taste on the tongue. The only tastes differentiated are salt, sweet, sour and bitter ; other tastes are combinations of these or are actually sensations of smell, not sensations of taste. Sweet things are tasted rather at the point of the tongue, bitter at the back. A heavy cold inhibits taste, in preventing smell.

The Eye

The *eye* is actually a mechanism for focusing impressions of light on the spread-out nerve endings of the optic nerve, called the retina. The spherical eyeball is protected against injury from chance blows by being well embedded in its bony socket. The fatty tissue that packs the socket is sometimes used up by illness and the patient is then hollow-eyed.

The front of the eye-ball is protected by upper and lower eyelids, which are lined continuously on their inside and over the eyeball by a transparent serous membrane, the *conjunctiva*. At the outer and upper corner of each eye is the tear gland, and if the eye is injured or the person is emotionally affected, tears wash across the eye surface and out through the tear-duct openings at the inner corners into the nose. Hence the value of blowing the nose to relieve the feeling of having something in the eye. The discharge of tears over the eye when some particle gets in, is an example of a reflex of happenings. Tears have a marked bactericidal effect.

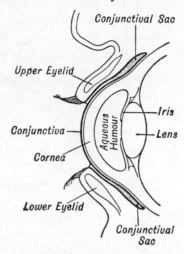

FIG. 112.—Diagram of a vertical section of the front of the eye, to show particularly the *conjunctival membrane* that passes over the front of the cornea and lines the eyelids. It is this membrane that is first irritated when any foreign body enters the eye.

Along the edge of the eyelids are the eyelashes, which help to protect the eye from foreign particles, and the openings of the *meibomian glands* that secrete fat along the eyelid to prevent friction and soreness from the constant touching of the upper and lower eye-lids in blinking, and also to retard the overflow of tears down the cheeks.

At the inner eyelid corner is the vestigial third eyelid. The outer *sclerotic coat* of the eyeball, that can be seen as the white of the eye, is exceedingly tough and strong, particularly at the back. To the outer surface of this are attached, towards the back, the three pairs of muscles that move the eye, their other ends being inserted into the bone of the eye socket. One antagonistic pair of muscles controls the turning of the eye to look inwards and outwards, one pair controls the upward and downward movement, while the third pair are set obliquely and help the work of the rest. All six contracting together steady the eye in movement.

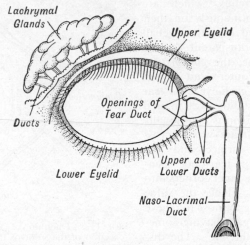

FIG. 113.—Lachrymal gland and tear duct of the right eye.

Anyone who has handled a camera has used an instrument made on the plan of the eye. The *lens* divides the eyeball into two chambers. In front of the eye, the sclerotic coat becomes transparent and rather more convex, and is called the *cornea*. The front chamber of the eye is filled with colourless watery liquid, the *aqueons humour*, which gives shape to the convex cornea, and, as it renews itself and seeps out, brings nourishment to the lens and iris and removes waste products.

In front of the lens is the *iris*, the pigment of which gives the eye its characteristic brown, blue or other colour. The iris is an involuntary sphincter muscle that reacts reflexly to light and regulates the amount of light that enters the eye. The black hole in its middle, black because it looks into the dark inner chamber, is the *pupil*. In the dark the iris retracts and the

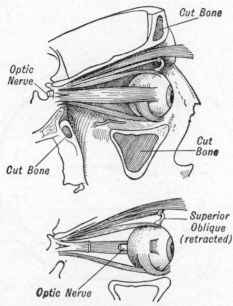

FIG. 114.—The three pairs of muscles that move the eye, being attached from the tough sclerotic coat of the eye to the eye socket. Unequal contraction of any pair of these muscles gives squint. Note the optic nerve (cut through) in each diagram. The supporting fatty tissues have been removed.

black of the pupil shows large, while in the light the iris shows more and the pupil is smaller.

If the light in a brightly lit room is put out for a couple of minutes, it is possible for neighbours to see in each other's eyes the difference in pupil size before and immediately after the dark period. In the same way, in using a camera, a large stop and a prolonged exposure is given to get in enough light to take a dim indoor scene, whereas a pin-head stop and a short exposure is necessary when taking a picture in the brilliant light of sunshine over the sea.

The iris does not react immediately to very wide light differences. On going into a cinema from daylight, people stumble at first, but after a few minutes the building seems comparatively light, the iris having adjusted itself to let more light into the eye.

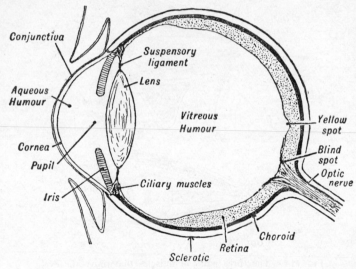

FIG. 115.—Horizontal section of the left eyeball.

Immediately behind the iris is slung the circular *lens*, held in place by the *suspensory ligament*, which joins the lens to the sclerotic coat. The inner chamber of the eye is held in its spherical shape by a colourless jelly-like substance called the *vitreous humour*. Inside the sclerotic coat is the *choroid coat*, which holds loosely the dull black pigment that, as in the inside of a box camera, prevents confusing reflection of light. The pigment is related to vitamin A. This pigment is used up in the light and renewed during darkness, and particularly in sleep. For this reason children should be trained to sleep in the dark. Inside the choroid coat lies the *retina*, the concavely expanded film of nerve endings of the optic nerve.

The lens bends the rays of light that come through it, so that they converge and focus on the sensitive retina forming a small image of the thing seen. A similar effect can be produced by moving an ordinary magnifying glass till the light is concentrated or focused into one clearly defined bright spot on, for example, a piece of paper.

When we look at anything over 20 feet away we do not need to alter the shape of the lens in order to focus. For anything

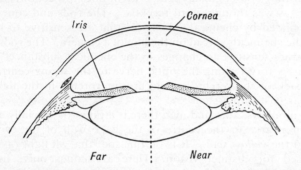

FIG. 116.—Diagram to show accommodation. The left side shows the form taken by the lens at rest and when looking at distant objects over 20 ft. from the eye ; the right side shows how the lens gets more curved to focus near objects. To look at distant objects, therefore, is comparatively restful because no effort to focus need be made.

nearer than 20 feet the *ciliary muscle* contracts, thus relaxing the suspensory ligament to make the lens just sufficiently more convex, so that rays of light focus on to the retina. This finely controlled power of alteration of the lens is called *accommodation*.

It is clearly less tiring to look at a distant than at a near view. Part of the value of an outdoor life and of playing games lies in the chance given for children's eyes to become strong by looking at distances natural to the eye. The German policy after the 1914–18 war of encouraging interest in sport was to some extent designed to combat the national tendency to short-sight, brought on by too much study and too little outdoor exercise.

The cornea and aqueous humor are responsible for about two-thirds of the bending of rays of light that enter the eye, but the importance of the lens lies in its being elastic and so able to alter its shape and thus focus the rays on the retina.

The retina, which looks like a milky opaque film, is made up of differentiated nerve endings called *rods and cones* from their respective shapes. The rods are for distinguishing black and white, that is, for seeing in the dark, and the cones for distinguishing colours in daylight. Light does not act directly on them, as was thought until recently. The rods and cones are surrounded by chemical substances that are sensitive to light, like the chemicals spread on the film of a camera. The rods and cones are sensitive to changes in the chemical substances, and impulses travel along the optic nerve to the seeing centres at the back of the cerebrum, and are interpreted in the light of similar past impressions.

In monkeys, apes and men there is a point of specially acute vision nearly in the centre of the back wall of the eyeball, called the *yellow spot*. It is on this spot that all light rays are focused for distinct vision. Here are cones only, tightly packed together, and a third of all the optic nerve fibres connect with this spot. If one thing, such as a flower petal is looked at steadily, one is conscious of the background and objects around the petal, but they are not clearly seen. A similar effect can be attained by focusing a camera on to an object in the foreground, when the background is less distinct, or in a cheaper fixed-focus camera, when the background is clearly defined, but nearer objects are blurred, or as we say, out of focus.

Animals that lack this yellow spot, of which the cow, horse, mouse and dog are examples, probably see all things comparatively blurred and without detail. On the other hand, an animal such as a rabbit has a finely developed brain area for detecting movement, which fortifies it against dangers that might prevent survival.

The human eye itself is quick to notice movement, though not so quick as a rabbit's. It is of interest to experiment,

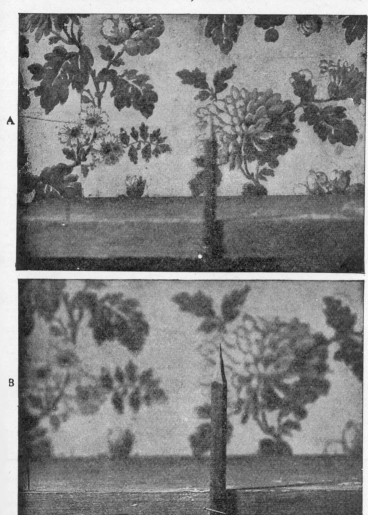

FIG. 117.—The effects of accommodation. A shows the eye focused on the wall-paper, B on the pencil. Sight defects often mean that objects seen are blurred, because the eye cannot be focused suitably. (*From Dell's " The Gateway of Knowledge "—Cambridge University Press.*)

while looking fixedly forward, to see how far back at the side of the head, first, the still fingers, and then the moving fingers of the hand can be detected. This ability is probably left over from that time when man or his evolutionary ancestors needed to be readily aware of moving creatures, both enemies and those that might be useful for food.

Where the optic nerve enters, the retina is insensitive to light

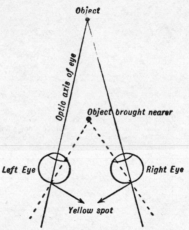

FIG. 118.—The turning of each eye inwards, so that the images seen by each eye are superimposed, is known as *Bifocal Vision*. It correlates with the arboreal habit of the Primates, and it allows of distance and thickness being estimated. Animals, such as cows and most birds, which have the eyes on either side of the head, lack bifocal vision. Marked defect shows as squint. (See Figs. 122 and 123.)

and the small area is called the *blind spot*. To demonstrate this make two dots, about three inches apart, on a piece of paper, close the left eye and look fixedly at the left dot with the right eye. Move the paper slowly nearer the eye from a distance of about a foot. The right dot will suddenly disappear because it has at that stage become focused on the blind spot.

Close left and look with
right eye here.

Actually, the image made on the retina is, as in a camera,

upside down and right side reversed to left, but the mind, in interpreting the information it receives, corrects these impressions for us. The retina retains impressions made on it for about an eighth of a second. Thus, falling rain-drops look like lines, and a rapidly flicked-by series of pictures give an effect of continuous movement, the factor that is made use of commercially in moving pictures.

In the more highly evolved animals the two eyes converge, so that they are both directed on to the same object. The nearer the object looked at, the more must be the *convergence* and the greater the degree of control and the work of the eye muscles. Children do not get complete control of this convergence until about seven years of age, which is an additional reason for their not doing fine work of any kind. Distance judging is done by the two eyes working together. Close one eye and *then* get someone to hold up a pencil a yard or more in front. Try to touch, accurately, the tip. The pencil is apt to be missed.

CHAPTER XXII

EYE DEFECTS—SPECIAL EDUCATION FOR THE BLIND

THE *teachers' responsibility in connection with defects of sight* is to understand and be able to recognise the main difficulties of vision that may be expected to occur in children. Thus they can protect the children from acquiring and increasing any defect, and early recommendations to go to a doctor for treatment can be made.

For distinct sight it is essential that the rays of light shall be so bent that they are focused on the yellow spot. In *long-sight*, because the lens or cornea or both are too flat, or more usually, because the eye is too short from back to front the rays of light are bent so that they would focus behind the yellow spot. Long-sighted people can see distant objects clearly but near objects less well. This is dealt with by wearing a convex glass, the shape of an ordinary magnifying glass, which bends the light rays inwards more sharply so that they are then focused on the yellow spot.

All children should be long-sighted at birth. By about 5 years of age, the eyeball should have lengthened from back to front to the normal eye proportions. If this lengthening continues, the child becomes short-sighted. Most myopia stops increasing when growth has stopped at 18 to 20 years of age. The long-sight of old age is due to loss of ciliary muscle elasticity.

In *short-sight*, because the lens or cornea is too convex, or more usually because the eyeball is too long from back to front, the rays of light are bent too sharply so that they are focused in front of the yellow spot. People with short-sight see near objects relatively distinctly, but distant objects are blurred. It is characteristic that they often tend to screw up

266

the eyes in an attempt to focus the rays to a point nearer to the yellow spot. The *cause of short-sight* is unknown, but the lack of inherited toughness of the eye tissues is a likely factor. There is however "practically no evidence" that tiring the eye muscles, as by reading, causes lengthening of the eye-ball and so increases myopia, as was once thought (*Health of the School Child*, 1946–47).

Short-sight is corrected by wearing a concave glass, which

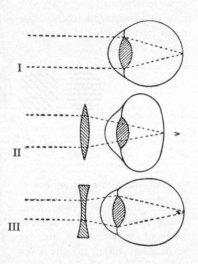

FIG. 119.— Diagram to show vertical sections of—
I. *Normal Eye*, in which the eye lens bends the entering band of light rays, so that they focus on to the yellow spot.
II. *Long-sighted Eye*, in which a convex lens has helped to make the light rays converge more sharply, so that they focus on the yellow spot. Without this extra lens, they would focus at the point shown outside the eye.
III. *Short-sighted Eye*, in which a concave lens bends the light rays outwards, so that the image is no longer formed in front of the yellow spot (as marked on the diagram) but on it.
Thus in long-sight the two lenses work in conjunction, while in short-sight they work in opposition.

bends the light rays outward, so that they ultimately focus farther back in the eye, on to the yellow spot. Short-sight is called *myopia*, and those showing the defect, myopes. It is a much more common defect in older children than is long-sight, and under adverse conditions and lack of treatment may tend to become progressively worse.

Astigmatism

Astigmatism is a condition of unequal curvature of the lens or cornea, and is inborn. It results in tiredness of the eyes when the pupil is doing only average work. In consequence the pupil suffers from headaches, rubs his eyes, frowns, holds his head on one side, and he may show all these signs if the astigmatism is severe. The condition can be corrected by glasses. Probably many people of normal sight have a slight degree of astigmatism.

Few people have equal sight in each eye. Cases of short- or of long-sight may also show degrees of astigmatism. If a person looks with one eye at a number of radial lines, the degree of astigmatism is roughly tested by the number of lines seen clearly, and not blurred. The eye defects of astigmatism may be compared to those defects that distort mirrors which make people who look in them appear too fat or too thin.

FIG. 120.—This shows the type of test used to discover *Astigmatism*. To the astigmatic eye the circles appear to be of unequal blackness.

New Views on Eye-tiredness

There has been a considerable shift of opinion in the matter of the effects of eye-strain. It is now held that "Seeing which takes place whenever the eyes are open can of itself do no permanent harm to the eyes" (*Health of the School Child*, 1946–47). Reading, for example, may, if the print is small or the lighting poor, tire the eyes rapidly and lead to loss of interest, but *not* to any permanent eye defect.

Analogously, prolonged running makes the leg muscles tired and painful, but no permanent ill-effects result.

If, however, teachers are to attain maximum results from their efforts, pupils must be able to see comfortably so that class room conditions need to be satisfactory from this point of view.

In the classroom *light* needs conserving in every possible way. It should fall from the left as the child writes, to avoid shadow being cast on what has been written. Light from the right makes a defined shadow, light wholly from behind throws a shadow over the whole work, while light from in front may well be too glaring.

Windows should run from 4 feet above the floor up to the ceiling, and shadows from mullions and blind cases should be minimised. Plants and other materials kept on window-sills should not be large enough to obscure the light. If obscured glass is necessary, fluted is preferable to ground, because it lets in more light. Sun-blinds, if they are necessary, should be of cream rather than of coloured material.

Dark colours, such as deep reds, browns and greens, absorb light, making lighting problems the more difficult. Thus walls and paint should be light in tone. White absorbs the least light, but is glaring and unrestful if unrelieved. Light grey or green walls are best, with, if necessary, the bottom 3 feet of the walls painted a darker colour. Light-stained wood desks are preferable to dark.

Reflections of any kind tire the eyes, so that desk tops should be wax-polished rather than varnished, and walls, paint, blackboard surfaces and the paper of books should be matt-surfaced and never shiny. A room wide in proportion to its depth tires the eyes, children sitting at the side having always to look at the board at an angle.

Desks must be adjusted to fit the children, so that good sitting postures for reading and writing are possible. Even with the best of desks children should be given frequent changes of position, as in change of work or relief drills, which, by making sitting less irksome, will enable better postures to be maintained.

Short-sighted people and children tend to hold their books close to the eyes, that is nearer than the conventional 10 inches. *No accommodation strain is thus caused* and such readers need not be prevented from doing this from the point of view of possible permanent eye damage.

Working continually with the eyes thus close to the book leads to poked head and round shoulders and for this reason needs to be prevented.

In addition, looking at objects with the eyes close up does keep the muscles of convergence in a continual state of tension and this may, in a short-sighted person, make him dislike reading and unwilling to try to read. The testing of such people for some degree of squint may be advisable.

Long-continued reading, as for six hours on end, is not found to damage the sight permanently in any way. In any case both children and adults have a defence against eye tiredness due to natural limited spans of attention.

Artificial Light

Artificial light is never as satisfactory as natural light, so fine work, such as sewing, is better done in daylight. Electric lighting is preferable to gas or lamps, because it does not flicker or heat the air markedly. Too much light, producing glare, can be harmful. Diffused indirect lighting, as by inverted bowls, is not so economical as direct lighting but it causes less eye tiredness.

Much can be done to improve light distribution by the judicious use of shades and arrangement of heights and placings of lamps, which need to be so spread that all desks get equal lighting. For this, central lights only in a room are insufficient. Desks just under them get glare, and those round the walls too little light. Light is measured by foot-candle-power, that is the light that a standard size and make of candle gives at a foot distance.

Building regulations specify 10 foot-candle-power for ordinary schools. *Fluorescent lighting* in schools is being tried. It gives higher intensity of light without increasing running cost—an intensity of possibly 30 foot-candles on the book. This is not too much when it is compared with good daylight which gives about 300 foot-candles (and with sunlight much more.)

A satisfactorily ventilated cool classroom braces up the eyes as it does the rest of the body, whereas a hot, stuffy atmosphere makes the eyes tire more readily.

In *writing*, the child at an early stage learns to make freehand symbols in sand with the finger; then to make letters, still freehand, with chalk or pastel, using wall blackboards. Script writing, because it compels the child to learn only one set of symbols for sounds instead of two, as in learning cursive writing, reduces nervous effort, and it is speedily done and is legible. From freehand work on the blackboard, the children would progress to using a soft black lead pencil and paper, but the writing should still be bold.

The only criterion for *size of writing* is that the child should be able easily to see what he writes and so he should, at all ages, use material giving sharp, clearly defined letters. Greyish lines such as those made with a steel pen or with thin chalk or crayon are to be avoided. " Feint " guiding lines in exercise books are not generally recommended because of the difficulty of their being seen clearly.

Books ought to be made to open flat to prevent a convex page, the reading of which tends to tire the eyes. The paper should be of sufficient thickness so that the print of the other side does not show through. In reading, the eyes skim along the top line of the type, recognising letters and word shapes from that.

Too long a line of type increases strain, $3\frac{1}{2}$ inches being about the best length. For clarity, the size and the spacing of the type matters. This book is set in 10 point. Type may be leaded. This slightly increases the space between the lines and makes for clarity and lessened strain. This book, in contrast, is " set-solid," but is quite readable for adults. Print should always be as black as possible, not grey.

School environment may be satisfactory for work using the eyes, and *home conditions* unsatisfactory. If the child's health and nutrition are poor, eye-tiredness occurs more readily.

Myopia—Short-sight

An inherited tendency to get short-sight with only slight strain may show itself in families, and children from such possible inheritance need particular care.

The *symptoms of short-sight*, besides a tendency to hold all work close to the eyes, include headache, inattention and dullness, insomnia, inflamed and watering lids, a tendency to rub the eyes, and the recurrence of styes. Often, but not always, short-sighted eyes are prominent, whereas long-sighted eyes may be rather deep set. Mistakes made in reading from the blackboard also suggest short-sight.

There are at least three types of myopia (short-sight) to be considered in children:

(i) Non-progressive myopia.

(ii) Myopia due to elongation of the eyeball which progresses steadily until growth is complete. This is inherited and is not produced by close work or by physical exercises. Children with this type of defect should be educated in the ordinary school unless their degree of myopia is too high.

(iii) Progressive myopia. Here detachment of the retina might occur, and education should be in a class for the partially sighted.

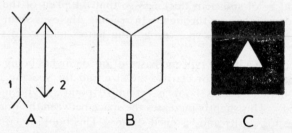

FIG. 121.—The process of seeing is not just physical. Interpretation by the mind is necessary. Everyone looking at Fig. 121 receives the same set of retinal images but in A is 1 or 2 longer; in B are you seeing the inside or cover of the book; in C do you see a white triangle on a black ground *or* a triangular hole in a black square?

Partially Sighted Children

Partially sighted children include myopes and non-myopes. All such children who can keep up with the work in an ordinary school should be educated there. They should have all possible help such as wearing glasses, being put to sit in the front and using a magnifying glass.

Partially sighted children who need special education should always be taught by methods involving sight and should not, as formerly, be educated with blind children.

The work of the special school for the partially sighted is to help the children to use the sight they have to the best advantage and not, as it once seemed, to prevent them from being educated, to save their sight.

Education of the Partially Sighted

Partially sighted children can be allowed to read any size of letters that they can see clearly and to hold books as close to their eyes as they like, provided they use both eyes. Eyestrain is not met with in one-eyed individuals. The size of the print will vary with the age of the child and the degree of short-sight, the younger the child and the greater the myopia the bigger and bolder should the lettering be if the child is to profit.

Normal sized writing should be taught to all children who can see it.

Art and handicraft materials difficult for the child to see should be avoided, not because of eye-strain but because the child should be able to do any work attempted to a high standard.

Exact measurement similarly may be impracticable for such children but, if they can do it, it is not harmful to the eyes.

These children can safely take part in normal Physical Training. Indeed, they need probably extra posture training to counteract and prevent stooping.

Children who cannot see to read 10 or 12 point print (this book is 10 point), can be enabled to do so by use of a lens. A magnifying power of $+3\cdot5$ is suitable for most children. Such a lens increases the number of books available to the partially sighted for reading and study.

Squint

An important and relatively lately acquired power in higher animals is that of *binocular vision* (Fig. 118). The two eyes are able to focus any object looked at, hence the two images seen, one on each retina, are superimposed, so that the brain receives the impression of one image only. This working of the eyes together allows distance and thickness to be judged accurately. From an evolutionary point of view, it correlates with a tree-living habitat, such as that of the Primates.

Binocular vision is made possible by the fine contraction of the three pairs of muscles which move the eyeball (Fig. 119), the control coming from the brain.

Squint is due to failure of the brain to control this fine muscle adjustment. The muscle that turns the eyeball inwards, towards the nose, may, for example, be stronger than that turning it outward, instead of their being controlled to pull equally and balance each other antagonistically. This produces a convergent squint with the eye turning inwards, a more common form than the divergent outward one.

Squint tends to occur first in children between two and five. If children concentrate too long on some close occupation, squint may be noticed. All children should be guarded from such prolonged strain, but particularly those showing any tendency to weak eye-muscle control and squint. It is school work that is most likely to produce such eye-strain.

Occasional temporary squint suggests the need for the removal of causes of strain, but if the squint persists, prompt medical advice is needed, because the squinting eye very quickly ceases to see clearly or at all. The brain, in fact, cuts out the confusing image it gets from the squinting eye. Unless treatment is begun without delay, the sight of the squinting eye will be permanently lost.

Squint may be produced by emotional disturbances in the child's environment, such as from the child feeling neglected after being pampered or because of disagreements among adults which the child senses without understanding.

Pronounced squint can be readily recognised, but it is well established that less marked deviations from complete binocular vision are relatively common and that they produce eye-tiredness and headaches.

Treatment of Squint

Treatment of squint consists of (i) correcting refractive errors by glasses; (ii) occluding the good eye so that the squinting eye has to work and is thus strengthened and (iii) training of binocular vision by exercises. The occluding of the good eye may be done by pasting a piece of black paper over the spectacle lens or by a special occluder.

A type of eye exercise used to re-train binocular vision is seen in Figs. 122 and 123. A stereoscope is used (Fig. 122), and when looking through this the eyes ought to be able to superimpose the two pictures in Fig. 123, seen respectively by the right eye and the left eye so that *one* picture is seen, in which there are three figures only, the seated figure in each appearing only once.

This " complete " picture can also, with practice, be " held " by the eyes, while the stereoscope frame is slowly moved to and away from the eyes. Sets of stereoscopic cards of graduated difficulty, for these exercises, can be obtained. Treatment for squint may also include the use of appropriate glasses.

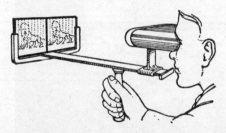

FIG. 122.—This shows one type of *Stereoscope*. Cards such as that shown in Fig. 115 B, in which the eyes see partly different pictures, are used to treat bifocal vision defects.

Orthoptic Clinics

This treatment is carried out in *Orthoptic Departments* organised by Eye Hospitals and by Local Authorities. Success depends on the intelligence and co-operation of the children and also of the parents. Treatment may need to be continued two to three times a week for at least a year in addition to the carrying out of home exercises.

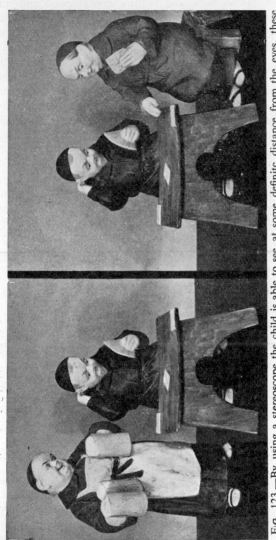

FIG. 123.—By using a stereoscope the child is able to see, at some definite distance from the eyes, these two pictures as one containing three figures, the two like figures being superimposed. With practice, this fusion picture can be retained while the steroscope frame holding it is moved slowly away from and towards the eyes. The set of cards, as above, are of graduated difficulty. Figures are used on the card as an incentive to interest. (*Photograph by S. H. Wilkes.*)

It is found that children below five are not able to co-operate fully and seldom obtain marked benefit. Children over seven have often acquired bad visual habits and give little response to training.

It is recommended that operation for squint should be deferred until after twelve, other methods of treatment having failed. Such an operation improves the child's appearance but the sight and control of the squinting eye is not restored.

Night Blindness is associated with shortage of vitamin A in the diet (see Chapter VIII).

Cataract is an opacity of the lens, and may be either congenital or acquired. An operation can be performed and if this is necessary in a child, the earlier the better, for then the retina will have normal stimuli during growth, and will develop fully. In some cases, the lens can be cleared by injection treatment.

External eye diseases are started by dust and dirt, by the after-effects of infectious diseases, particularly measles, by contagion from using common towels, by injury in play, and by venereal disease.

Stye

Stye is the inflammation of certain meibomian glands along the eyelid edge. Three factors possibly help to produce styes ; (i) the child may be run-down in general health, (ii) there may be eye-strain, or (iii) the eyes may have been rubbed with dirty hands, and so infected. Recurring styes, therefore, suggest the need for glasses, as well as a tonic and a holiday. Mercuric oxide—golden ointment, which can be bought from a chemist for a few pence is useful. Sold as a patent medicine, the same quantity costs about half a crown.

Blepharitis

Blepharitis, the condition known as " sore eyes," starts as redness and thickening of the eyelids, and may go on to ulceration and permanent loss of eyelashes. It is often associated with visual defect, and dust may be an exciting cause. It occurs much more among the children of manual workers than among those of clerks and shopkeepers. Poor nutrition and ignorant home care accentuates the difficulty of cure, which may take many months ; when cured it tends to recur. The condition may start as an after-effect of measles.

The eyelids are treated by bathing with an alkaline lotion, such as bicarbonate of soda and water, followed by the application of a mild antiseptic ointment. Defects of sight must be treated by glasses. On occasion, transference to an open-air school with the chances of cod-liver oil, milk, plenty of sunlight and a change of regime will be necessary.

Pink Eye

Conjunctivitis or Pink Eye is inflammation of the lining of the eyelids, and may be associated with blepharitis. This, unlike blepharitis, is extremely infectious, and can be conveyed on dirty hands or by using common towels or from badly tended swimming baths. The eye looks pink and is congested, and there is swelling of the eyelids and a discharge of tears and matter (pus), so that on waking in the morning the lids adhere. There is also a continual feeling of having something in the eye, caused by irritation of the nerve endings of the conjunctiva, and light causes discomfort.

Treatment is by Albucid drops applied hourly. The condition generally lasts about a week. Exclusion from school of even the mildest cases is essential. To bandage the eyes, although it may make the patient comfortable, is wrong, for the bandage keeps the pus and germs in, and encourages them to incubate under the lids.

Keratitis

Phlytenular Conjunctivitis—Keratitis—appears as small blisters or blebs on the edge of the cornea. It is difficult to get the child to open his eyes because of the acute pain. The blebs may ulcerate, and sight is then permanently damaged by the resulting opaque scars on the cornea that result. The disease occurs mainly at about five years of age. It is thought to be of tubercular origin and is connected with malnutrition and decay of teeth, for the cranial nerve that supplies the teeth sends twigs to the surface of the cornea and the blebs occur on the endings of these twigs. Dental treatment must accompany care of the actual eye condition. The general health should be built up by a generous diet and artificial or natural sunlight treatment as a tonic (see Chapter VI), and possibly attendance at an open-air school. Such measures also help to prevent relapse.

Ophthalmia of the New-Born

Purulent conjunctivitis, also called *Ophthalmia Neonatorum* or ophthalmia of the new-born, is an infection that most frequently occurs in babies' eyes which are infected during birth, a germ from the mother attacking the eyes. It is associated with the presence of the venereal disease, gonorrhœa, in the mother (see Chapter XXVIII). It can rapidly destroy sight, and is responsible for one-quarter to one-third of the blindness in English and American schools for the blind.

The use of sulphonamides has greatly decreased the incidence of blindness and of impaired vision following ophthalmia neonatorum. In the five years 1934–8, immediately before sulphonamides became the treatment of choice for gonococcal ophthalmia, of 20,726 cases of ophthalmia neonatorum notified in England and Wales, 157 resulted in impaired vision and 38 in blindness. In the five years 1939–43, during which treatment by sulphonamides became a matter of routine, out of 21,326 notified cases, 55 resulted in impaired vision and only 9 in blindness.

The Midwives Act (1900) greatly reduced the incidence of the disease by the ruling that all babies' eyes shall be washed out with a disinfectant, such as weak silver nitrate, immediately at birth, and that, on the least eye inflammation appearing, a doctor must be called in. For a midwife to have a case of the disease is now considered to be carelessness, and her name may be struck off the roll of registered midwives (as doctors or solicitors may be struck off their registers) for professional misconduct. Older children, particularly girls, may catch the disease from nursing babies who have it.

Sight Testing

Vision Tests for people who can read are chiefly made by Snellen's Sight Tests, a card of letters of varying sizes, each size being such as can be read at a set distance from the card in a good light by a normal eye. The child stands, back to the light, 20 feet or 6 metres from the card, on which a good light shines, and with one eye obscured by a card held in front of it tries to read the 20-foot line of letters. On failure, the child tries to read the 40-foot line of type (12 metres), and so on progressively. The results are recorded as a fraction, which may be expressed as $\dfrac{\text{where child stands}}{\text{what child sees}}$, and the eyes are noted as R.V. and L.V., that is, right and left vision.

Thus, if a child at 20 feet from the card reads the 20-foot line, his vision for that eye is $\frac{20}{20}$, or $\frac{6}{6}$ if using metres, that is, to that extent, normal. If he can see only the 40-foot letters, his vision for that particular eye is $\frac{20}{40}$, suggesting short-sight. If, on the other hand, he can when standing 20 feet from the card read the 10-foot line of type, the result is expressed as $\frac{20}{10}$, and suggests long-sight. If the child habitually wears glasses the test should be made with them on. The card should be put away between use or the children may learn the letters in order by heart.

Such letter tests cannot be used for children under six, who can be tested by Cohn's Type, capital E's in different positions, the child being required to state which way each points.

Charts showing trains or steamers going, by their smoke, to the left or right are used to test the eyesight of people who cannot read letters.

It is obvious that for enjoyment of life, for success in work and for attractiveness of personal appearance, sound eyes are extremely valuable.

Chemist-opticians who test eyes and supply glasses, cannot, by their limited training, understand the eye itself and its relation to the whole body as can a qualified medical eye specialist. Opticians are not allowed by law to use, in examining eyes, certain drugs to dilate the pupil or to paralyse temporarily the ciliary muscle as a qualified doctor does, so that examinations by opticians cannot be complete. Teachers should both bear this in mind for themselves and should urge upon children and parents the need for specialist's advice about eye defects.

In addition, glasses given by partially skilled practitioners may be only approximately correct, and if they are, for example, too strong the eyes may become used to having too much help and the sight be thus weakened or strained unnecessarily. Buying glasses by means of sight-testing cards at a cheap store is definitely harmful. Most people probably have some degree of astigmatism which may need correcting, as well as the short- or long-sight for which they may seek help.

These different defects, such as astigmatism plus long- or short-sight, need to be corrected when lenses are cut.

Children should be supervised so that they wear their glasses regularly ; bent frames should be adjusted, for the glasses are made to be

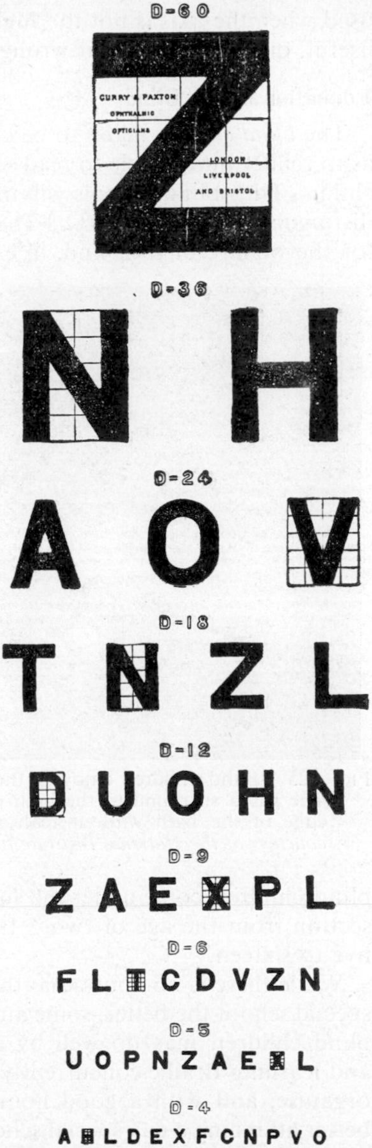

FIG. 124.—A Sight-testing Chart, a quarter of full size.

used when the axis is not too high or too low, and may be less useful, or even harmful, if wrongly worn.

Education of the Blind

The *blind child* is taken to be one whose sight is so defective as to render him unable to read school books used by a normal child. Thus blind schools will include some children who can distinguish light from dark. There exist now area committees for the welfare of the blind, in every part of the country, and

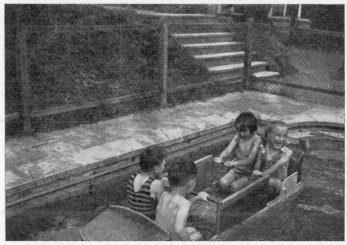

FIG. 125.—Blind children enjoying themselves in their swimming bath. The gated surround to the bath prevents them from getting to the edge of the bath without realising the need for extra care. (*By courtesy of the National Institute for the Blind.*)

blind children come under the surveillance of the child welfare section from the age of two. Education is compulsory from five to sixteen.

While there is no doubt that the earlier a deaf child attends a special school the better, some authorities advocate that certain blind children may do well by attending an ordinary school and learning Braille concurrently. Actually, this is difficult to organise, and with a good home, a blind child seems to be better attending a day special school, with transference possibly at eleven to a residential school for vocational training.

In the *Special School for the Blind* the children learn to read by the Braille system of feeling raised dots in an oblong, $\vcenter{\hbox{$\cdot\;\cdot$}}$, arranged in different positions and with different dots omitted for different letters. Braille writing is done with a blunt awl and a perforated ruler, and machines are used to write Braille and Braille shorthand. For arithmetic, special boards perforated with star-shaped holes which give eight positions representing numbers are used, and for geometry and geography raised diagrams and relief maps.

By means of the *optophone*, a blind person can read, with practice, the print of an ordinary book or newspaper. Light passes over the print and is translated into vibrations registered on a perforated disc rather like a gramophone record and heard by the blind person through earphones. By a still more recent French invention, light passing over the type of an ordinary book enables the blind person to feel raised shapes corresponding to the type over which the light passes.

Blind children need vigorous physical training, skipping, games, dancing and swimming. Besides promoting circulation and producing sturdy growth and good posture and a firm unhesitating walk, such activities give confidence in overcoming timidity and caution, natural to the untrained blind. Balancing exercises are of particular value.

Sprint races, the child holding a handle loosely attached along a taut wire to mark the course, and cricket, in which a broken wicket is marked by a bell ringing, show some possibilities. Such work gives emotional and social outlet. Blind children's playgrounds or halls need to have the outer boundary paved differently from the playing area, so that the feet, feeling concrete instead of board or gravel instead of grass, recognise the need for care.

Vocational training work includes for boys basket and mat making, chair caning, piano playing and tuning, and, for girls, knitting and typing. The possibilities, however, depend on the individual. Some exceptional blind boys and girls have done well at universities. In schools for the blind there should not be more than fifteen children to a class.

CHAPTER XXIII

HEARING—SPECIAL EDUCATION FOR THE DEAF

SOUND is produced by a series of vibrations of the air; it consists of waves moving outwards from some objects in motion, just as a stone thrown into a pond makes a widening circle of rhythmical ripples that become continually slower and less marked. The ear collects certain sounds and transmits an impression of them to the brain, and the mind interprets them —" that's the bell," or " paper being torn," or " the chink of cups."

The mechanism of the ear is set in a space deep in the bone of the skull, and is in three divisions, the outer, middle and inner ear chambers. Outside the quarter-inch diameter of the outer ear, which can be seen in a skeleton, is the cartilaginous pinna, which in man is of little use now.

The *outer ear* is a narrow bony passage bounded at its inner end by the resilient outer drum, which closes the passage completely. The walls of the passage excrete a bitter, poisonous wax, discouraging to insects that might happen to get into the ear.

The *middle ear* is a small unequal space in the temporal bone. From the middle of the inner side of the outer drum is attached the tiny hammer bone which connects with the anvil, and then the stirrup bones. The stirrup bone fits again over the *little oval window*, the name of the inner drum that communicates with the inner ear. Thus the middle ear is itself a closed chamber, except that it is connected with the throat by the *Eustachian tube*, that opens rather to the back of the posterior nares of the nose.

The Eustachian tube is lined with mucous membrane as is the mouth, and usually the walls of the tube are in apposition. If the nose is pinched and the cheeks blown out, air can be felt being forced into the middle ear by these tubes. By letting air into the middle ear, the air pressure on either side of the outer drum is kept equal. Adenoids cause deafness because they press on the Eustachian tube and partially prevent this entrance of air to the middle ear cavity.

The *inner ear* is an irregular space in the bone, and is filled with a colourless liquid into which nerve endings of the auditory nerve protrude. Sound vibrations shake the outer ear

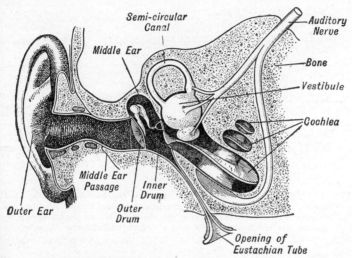

FIG. 126.—Semi-diagrammatic section of the right ear.

drum, which passes the vibrations along the three little bones to shake the inner drum. This moves the liquid in the inner ear just as tapping a glass containing water makes the water inside shiver. Nerve endings, moved in the movement of the liquid, transmit impulses.

The inner ear is in three divisions, the *vestibule* with the *cochlea* and the *semicircular canals* on either side. The *cochlea* is the part that distinguishes sounds. The inside is shaped like a coiled snail shell in a dwindling spiral. This spiral is divided into three compartments by partitions that are continuous throughout its length. On the partition emerge the end organs of the auditory nerve, with hair-like stiff protrusions on the upper face. They are, as it were, slung on an elastic membrane with a stiff shelf over-hanging them. When the inner drum is shaken by sound waves, the liquid within is moved and the nerve endings of the cochlea are bumped against the part of the shelf above them. This excites them to send impulses, translated as sound, by the auditory centre in the brain.

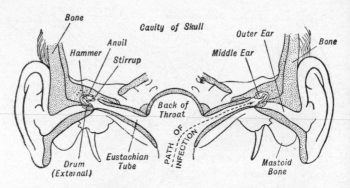

FIG. 127.—Diagram to show *the position of the Eustachian Tubes* that connect the two middle ear chambers to the throat or pharynx. Infection from a septic throat or the tonsils can travel up to the middle ear to cause abscess and a degree of deafness.

It is held that different nerve endings are probably sensitive to different sounds, for example, that different nerve endings would be stimulated by a high shrill note on a violin from those stimulated by a low growl. Both these sounds would shake the liquid in the cochlea, but only certain cells would be tuned to respond to the particular variety of vibration.

Man can hear only a certain range of sounds. Whistles designed by Galton can be bought, the note of which is pitched so high that while a dog can hear it his master cannot. Similarly, not everyone can hear a bat's squeak because of its high pitch. The sirens of some luxury liners are similarly pitched too low for passengers to hear them.

The vestibule and semicircular canals have to do with sense of position and movement of the body—body balance. The three *semicircular canals* are set in planes at right angles to each other. If the body spins round, the liquid in the canals is slightly left behind, and so nerve endings in it register the extent of this drag and the brain co-ordinates adjustments of the body position accordingly.

Giddiness after turning round is due to the fact that the liquid in the canals has caught up with the rotation of the

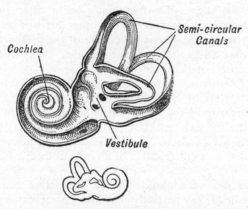

FIG. 128.—The interior of the left bony labyrinth or inner ear. The right bony labyrinth is shown in its natural size.

body, and when the body stops it goes on, and it is not until it has slowed down again that adequate power of balance returns. It is continued upset of the semi-circular canals that causes sea-sickness.

In the *vestibule* there are patches of nerve endings against which tiny grains of lime called *otoliths* press at any movement of the head, and thus show its position in relation to the vertical.

A *sense of position and balance*, therefore, depends on the working together of the end organs in the muscles, the cerebellum and the ear, the control being by habit and mainly

10*

unconscious, though, where necessary, conscious through the brain and mind.

Deafness

Deafness may be of the outer, middle or inner ear. That of the outer ear is usually due to concretions of wax which close up the passage to the drum. The careful syringing necessary to remove this should be done by a doctor or trained nurse, lest the outer drum be inadvertently damaged. For the same reason it is dangerous to poke hard instruments into children's ears to clean them. Deafness may occur after swimming, because water that has entered the outer ear has been unable completely to escape, possibly because of the presence of wax. Impetigo may affect the outer ear passage. Wax in the outer ear may cause cough.

Middle ear disease—otitis media—is the most likely form to affect children seriously, and so the most important to teachers. The cause is usually the spreading of septic infection from the throat to the Eustachian tubes. Such infection may be due to decayed teeth or enlarged septic tonsils, or to a septic throat condition left as an after-effect of an infectious disease, such as scarlet fever or measles.

The presence of adenoids or the congestion caused by a cold in the head may partially close the Eustachian tube at its lower end, so that air cannot enter to equalise pressure on either side of the outer drum, thus causing deafness. Earache in a child is a danger sign of middle ear infection, and should never be considered lightly.

In *otitis media* the mucous membrane lining the middle ear cavity becomes inflamed. If an abscess forms, the outer drum may be perforated and a purulent discharge be given off from the outer ear.

This condition of discharging ear—*otorrhœa*——should receive immediate treatment. If it becomes chronic (i) it may result in the breakdown of the bones of the middle ear and in permanent deafness. (ii) In the mastoid bone, which can be felt as a prominence behind the ear, a mucus-lined antrum, or space, in the bone communicates by a small opening with the middle ear cavity. Bacteria may spread into this antrum from the middle ear and cause a mastoid abscess ; this condition may require immediate operation. (iii) An abscess in the middle ear cavity may erode the temporal bone, causing meningitis (inflammation of the linings of the brain) or brain abscess.

Treatment of otorrhœa (discharging ear) aims at cure without operation, that is, by conservative methods. Cleansing and insufflation of the ear with iodised boracic powder is of value. For more stubborn cases *zinc ionisation* is useful. A zinc sulphate solution is introduced into the middle ear cavity via the perforated drum, and a weak electric current causes zinc ions to be liberated to penetrate the tissues and kill the bacteria. One such treatment often effects a cure but three to four may be necessary. This work is carried out in the school clinics.

It can be readily recognised that signs of ear defect are specially important. In contrast, eye defects may be partially remedied by glasses, but with deafness, cure or even ready alleviation of the defect is difficult.

Inner ear deafness is not common during school age. It may result as a rare after-effect of mumps, scarlet fever or other infectious diseases.

Prevention of Deafness

Prevention of deafness in school children largely depends on the early and careful treatment at home or at the clinic of throat and nose defects, such as adenoids, enlarged tonsils or septic throat conditions following infectious diseases. All measures that raise a child's resistance against the common cold or forms of chronic catarrh and which induce habits of mouth breathing, are useful ; the general inference is that the child must have good home conditions, food, sleep and care.

Statistics show that middle ear deafness has a definite connection with poor housing conditions. Children whose families live in one room are more likely to show middle ear deafness than those occupying two rooms, and these again than families with a whole house to themselves. Squalid conditions, in fact, go with poor health, which shows in one of many ways such as sore throat, which again leads to middle ear infection.

Deafness may also be associated with congenital syphilis, tuberculosis, concussion, and the effects of blows on the head.

Recourse to quack remedies for deafness, by delaying skilled treatment, lessens the chance of cure and absorbs money better spent otherwise. One patented deafness remedy consisted of the rubbing of an ointment, mainly vaseline and worth about one penny, on the *outside* of the ear, a form of treatment which the patentee must have known to be useless and, in essence, fraudulent. The selling price was ten shillings.

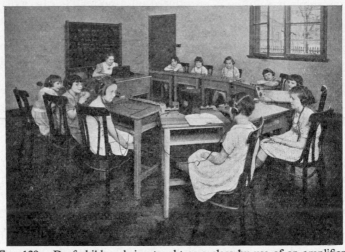

FIG. 129.—Deaf children being taught as a class by use of an amplifier and earphones. Note the children's interested natural expressions. (*By courtesy of the Royal Residential Schools for the Deaf.*)

Besides earache and discharging ears, other signs of ear defect are continual shaking of the head (particularly in infants too young to speak), lack of interest that seems superficially like dullness, misunderstanding of verbal directions, poor spelling and complaints of noises in the head.

Testing of Hearing—The Audiometer

The most accurate way of *testing the hearing level* is by the electric apparatus called the gramophone audiometer. The school nurse can test some forty children—each ear separately —in twenty minutes. Each child wears earphones connected with the audiometer on which a special record is played. The intensity of sound—numbers—decreases gradually to a whisper, then increases quickly to a maximum and again decreases. This variation occurs four times in each record, two series spoken by a man's, and two by a woman's voice. The numbers used are varied to prevent learning by heart. The children write down the numbers they hear. The test has the advantage of being standardised and of being impersonal. Cases of deafness which might be otherwise overlooked are likely, by this method, to be discovered.

How Deaf Children are Classified

It is recommended that deaf children should be classified not by their degree of defect but by the type of education by which they can profit.

Grade 1 includes the slightly deaf who, without *any* special arrangements, can profit by the work of an ordinary elementary, secondary or technical school.

Grade 2 children have naturally acquired speech but need some special facilities. Grade 2A can work in ordinary school classes if they sit in the front or use a hearing aid, or learn lip reading. Grade 2B need " special school " tuition.

Grade 3 children need to be taught by methods for the deaf who have never acquired natural speech. These include the totally deaf.

The basis of teaching for all the mentally normal deaf is by *lip-reading*, by which the deaf person understands spoken words, not by sounds, but by the shaping and movements of the lips and face muscles. Deaf people also can only hear their own speech imperfectly, if at all, and speech defects are common. To counteract this and learn speech, the child not only watches lip movements, but touches and tries to imitate the muscular movements of the teacher's mouth and neck, as he makes specific sounds.

Some Grade 2 children can be put into smaller classes— about twelve per class—in an ordinary school, with, if possible, a specially trained teacher who speaks slowly and clearly.

Lip-reading will help these children in school and in life. They can attend a number of the lessons of the ordinary school. Separate classes for ages seven to ten and eleven to fourteen are advisable, with further age divisions as far as can be arranged.

Children known to be deaf cannot start their special education too young. If they do not attend until seven, they have lost the most valuable years for speech training. They ought to start to be trained at two years of age, and the Education Act, 1944, provides for this.

Grade 3 includes children deaf from birth or who became deaf so soon after birth that they have never heard speech. The ideal for all such deaf children is to live at home and

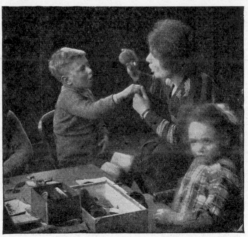

FIG. 130.—Teaching a deaf and dumb boy to talk by lip-reading. (*From the Special Services of Education in London (University of London Press, Ltd.), by permission of the Education Department of the London County Council.*)

attend a special school for the deaf, at any rate until the last year or so before they leave school, when a residential school may give a better chance of vocational training. Whether the child lives in a rural or urban district partly conditions this. Boarding out of children with approved foster parents may be arranged.

In schools for the deaf, children are graded partly by age and scholastic attainments and partly by their lip-reading ability. Besides lip-reading and speech, they learn the ordinary primary school subjects, but with no more than ten pupils to a class. Teachers of the deaf need infinite patience and resource, backed by special training in technique.

Few, if any, children are dumb from defects of the organs of speech. They are only dumb because they have never heard speech. Occasionally the larynx and vocal cords have been injured by ignorant quacks, who have attempted to treat the dumbness (by interfering with the larynx) instead of the real cause, the deafness.

Deaf children tend to be timid from continually misunderstanding directions and making mistakes. They do not call out naturally during play, and have often poor chest and lung development. They need to take part in regular and well-coached physical training and games, preferably with normal children, so that they get out of breath and are compelled to breathe deeply. Success in games also develops selfconfidence and bodily skill. Bubble blowing for younger deaf children makes for deep breathing and chest development.

After about thirteen years of age some half of the school time is given to vocational training for subsequent wage earning. Cabinet-making, tailoring, book-making, bakery, printing, photographic process work are possible for the boys ; cooking, baking, dressmaking, millinery, bookbinding, some librarian work and laundry work for girls. The deaf cannot take up work in agriculture or among traffic.

Deaf children who are normal mentally but who are also blind or physically defective, must be educated as far as their individual difficulty allows. The *mentally defective deaf* are the only class still taught by " deaf and dumb " alphabet system of hand signs. Hand signs are relatively easy for deaf people to use, but if mentally capable children are allowed to use them, they may well be less anxious to learn the more difficult but more useful lip-reading. By hand signs the deaf can only communicate with each other, whereas lip-reading allows them to mingle with relative ease with normal hearing people.

It should be noted that it is the legal duty of the local education authority to provide education for deaf children in their area. After-care committees and old scholars' associations in special schools follow up the deaf adolescent after he has left school. They supervise his working conditions, find him suitable work and encourage him to be a self-respecting and self-supporting citizen.

CHAPTER XXIV

SEX PHYSIOLOGY AND TEACHING

WHETHER or not the need to give sex instruction devolves on the teacher, every teacher should have some knowledge of the physiology of sex and of the child's sex development and interest in sex, and should have reached a considered view-point, unimpeded by prejudice and emotion, on the reasons for, and the stages of teaching in sex matters.

Up to now all organs considered have had to do with the balanced working of the individual, the muscles to make movement, the digestive organs to convert food for use. The work of the sex organs benefits not only the individual by internal secretions but also the race.

In the higher mammal development the male deposits sperm in the female sex organs, the ova that are ripe there fuse each with a spermatozoon, and each fusion, called a zygote, grows into a new individual, nourished inside the maternal uterus or womb until in due time it is expelled at birth.

The reproductive organs, in a woman, consist of a muscular pear-shaped bag about 3 inches by 2 by 1, the *uterus* or womb, which opens by a passage about 4 inches long, the *vagina*, into the external genital organs. At the upper wider end of the uterus there lead off on either side the two narrow Fallopian tubes, each of which opens near its ovary, of which there are two, right and left. The uterus lies between the rectum or gut at the back and the bladder in front, and is kept in place by tense elastic ligaments.

The *ovaries* are oval bodies about 1 inch long. At birth, each one contains some 32,000 ova, which lie quiescent until the onset of puberty and menstruation, the name given to the monthly period, at about eleven to fourteen years. Once menstruation has started, an ovum or single egg cell, just

295

visible possibly to the naked eye, ripens and is released once every month, alternately from each ovary, and passes impelled by the rhythmical waving of cilia down the Fallopian tube into the uterus and eventually, if it is not fertilised, out of the body through the vagina. This occurs between the periods of menstruation. This regular periodical ripening of ova continues until the woman is forty-five or fifty when menstruation ceases at the period of life known as the climacteric.

In the man spermatozoa are formed in the two *testes* that correspond to the ovaries in a woman. The testes are contained in the scrotum, a pouch which holds them at the back of the penis. A spermatozoon is relatively to an ovum very small, with a thin whip-like tail of protoplasm to help movement. The testicular fluid, containing some millions of spermatozoa, passes from the testes by a long narrow coiled tube to be stored, eventually leaving the body through the urethral tube of the penis. In the course of the sex act (coitus) the penis of the male, becoming engorged with blood and stiffened, is inserted in the female vagina, where an ejaculation of sperm is made. These millions of minute spermatozoa make their way by their lashing tails up the uterus until, it is supposed, in the Fallopian tube, one of them meets a descending ovum. The sperm and ovum fuse, and the ovum is no longer susceptible to other sperms encountered, which eventually die.

The fertilised ovum divides rapidly into two, four, eight, sixteen cells, in the meantime descending to the uterus. Here it fixes itself into the uterus wall—the placenta or after-birth—and thus, being able to get food from the mother's blood-stream, continues to grow for nine months, enclosed, as the fœtus develops, in water-holding membranes that guard against jars.

The elastic muscular walls of the uterus expand to the fœtus' increasing size, and eventually at birth contract to expel it, together with the umbilical cord and the placenta, which is attached to the uterine wall. The most usual position for the fœtus in the uterus is curled up upside down, so that the head is born first. After birth it is important for the mother's future health for the uterus and abdominal muscles to have sufficient time to contract fully, before the mother gets up again.

From the individual's view-point the ovaries and testes are important in that they give out internal secretions or hormones from their interstitial and other tissues. These secretions work with the ductless gland secretions to regulate sex characteristics and rhythms, such as the growth of hair at puberty and the breaking of the voice in boys and the development of breasts and of the menstrual period in girls ; the development of the characteristically male or female shapes of body probably depends partly on these hormones. A eunuch from whom the testes have been removed, keeps a high-pitched voice, tends to have female depositions of fat round the hips, and is indolent and less dynamic and manly of temperament than normal.

Sex Education

While most authorities on the upbringing of children—medical, parental, educational—do now agree that children should be instructed in sex matters (and not be left to find out by chance or inaccurately from precociously guessing juveniles), there is still a good deal of division of opinion as to when such instruction should be given, what should be taught and how, and who should be responsible for it.

The mean seems to be to tell the child as much as it asks, when it asks, taking care to be unemotional and easy of manner about it. While religious appeals for control of sex excesses may be useful in adult life, any mixing of what is mere scientific fact with the suggestion that the subject is specially sacred, or wonderful, or a matter of fear, is to be avoided. It is actually an imposing of adult standards on a child who has not reached that stage of thinking. While, too, the development of the fœtus is wonderful, it is not more so than is breathing and digestion in their degree, and no one would be tempted to sentimentalise such processes.

The earliest questions generally come at about five years of age, when children want to know where babies come from, and they should be told quite simply that the baby develops inside the mother's body. Stories about storks or gooseberry bushes or doctors' bags ultimately destroy confidence and should be avoided. The father's part will probably not be asked about till nine or ten, but when the child asks it should be told.

Undoubtedly the most appropriate source from which such information should come is the child's parents, and teachers should not give sex instruction without consulting the parents' wishes in the matter. Not all parents, however, feel competent to give such instruction. It is apt to be left, because of such uninstructed embarrassment, for the child to find out haphazard, thus inflicting considerable unnecessary worry and shock that may prejudice ease of feeling towards sex matters even into adult life.

Failing the parent, instruction by a doctor or an experienced teacher suggests itself. Solemn private talks, however, are rather to be avoided. Class instruction methods have been used with success. The Birmingham Education Authority employs peripatetic teachers of hygiene to give instruction in health and sex teaching to older girls who are about to leave school. By this age, of course, the actual facts of sex would certainly be known.

As to methods of approach in giving instruction, that through the teaching of botany and nature study, with the plants' reproduction with stamens and ovaries, or of teaching biology with the reproduction of amœba by division, but with no mention of reproduction when the frog is reached, is but begging the question. The hope apparently is that the child will guess, but such vague guesses only lead to worrying curiosity, which seems wrong.

Such a guess as to the method of human reproduction, if it is made, will have to be confirmed before satisfaction is felt, and it is likely to be confirmed by some half-knowing sniggering adolescent or adult, making the whole matter seem doubtful. This offering of half-knowledge seems but a cowardly evasion on the part of responsible adults, and is to be deprecated.

Similarly, children ought not to have to go to the Bible or to unexpurgated editions of Shakespeare and other classics to try to satisfy a natural curiosity. It is undesirable that such classics should be associated for life with the memory of an emotional difficulty.

A possible course is to put into the hands of the child or adolescent books giving sex information which can be read and afterwards possibly discussed individually. Many such books are now available. Some will be found listed in the bibliography. Such books are not supposed to form a basis for class instruction, because children of the same chronological age are at differing stages of development and interest in the matter. A parallel line of information can be given by keeping pets, mating them and superintending the births of litters.

Most school biology courses now include some human physiology and routine teaching about the sex organs.

However children are to get reproduction information they should get it easily and as unmixed with emotion as are the answers to most of the other questions they ask. Once they know, they need not worry about it, and it will probably not be thought about more than any other of the many new problems and facts in which children are interested. Interest in sex is only natural and right. It is not prurient, and it is only to sentimental sex-worried adults that it seems so—not to children.

The Adolescent Boy

Apart from the mechanism of reproduction, every adolescent boy and girl has a right to information about the changes that occur in themselves at puberty and to suggestions about health.

In the boy, at puberty, the spermatic fluid which has ripened in the testes is stored up and the first ejaculation of this milky fluid probably occurs involuntarily in sleep. This is normal and causes no physical disturbance, but if a boy has not been warned beforehand and perhaps reads quack advertisements which suggest vague terrifying illness, considerable unnecessary worry may be caused. Such emissions occur at intervals of from one to six weeks. If they occur oftener over a prolonged period, the need for a doctor's advice is indicated.

The Adolescent Girl

Menstruation, in the adolescent girl, is the result of the monthly engorging of the uterine walls with blood, accompanied by shedding of the mucous membrane of the wall. The discharge occurs usually in twenty-eight day cycles from the beginning of one period to the beginning of the next, but any cycle from twenty-four days to thirty-two is normal for health. Deviation in the particular individual's rhythm is what matters rather. The discharge usually continues for from four to five days, but again anything from three to seven days is normal. Many girls on first leaving home miss one or even several periods. This is due to change of environment as from a country to a town life, and gives no cause for alarm. The period eventually re-establishes itself.

Girls should be told about the incidence of the period *before* the first period happens. To know a month or so too soon does no harm, whereas the shock and disgust of such an unexpected and uncomprehended difficulty may well colour the girl's outlook for years. Menstruation should be represented to the girl, positively, as a promise of growing womanhood and of correctly balanced and normal development, such as every one would wish. It should not be depicted (as it has sometimes unfortunately been) as a purposeless monthly time of unpleasing disability to which women and girls are apparently subject, nor should such biased euphemisms as " being unwell," " having a pain," " sick time " be used to mention it.

The discharge is natural, a sign of good not of bad health, and in healthy girls should cause no disability or pain or alteration in a normally sensible way of health life. In the past a certain amount of disability felt at that time has almost certainly been due to suggestion, to the fact that girls and women had always been told that they would expect to be ill every month, and that they could legitimately claim special consideration for themselves at their period time. Psychological theory shows that to be ill is one way by which unimportant people try to make themselves appear to be important.

With the entrance of women into the labour market, combined with more accurate research into menstrual problems, it has been found that many women have no pain, that much menstrual pain is avoidable by better understanding of health habits, and that medical treatment can be had for real cases of disability. It is time to substitute scientific knowledge for old wives' tales here as elsewhere in health matters.

Most of the passing pain and sense of heaviness that occurs before and at the beginning of the period is due to the congestion of blood in the uterine walls, and once the flow is started, the pain goes. Occupations in which there is much sitting or standing (as opposed to walking), overtight clothing and constipation tend to increase pain. Body and trunk movements, such as in doing housework or playing reasonable games, would tend to increase the flow and relieve congestion, thus minimising pain, whereas the former common practice of resting during the period would make for continued congestion and pain.

Statistics show that women of the so-called working classes in whose lives physical work plays an important part, suffer from dysmenorrhœa (pain at the period) rarely, whereas the more sedentary middle-class woman has been fairly often subject to it. Games and fewer maids, however, have made it socially correct for the middle-class woman to be more physically active, and her menstrual health level has improved in consequence. A warm bath or hip bath also lessens congestion and minimises pain.

Constipation, by the pressure of the hard fæces in the rectum on the congested uterus, causes pain, and care not to be constipated at the period time, as at every other time, will do much to relieve discomfort and the need for self-pity. Regular, restful sleep in an airy room with the windows open wide is also of indirect value. For any recurring disabling pain at the period a doctor, preferably perhaps a woman, should be consulted.

One important aspect that should be specifically brought to the notice of adolescent girls is that there is no danger in washing during the period, and that a girl or woman obviously needs to wash more, not less, at such times if she is to be comfortable herself and inoffensive to her neighbours. All regular habits of washing and bathing can be continued without any danger and with advantage to the girl herself. It is also important to change towels frequently.

Many girls take part in games during the period, but others

refrain from doing so because of the difficulty of not being able to change frequently enough, with the resulting possibility of chafing the thighs. No games field for girls should be considered complete that lacks offices and the chance to discard used towels in sanitary bins there after changing. Also at no time should girls have to retain urine in the bladder over the long period of going to and from a games field and playing excitingly there.

No girl should be forced to take part in games during the period, and arrangements for staying out should be made easy and unobtrusive. Actually, a good many girls and women do play games with continued enjoyment and benefit. Some authorities would limit games playing to what might be called obvious " soft options." It seems rather that no games at any time should be played past fatigue point, but this limit should be judged by those responsible for the games and should not, as far as adolescent girls are concerned, be a matter for their personal decision. Games, then, can be played with unself-conscious vigour at all times while they are played. Actually, no one likes half-hearted play, which lacks emotional stimulus ; a well-contested game and a rest afterwards is always more satisfying, and once a woman is old enough to settle her own playing, she will have learnt by then her own limitations.

Chapter XXV

MENDELISM AND HEREDITY—EUGENICS

THE unit of living tissue is the single cell, and though there are larger and smaller cells and cells of widely differing function and shape, the cell can never grow beyond a certain economical size. Where growth or replacement of wounded tissue is needed, this must be effected by the continued division and re-division of cells.

Under a microscope, the cell is seen to be made up of colourless jelly-like protoplasm with a less opaque undifferentiated central part, the nucleus. When a cell is about to divide, two spindle points appear in the nucleus, and move to each side. From these points cobweb-like threads radiate out to the nucleus on either side. The nucleus, meanwhile, is in a twisting, writhing state, and a number of denser, stubby rods called *chromosomes* differentiate themselves and arrange themselves in a circle round the equator of the nucleus, the cobweb-like threads to the spindle points at each side connecting to the chromosomes. To arrive thus far ready for division takes about eight minutes.

Each chromosome now splits down its length, and the halves are pulled apart to either end of the nucleus. It takes from five to ten minutes for the chromosomes to separate completely at either end of the nucleus. Meanwhile, for perhaps a further six minutes, the whole cell bubbles and seethes, a waist appears in the cytoplasm and the nucleus divides and forms two cells. The process, called *mitosis*, takes about thirty minutes, and the re-conditioning of the new nuclei a further two to three hours.

The striking point about this division is the way in which the chromosomes are bisected longitudinally so that each cell gets a complete set of chromosomes. The number of chromosomes present in the cell of different species is the same for all

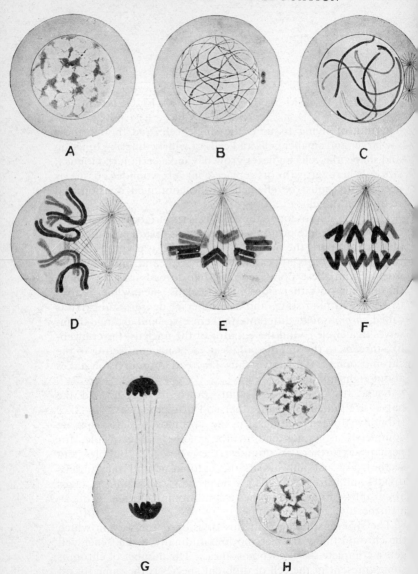

A   B   C

D   E   F

G   H

the individuals of one species. Thus the human nucleus has always twenty-four pairs of chromosomes, the mouse twenty pairs, the fruit fly Drosophila, on which much research concerning chromosome function has been done, four pairs (see Fig. 133).

Reduction Division

Chromosomes then, are present in homologous pairs and are constant and individual in shape and in character, some, for example, round, some rod-like or in the form of a j, some v-shaped. There exists only one exception to the constancy of chromosome numbers in each cell, and that is in the sex gametes, the ovum in the female and the spermatozoa in the male ; each contains a complete half set of chromosomes.

During the formation of either sperms or ova, in a process spoken of as the *reduction division*, the chromosomes arrange themselves in pairs round the equator of the nucleus, and instead of splitting longitudinally as in ordinary division, one whole chromosome of each pair is drawn to one side of the nucleus and the other to the other side. Cell division proceeds as usual ; two cells are produced, each with half the normal number of chromosomes, for example, twenty-four in man, four in drosophila (see Fig. 132). Each of the new cells thus formed is a potential sex gamete (Fig. 138), a sperm or ovum, according to the sex of the parent.

Hence, in the formation of any new individual, one chromosome of each like pair is contributed by the male parent and the other by the female parent, that is to say, in the fusion of the male and female gametes, each gamete will bring half the normal number of chromosomes to make up the full complement for the offspring. The chromosomes are of particular interest, because it is through them that inheritance of qualities of all kinds takes place. The units of inheritance of particular qualities are called *genes*.

FIG. 131.—Diagram of cell division. A, resting nucleus ; B, early nuclear activity ; C, formation of chromosomes ; D, arrangement of chromosomes on spindle ; E, chromosomes on equatorial plate ; F, separation of split chromosomes ; G, reformation of nuclei ; H, daughter nuclei completed. (*From Agar's " Cytology "—Macmillan & Co., Ltd.*)

Mendelism

The laws that govern inheritance of characteristics were first

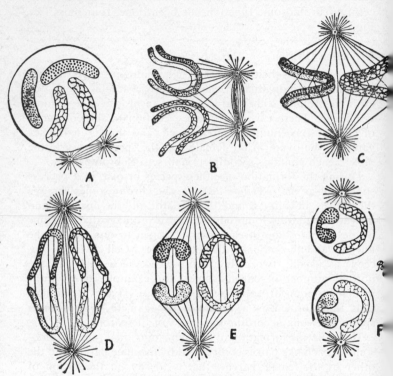

FIG. 132.—Diagram showing the reduction division of a nucleus with four chromosomes. A, showing two pairs (dotted and lined) of corresponding chromosomes and the early formation of the spindle ; B and C, showing corresponding chromosomes lying side by side ; D and E, separation of *whole* chromosomes to opposite poles ; F, formation of nuclei, each with half original number of chromosomes ; one of each pair of corresponding chromosomes has entered each nucleus. (*From Wenyon's " Protozoology "—Baillière, Tindall & Cox.*)

discovered by the Abbé Mendel, an Austrian monk, who experimented mainly with such easily controlled plants as peas over a period of years, publishing his results first in 1866.

Little notice was taken of them until, thirty-five years later, after his death, his results were re-discovered and have been made the basis of research and advance that are still going on.

As an example of the way in which these laws work, take the case of a pure-bred, splashed-white fowl mated with a pure black. All the offspring of the next generation are bluish-black, that is, hybrid and unlike either parent. If two of these bluish-black generation are again mated, the offspring contain different types, of whom 25 per cent. are splashed-white, and bred together never produce any but splashed-white fowls ; 25 per cent. are black and breed pure similarly, never showing any splashed-white or bluish-black offspring, while 50 per cent. are the bluish-black of the generation before (Fig. 134).

These bluish-black, bred together, always produce similar proportions, that is, 25 per cent. pure splashed-white, 50 per cent. bluish-black and 25 per cent. pure black, or in the proportion of $1:2:1$.[1]

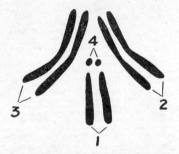

FIG. 133.—Drawing of the four pairs of chromosomes of *Drosophila*. (*After Morgan*.)

Similarly, if a pure red snapdragon flower is mated with a pure ivory, the resulting generation is all pink, but this generation mated together gives red, pink and ivory in the proportion of $1:2:1$, the pinks mated again always giving this proportion:

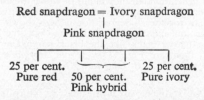

[1] It must be clearly understood that all these results are statistical, that is, the larger the number of cases considered the more clearly do the expected proportions appear and hold good.

Here a red mated with a pink in the third generation would give red and pink flowers only, and an ivory and pink, ivory and pink flowers only. It is of no importance whether any

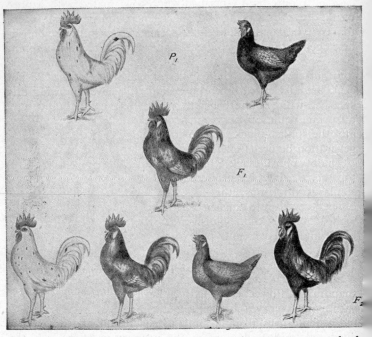

FIG. 134.—Diagram to illustrate *the results of crossing two pure-bred strains of fowls, splashed-white and black*. P_1 the parents. F_1 the first hybrid generation, all individuals of which are alike, of a bluish-black shade. F_2 the second hybrid generation, derived from mating F_1 individuals together. Segregation is here shown, there being on the average one-quarter splashed-white like the splashed-white parent, one-quarter black like the black parent, and one-half blue like the F_1 (compare Fig. 135). (*From Morgan's " The Physical Basis of Heredity "—J. B. Lippincott Co.*)

qualities, as of redness or whiteness in snapdragons, or of splashed whiteness or blackness in fowls, comes from the male or female gamete. The proportions and certainty of inheritance are the same.

Mendel, in experimenting with pure lines of peas, mated a pure tall strain with a pure dwarf strain of pea, and found that in the next generation all peas were tall.

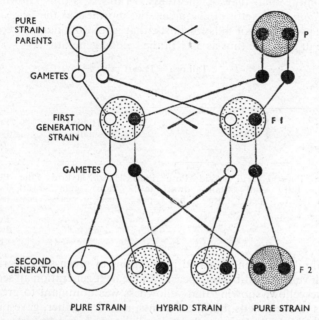

FIG. 135.—Diagram to show *how the Mendelian conception of hereditary units (factors, genes) explains the foregoing results* (Fig. 125). The organisms are represented as large circles, the genes as small circles within them. In the gametes, only the genes are represented. Unshaded represents splashed-white; black represents the gene for black, and close dotting visible black; sparse dotting represents visible blue. (*From Goodrich's " Living Organisms "— Clarendon Press.*)

Dominant and Recessive Characteristics

On mating this generation together he got three tall peas to one short pea. The short peas bred true together and never produced any tall peas; of the talls, one-third bred true together as talls, while the other two-thirds fertilised together, produced pure tall, hybrid tall as themselves, and pure short in the same ratio, that is 1 : 2 : 1.

This, it can be recognised, is the same ratio of inheritance as the red, pink and ivory snapdragon, and of the splashed-white, bluish-black and black fowls, but the quality of tallness comes out more than that of shortness. Tallness is thus known as the *dominant* factor or characteristic, shortness as the *recessive*. The proportion of talls to shorts, that is, of dominant to recessive in type, are thus as 3 : 1 in the second generation.

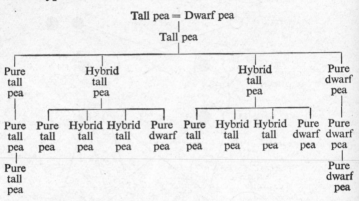

Similarly, Mendel mated pure strains of green seed-bearing with yellow seed-bearing peas. In the next generation all seeds were yellow, showing that yellowness was dominant to greenness in such seeds, but these plants, mated together, gave pure breeding yellow seeds, hybrid yellows and green seeds and pure breeding green seeds in the proportions of 1 : 2 : 1, the 50 per cent. hybrids all showing as yellow seeds in the second generation.

Thus in man, curly hair is dominant to straight, brown eyes to blue, the Hapsburg lip to the normal lip. Though many qualities in man have been recognised as dominant and as recessive, it is obvious that wideness of inheritance laws and taste against inbreeding, and the slowness of the passing of generations make certainty of inheritance and proportions of inheritance the less easy to foretell. It is possible that in man, as in other animals, a recessive gene may remain hidden, as it were, in the chromosome inheritance over a number of generations until mated with someone with a similar recessive gene, when the quality will show itself in some of the children. Mental defect is thought to be a recessive character of this nature (see Fig. 139).

In some pairs of characteristics the dominance of one over the other is not complete. Thus, if a pure white leghorn cock is mated with a brown leghorn hen, the next generation of hybrids are white with flecks of brown feathers. That is to say, the " recessive " brownness reveals itself in a few brown feathers.

In considering two pairs of factors, the proportions sometimes seem to differ, but this is only apparent. If, for example, a pure strain of smooth black guinea-pig is mated with a pure strain rough white guinea-pig, black being dominant to white and roughness to smoothness, in the first hybrid generation all offspring are rough blacks, that is, the two dominant factors have come out. If these rough blacks are mated together, out of every sixteen offspring, nine will be rough black, three smooth black, three rough white and one smooth white. Either character taken separately thus gives a proportion of three dominants to one recessive. (Fig. 136.)

These proportions hold for any similar two pairs of dominant and recessive characters so mated. Obviously, every living thing has many more than two pairs of characteristics ; every mental or physical aptitude or capacity or lack of it, the endocrine gland balance, appearance and colouring, tendency to prefer certain interests or work, to prefer and be able to digest or to be upset by certain specific foods, to contract or resist certain diseases, longevity, everything about the animal is settled to some extent by its heredity. As will be seen later, however, a poor environment may hinder partially or completely the development of inherited tendencies to their full.

The proverb about the difficulty of making a silk purse out of a sow's ear recognises the futility of teaching highly skilled work or activity to anyone lacking inborn aptitude and interest. Thus the average person can play tennis well enough to take part in a game, or understand mathematical processes sufficiently to regulate his business with foresight, but people with inborn aptitudes for either tennis or mathematics are worth

11

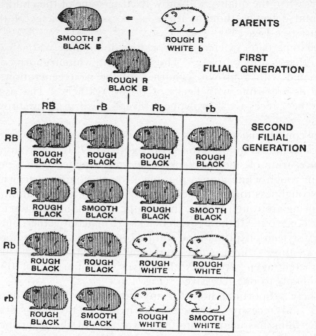

FIG. 136.—*Inheritance of Characteristics.* When a pure smooth black guinea-pig is mated with a pure rough white guinea-pig, the first filial generation are all black rough guinea-pigs, showing that these two qualities are the dominant ones of these four. The letters R and B are used in the diagram to represent roughness and blackness, and r and b absence of these qualities, which show as smoothness and whiteness. Thus each individual of the first filial generation has four possible qualities, RBrb, and there are four possible combinations, RB, rB, Rb and rb, and sixteen different mixtures, as it were, of individuals as to these qualities. Those having RBRB when bred with each other, can never show any white or smooth animals. Similarly, those showing rbrb can never show any roughs or blacks. In all other combinations of qualities, it can be seen that always any dominant characteristic comes out. Thus the proportions in the second filial generation of rough blacks, smooth blacks, rough whites and smooth whites would be 9 : 3 : 3 : 1. If three pairs of dominant and recessive characters are in question, as, for example, in guinea-pigs, black and white, rough and smooth and long and short hair, there will be sixty-four different combinations of characters possible in the second filial generation. This diagram is drawn after an exhibit at the German Hygiene Museum, Dresden.

additional and specially expert training. They set a standard for others in their particular field of ability.

Mathematical Laws of Chance

It must be emphasised that fertilisation is a random process, obeying the recognised *mathematical laws of chance*. This means that the larger the number of cases considered, the more nearly the predicted proportions hold. Thus, 5000 parental pure-line guinea-pigs bred together would give results more nearly of the predicted proportions than if only fifty were used (see Fig. 136).

A standard example of the law of chance is seen in the results of tossing two pennies. There is obviously twice as much likelihood of one penny turning up " heads " and the other " tails," as of getting both " tails " or both " heads." In 10,000 " tosses " the proportion of 1 : 2 : 1 is certain to show, but not in only 10 " tosses," where each " toss " has more relative power to upset the results.

Chromosomes are present within the nucleus in homologous pairs and are specific, that is, pair A, A' are different from pairs B, B' and C, C'. Each such pair of chromosomes carries a specific series of " twin " genes, that is, one " twin " on chromosome A and the other on chromosome A'. The genes occur in a definite linear order like beads on a necklace ; they are the fundamental units of inheritance. Examples of characters arising from such " twin " genes are black or white coat ; and rough or smooth coat in guinea-pig ; tallness or dwarfness in peas ; brown or blue eye colour in man.

That the *genes* are arranged linearly on each chromosome, has been discovered from phenomena which occur and can be seen only at the Reduction Division. At this stage, the homologous pairs of chromosomes lie side by side, and they may get twisted together, so that, when they are pulled apart in the actual division, they break, and part of each chromosome changes place with a similar part of its partner. Thus there is an exchange of a block of genes.

Genes themselves are too small to be seen microscopically but their relative positions and functions can be deduced.

This is done by breeding experiments, for which the quickly-breeding Fruit Fly, *Drosophila*, has been extensively used.

Certain characters, for example, are known to be linked in *Drosophila* ; that is, they are present together on a specific chromosome and they appear in the adult together. When, however, a character x appears in an adult with a character y, a combination which does not ordinarily occur, then it is deduced that a break has happened in the chromosomes concerned, to produce this (Fig. 137).

It can be readily seen that genes farther apart on any chromosome are more likely to get separated than are those nearer together, and the relative frequency of breaking between any series of genes is thus a measure of the relative position of the genes on the chromosome. By elaboration of these methods it has been possible to estimate the relative position of some hundreds of pairs of genes on the four like pairs of chromosomes of *Drosophila*, and from these to construct chromosome " maps," showing the relative position of the known genes on their chromosomes. From these and similar experiments, it is inferred that genes are arranged in a similar plan on the chromosomes of all plants and animals.

Sex Determination

Many theories have been put forward as to *the cause of sex*. This research in relation to inheritance has established the fact that sex is settled by the presence or absence of special sex chromosomes, of which the larger is termed the X, the smaller the Y chromosome, or the Y chromosome may be absent. The female gamete, the ovum, always has the large X chromosome in it. The male gametes, formed during the reduction division, are of two kinds, those having together with the twenty-three other chromosomes a large X chromosome, and those having with the twenty-three other chromosomes a small Y chromosome.

When a sperm with a large X chromosome fuses with a female gamete, the resulting zygote cell then has two X chromosomes in it, and such zygotes always develop into females. When, however, the sperm lacking the X chromosome fuses

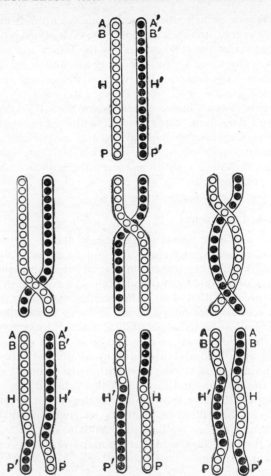

FIG. 137.—Diagram to show *how the two members of a chromosome-pair may exchange sections with one another*. When the two corresponding chromosomes pair up (top figure), they may twist round each other in various ways (middle row). They appear to break at the points of crossing and to join up again in new arrangements (lower row), but usually so that each chromosome contains one of each kind of gene. Such twisting of chromosomes takes place in the course of reduction division (see Fig. 132). (From *Wells, Huxley and Wells'* " *The Science of Life* "—*Cassell & Co., Ltd.*)

with a female gamete, there is only one X chromosome in the resulting zygote, and such a zygote always develops into a male. Thus the sex of the child is fixed by the father and not by the mother. (In some forms—birds, newts and some insects—the female is the bearer of the two kinds of gametes instead of the male.)

Roughly, twenty-one boy babies are born to every twenty girls, and it is thought that probably the sperms lacking the X chromosome are specially active and mobile and so effect fertilisation more often. Against this boys are rather less resistant to difficult conditions than girls, both in embryo and during upbringing.

Sex-Linked Characters

Beside the gene deciding sex, the X and Y chromosomes carry other genes, and these are said to be *sex linked*, and inheritance of them varies from that of other normally placed genes. Colour blindness is an inability to distinguish between red and green, both looking a dull neutral shade, and it appears to be a recessive sex-linked factor, showing more in boys than girls. Shull suggests a possibility that baldness is thus sex linked, being dominant in men and recessive in women.

There are obviously an enormous number of types of life, plant, animal, insect, fish, even within the limited experience of any one person, and the theory of evolution premises that all types of life have grown and developed out of other life. The species best fitted to profit by its environment tends to live, whereas the less well adapted tends to die out.

How then is it suggested that the many variations of animal and plant forms have come about ?

Variation

Variation may be due to the *action of environment* on growth. Beans of a pure stock, which are self-fertilising and therefore useful for such research, give, in every generation, a certain constant average size of seed. If one bean of this stock is grown in good conditions of soil, moisture, sun and air, and another in poor conditions, the former plants will be bigger and stronger than the latter and will probably produce bigger seeds. When these seeds are planted, however, the resultant plants give seeds of only the same average size as the original stock, and the seeds of the plant grown in poor conditions similarly produce plants giving seeds of a similar average in size, not smaller. The genes passing on the quality of size are, in this case, unaffected by the good or poor conditions in which the parent lived.

A man who loses a limb from an accident would have fully developed children, because he would pass on genes carrying the inheritance of an average body ; a man, however, born with a defective limb might pass the factor producing such a limb on to his children or through them to his grandchildren, and so on, producing a proportion of congenital deformity. Thus acquired characteristics due to environment are not inherited, because the genes carrying inheritance are unaffected.

There has been handed down from the last century a controversy between conflicting authorities as to whether acquired characteristics are inherited or not. Lamarck held that they were, but Mendelism and the work done on chromosome inheritance tends to prove that they are not. Research in the matter is still proceeding.

Mutations

Variations due to changes or jerks in the genes or to chromosome abnormality, that is, changes in chromosome inheritance, are called *mutations*, and the fresh types of life that result persist, if the change helps the animal or plant to survive, or at least does not hinder survival.

A Massachusetts farmer, for instance, in his flock of long-legged sheep had born a short-legged crooked-backed ram. As he was much troubled by the long-legged sheep escaping by jumping surrounding hedges, he discarded his long-legged rams and bred from this short-legged ram. By continually breeding from short-legged types he eventually got a whole flock of short-legged sheep that needed less tending to keep them suitably penned.

Such mutations of genes continue to affect the following generations. Not all such mutations are useful or successful. The first need of an animal is food. If a mutation made off-spring quicker and more adapted to reach its food, or better able to survive a shortage, such types would be the more likely to persist. It is, of course, impossible to follow out mutations that occur in wild life, but all plant and animal types that it has been possible to study carefully are found to be throwing mutations, *e.g.* drosophila, wheat, maize, peas, mice and shrimps. Much more frequent and violent mutations than usual resulted from flooding drosophila with X-rays of varying strengths ; too strong doses, however, produced sterility.

Hybrids

The word *variation* used in connection with the theory of heredity has acquired some vagueness of meaning. Variations of types of life can also occur from hybridisation, *e.g.* in the mating of the red and ivory snapdragons, and getting a pink flower. The essential thing is that changes so caused are not inherited ; they are not passed on to succeeding generations. Selected hybridisation of maize produced plants that grew taller and gave more corn, but continual self-fertilisation of these hybrids led to a progressive decrease of height and yield. Not all hybridisation, however, makes for a stronger stock even at the first cross, and in addition some hybrids are sterile.

An advantage of sexual rather than asexual reproduction is that it makes continual recombinations of genes possible, and by thus increasing the likelihood of variety of types it benefits the race.

Economic Values

The practical values of a knowledge of inheritance can be readily recognised in the improvement that has been made in domestic strains, both of plants and animals, when compared with wild strains. The cow is bred for giving large supplies of milk or for producing beef ; the sheep for heavy fleece of wool and for mutton ; horses for heavy dray work, for lighter hunting, and lightest of all, for racing. Such strains need protection. The lowland sheep with large body and heavy fleece could not, if unprotected, long survive the attack of

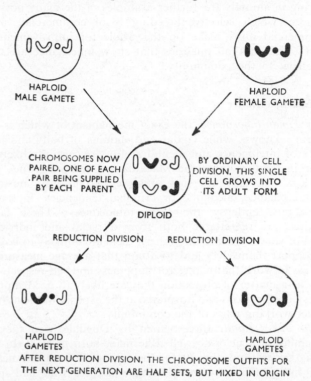

FIG. 138.—This diagram aims at showing how chromosomes from each parent are reassorted, so that new types are produced. It is, of course, only a generalised and hypothetical example, and does not represent any specific animal or plant. Actually there could be 16 different sets of the four chromosomes after the reduction division has taken place, but for convenience only two are shown.

flesh-eating animals. Their main natural protection lies in nimble flight, an ability now sacrificed to commercially useful bulk of body.

" Rust " is a fungus that affects wheat, spoiling the crop.

11*

By controlled fertilisation it has been possible to evolve a kind of wheat which, like poor yielding wild wheats, resists rust, but which also yields heavily. Egg-laying in hens, and fur-bearing in animals are further examples of the many possible ways in which selective breeding is of commercial value. Commercial aims make on the whole for improvement of stocks, but not all qualities that show inheritance are thus beneficial to the community.

Human Inheritance

In *human inheritance*, the exact mechanism of which is not yet fully known, while vigour and stamina of body and high grade of intelligence and mental ability are certainly likely to recur in families (note the Macaulays, Cecils, Darwins, and Huxleys), so also are such qualities as insanity, unstable mental balance, alcoholic or criminal tendencies, looseness of morals, epilepsy and feeble-mindedness. These latter qualities are regrettable both from a racial and individual point of view. People who inherit them are unlikely to be able to support themselves and to attain that average measure of success in work that makes for happiness and self-respect. If only as a matter of protection they are likely to need support (in asylums, prisons and hospitals) at the expense of the normal harder working parts of the community.

The Jukes family (investigated by Dugdale) were the five daughters of a ne'er-do-well fisherman, born in 1720. In five to six generations (by 1915), their progeny included nearly 2100 individuals, of whom 310 were paupers who had spent more than 2300 years in workhouses, at least 378 of the women were prostitutes, 181 were victims of alcoholism, and 118 were criminals, of whom 7 were murderers. They were estimated to have cost the State £500,000, and the expense still continues.

About 1770 *Martin Kallikak*, a young Quaker of respectable middle-class English ancestry, had a son by a feeble-minded girl, from whom descended 480 individuals, four-fifths of them feeble-minded, epileptic or criminal, and many of the women prostitutes. Later, he married a Quakeress of his own class and of similar stock, and through their eight normal children, they had 496 descendants, of whom, though a few were alcoholics, none were mentally defective and the majority were intelligent, useful citizens, who not only cost the community nothing, but made wealth for it. Several rose to be judges and citizens of similar eminence in other professions. It is of interest that the one feeble-minded illegitimate child pro-

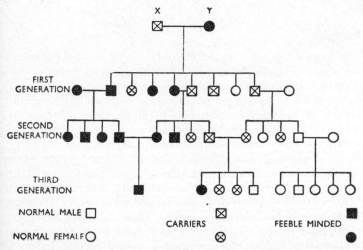

FIG. 139.—*The passing of feeble-mindedness as a Mendelian recessive.* An apparently normal man carrying genes of feeble-mindedness (X), marries a feeble-minded woman (Y). In the first generation, approximately half the children are defective and half are carriers. In the second generation, the marriage of two feeble-minded people gives only feeble-minded children. The mating of a normal with a carrier gives half normal and half carriers, but if a normal marries a normal, all the children are normal, as in the third generation.

duced almost as many traced descendants as the eight legitimate children.

Sir Francis Galton studied the family inheritance of men of genius and of the English aristocracy over a series of generations. He pointed out the ultimate ill-effects on any stock of arranged marriages with heiresses, who brought money and land but not physical and mental vigour. The subsequent generations, though rich materially, often lacked initiative and stamina and some died out. The women also were possibly heiresses because they came of families of low fertility, and this quality they would tend to pass on to their descendants. He urged that for partners of a projected marriage to bring to it a family record of physical fitness, intelligence and mental ability and achievement was of far greater ultimate value for success and happiness than the bringing of great wealth.

Eugenics

It was Galton who created the study of what is called *Eugenics*, the study of racial betterment through agencies under social control. It is of the first importance for a strong successful national life to have a people of robust body and high mental ability, of hardiness, initiative and courage, who will pass on these qualities to succeeding generations.

History gives many examples of the depletion or improvement of national quality by alterations of germ plasm. The Spanish colonies, in attracting Spaniards of adventurous spirit, initiative and courage to Central and South America, depleted Spain of their vigorous descendants, and that country has since been of lessened national vigour. These colonists, however, took few Spanish women with them, and by inter-marrying with native Indian races, formed a hybrid race of lessened vigour and ability. Generally speaking, the crossing of races nearly related in stock, as the English and Scandinavians, tends to make for a stronger and more efficient type, whereas crosses between widely differing stocks, such as between whites and negroes, results in a less virile progeny, weaker both mentally and physically.

The " Pilgrim Fathers," who emigrated with their families to America to escape religous tyranny, had in them the urge and vigorous purpose to risk unknown dangers and hardships for an ideal, and while the loss of their germ plasm was a serious one for England, these qualities were of particular value in the founding of a new nation. The American nation has adopted a limited quota system to check the introduction of germ plasm of negro and South European stocks. Such stock provides cheap labour but gives comparatively feckless, lawless citizens of limited intelligence, who need continual expensive State mothering, and this is not a source of ultimate national strength.

In the 1914–18 European War, the voluntary enlistment system in this country of the earlier years meant that the men of better physical types and more adventurous temperaments, particularly useful to a nation, tended to be killed first, thus depleting the national strength not only immediately but also through the loss of their descendants.

Artificial Selection

During the last century in civilised countries, artificial selection has more and more replaced natural selection as far as man is concerned. The rough method of preserving the mental and physical fitness of the race by the survival of the fittest is no longer in operation. Medical research with its discoveries about the value of sanitation, and the methods of preventing the spread of infection, has found how to stop epidemics and to supply immunity from infections ; it has also increased our knowledge about the proper care of babies, so that progressively more babies born survive to become adults.

A more humane view of the value of the individual has resulted in the regulation of working hours and conditions by the Factory Acts. Better housing, maternity welfare schemes, health insurance, and the school medical service are further examples of measures aimed at social amelioration, soon to be crowned by a national scheme of social insurance in full operation. The disability of the insane, formerly considered rather to be personally blameworthy, is more intelligently studied and treated, and the treatment of criminals is becoming more humane and understanding.

In the early part of the last century some 200 offences, such as petty theft, were capital offences punishable by death. This and the severe treatment of the insane must have removed and prevented from propagating much poor quality germ plasm of of the mental defective type, which is now given full scope.

Indeed, all factors, making for lessened stringency and danger in living, have meant that more weaklings have survived to have children themselves fecklessly and to pass on poor germ plasm. The quality of neurones of such defectives can be made the most of by education but cannot be improved beyond the limit set by their inheritance. To give a specific example, the average cost of education for a normal child in 1938 was £12 a year against that for a mentally deficient child of £78.

While the State cannot, in its own interests, do too much in health care and education during childhood for its children of good inheritance, the increase of mental defectives in relation to the whole population makes it seem more and more necessary that such socially inefficient people should be prevented from passing on their defect. Berry and Gordon suggest that the aim might well be to review the school population for possible defectives at eleven, before puberty, and to prevent propagation by segregation into self-supporting colonies, with the possibility of judicious sterilisation.

Biologists contend that politicians tend to act, as far as social legislation is concerned, as though acquired characteristics, fostered by costly education schemes for people of social inefficiency, were inherited. Actually, the germ plasm remains unaltered and the problem, under such handling, cannot but recur for expensive solving generation after generation.

Chapter XXVI

ALCOHOL IN RELATION TO SOCIAL PROBLEMS

In considering questions related to alcohol, almost everyone tends unthinkingly to approach the subject with an already formed prejudice in favour of or strongly against its use. It is important that teachers should try to preserve an outlook based on the scientific facts, and to distinguish between such proved facts and the opinions based on family or religious loyalty or personal likes or dislikes held by themselves and other people.

Alcohol is made by the fermentation of a carbohydrate such as sugar, and it is present in all alcoholic drinks. Beer is made from malt, which is barley in which the seed has germinated, wine from grapes, cider from apples, gin from rye or potatoes, and rum from molasses. In the process of fermentation, characteristic flavours are produced, but the effects of all these drinks is due to the alcohol in them.

Pure alcohol is a colourless liquid with a characteristic smell. Alcohol is much used in industry and for fuel as methylated spirits. Alcohol takes up water from the body when it is drunk, so that instead of quenching thirst it makes people more thirsty, which is advantageous for brewing interests.

Pure alcohol burns the mucous membrane and so cannot be drunk undiluted. Bottled beer contains only from 3 to 7 per cent., port 10 to 15 per cent., while spirits, such as brandy rum, whisky and gin, contain from 40 to 60 per cent. of pure alcohol. Thus light beers and wines containing from 3 to 5 per cent. of alcohol are preferable as drinks to diluted spirits, such as whisky.

The effects of alcohol, to be considered first, are those resulting from taking moderate amounts of alcohol on a normally healthy body. Habitual excessive drinking is a pathological symptom. Drunkenness is no longer fashionable as it was perhaps even fifty years ago, but is recognised to be the result of weakness and lack of control.

Alcohol and the Nervous System

The most obvious early effects of alcohol are seen in *the nervous system*. Alcohol is a narcotic poison of the same kind and acting in the same way as ether and chloroform, doses of which have a progressively deadening effect on the synaptic junctions.

The latest development of the brain has taken place in the cerebral cortex. Corresponding to growing elaboration of the brain can be traced the growing elaboration of mind, resulting in increase of intellect, will-power and powers of self-criticism and self-control. It is these higher mental powers that are first affected and dulled by alcohol. Thus, contrary to popular opinion, the action of alcohol on the brain and mind is to depress and not to stimulate it.

A moderate dose of alcohol thus makes the drinker less imaginatively aware of his surroundings and of what is expedient behaviour. He becomes more talkative, laughs more loudly and without due reason, airs his opinions more readily and is uncritically satisfied with his own work and actions. He may tend to reveal matters he would really wish to keep secret, to disregard caution, physical and social, to infringe rules and conventions usually respected, and he may become argumentative and readily quarrelsome. "Dutch courage" is a popular expression for the relative lack of imagination and increase of rashness that comes from taking a dose of alcohol, as before making a speech. Thus even the moderate drinker seems more noisy and talkative, and, in a loose sense, stimulated, but actually this is the result of the dulling of his powers of self-criticism.

As the effect of alcohol on the brain becomes progressively more marked, there is a dulling of the power of skilled movements, which become relatively clumsy and slow to react to a stimulus. A standard experimental method of testing this is that in which a man is directed to touch, with a pencil, dots as they come into sight on a revolving drum. After taking a moderate dose of alcohol, such as a wine glass of port or sherry, the touching of dots is less accurate but the man being less self-critical thinks that he has done better after the alcohol than before.

Thus alcohol, because it blunts self-criticism, may be used as a weak way of evading thought about personal worries, anxieties, deficiencies and home discomforts; the drinker seeks temporary relief in the narcotic effects of alcohol. The feeling of careless well-being that alcohol gives is termed *euphoria*.

Alcohol increases the length of reflex reaction time, for example, the time between the tapping of the knee and the reflex kick in the knee jerk reflex. This loss of *speed of reflex reaction* makes motor drivers who take even moderate amounts of alcohol less safe in emergencies. Not only do they perceive the danger more slowly and take action to avoid it later, but also their sense of well-being makes them feel more and not less confident and so more inclined to take risks.

Alcohol is detrimental to maximum *efficiency in muscular work*. In the South African War, on long forced marches, soldiers who drank much alcohol fell out first. Habitual moderate drinkers recuperate less rapidly from muscular fatigue than do teetotallers.

Heat Loss and Alcohol

Normally, if the air around is cold, the body automatically protects itself from undue *loss of heat* by withdrawal of the blood from the skin and extremities. Thus, compared with the organs and deep parts of the body the skin surface is cold ; but the deep temperature remains constant at $98 \cdot 4°$ F. Shivering is a reflex muscle-contraction method of generating heat and squeezing yet more blood to the deeper parts of the body, and also it may lead the individual to warm himself by running or walking.

A moderate dose of alcohol causes dilation of the arteries taking blood to the skin, which becomes flushed and inclined to perspire. The effect is essentially that of a hot bath. The skin feels a warm glow, but the body loses heat. To take a nip of alcohol " to keep out the cold " makes the body feel warm by this flushing of the skin, but actually more heat is lost and a rapid lowering of resistance to disease germs, with the likelihood of chill and pneumonia, results, unless the drinker keeps in a warm place.

Chronic alcoholism reduces the *body's power of resisting infections*. Slight doses appear to matter neither way, but alcohol does not strengthen resistance. Habitual drinking to excess is recognised to be a factor in lowering resistance to tuberculosis germs, directly by weakening the body and indirectly by wasting money that ought to be spent on necessities.

" The pregnant woman taking alcohol," says Dr. Truby King, " poisons the fœtus, damaging the brain nerves and other tissues." Contrary to popular belief, alcohol is not good for *nursing mothers*. It passes into the mother's milk, and so it stunts and retards the growth of the baby's body and mind, children being even more susceptible to its effects than are adults.

Alcohol can be burnt in the body as sugar can, so that technically in the body it can be classed as a food. Unlike sugar, fat and other foods it cannot, however, be stored. It has much less food value than tea with its milk and sugar. There is no proved foundation for its popular reputation as a body builder or blood former, nor does it increase the body's power to work, though it does blunt the worker's perception of his own poor work.

As a medicine, alcohol has its value and uses, but the recognition that it is a narcotic and not a stimulant has made it very much less used than formerly. In the last thirty years there has been, in hospitals all over the world, a marked decrease in expenditure per head on alcohol and a corresponding increase in the milk bills. Alcohol is not recommended as a stimulant in the official First Aid manuals.

Expectation of Life

While some differences of opinion still exist about the exact effects of varying doses of alcohol, there is no doubt that abstainers have a definitely greater *expectation of life* than non-abstainers. For example, at 20 the general expectation of life for men is 43 years, whereas for Rechabites, a Friendly Society in which the members are abstainers, the expectation of life for men at 20 is $48 \cdot 8$ years. So definite is this that Life Assurance societies can afford to give abstainers cheaper terms for assurance than are given to non-abstainers. On the other hand, many Life Assurance offices charge specially heavy terms to public-house keepers and their servants, because their expectation of life is definitely shorter than the normal average for other workers.

In the period 1910–12, while the deaths from alcoholism for all males was 7 per 1000 and for clergymen of all denominations only 2 per 1000, the death-rate for inn-keepers was 50 per 1000.

The problem whether to drink moderately or not at all is one for each individual to decide for himself, but the effect of moderate drinking is not probably any more harmful than moderate smoking and probably less harmful than habitual over-eating. There is no doubt that immoderate drinking is harmful, and it is because moderate can so insidiously become immoderate drinking that the social problems raised by alcohol have continually to be considered.

People working in the making and selling of alcohol, brewers, distillers, and licensees and their employees, are spoken of collectively as " the Trade," and it is naturally " the Trade's " first concern to sell as much alcohol as possible and to make as large a profit as possible for its shareholders. A " tied house " is a public-house which belongs (unlike a " free house ") to a brewery, the manager of which is paid in proportion to the amount of that particular brewery's wares sold. It is thus to the interest of the manager to encourage drinking as far as he can while keeping on the right side of the inspecting police, particularly as if the house sales fall he may lose his work.

A movement for *improved public-houses* seeks to make licensed premises not just places where a man stands and drinks, but places where a man could take his wife and family, get food and play games, hear music and not feel compelled to keep on ordering drinks so that he may be allowed to remain. The 1932 Report of the Commission on Licensing deprecates what it calls " vertical drinking " at a bar, and it advocates improvement of hotel premises and the paying of the manager in proportion to the catering rather than the drink trade he does, possibly by a proportional rebate in the cost of the licence.

Education for Leisure

While, however, regulation of the consumption of alcohol is essential, the better way still is to reduce the need for and interest in drinking, by education, by the provision of counter-attractions and by improving social conditions. Picture houses, though often abused as expensive and lacking in taste, have given people somewhere to sit for an evening, warm, dry and comfortable, at a set price, when perhaps formerly these people would have been in a public-house having to buy a series of drinks to keep their right to be there. The National Playing Fields Association movement and the Keep Fit and Youth movements increasingly offer health-giving counter-attractions to the invitation of the public-house.

Housing reform is an indirect way of tackling excessive drinking. In slums in Manchester, for example, in one room were living a man, his wife, sons aged 18 and 9, and daughters 16 and 12, six people in all, while in two rooms were living a man and wife, sons aged 20, 17, 14, and 12, a married son and his wife and two babies. It is little wonder if, with such living conditions, people do retreat to the cosy friendliness of the public-house and spend too great a proportion of wages there.

Education should include training in the use of leisure and direct teaching on alcohol consumption. Ideally adequate education and environment should give everybody a number of interests and hobbies that they want to work on in their spare time, and if people are thus occupied they will not have to manufacture amusements and try to gain a feeling of being smart by continually drinking.

The work of the Boy Scout and Girl Guide Associations, among other things, does much to help adolescents to find for themselves useful and satisfying interests.

Teaching about Alcohol

Teaching about alcohol should be given to all adolescents and should stress rather the positive values of temperance, the health and happiness and additional chances of fulfilling ambitions and of being a useful citizen, than the negative lurid side in which the teacher tries, consciously or unconsciously, to frighten the child by descriptions of revolting illnesses that result from drunkenness and the morbid horrors of a drunkard's home. Such negative teaching also tends, if the children go home and repeat what they have learnt to a temperate drinker, to earn scorn and derision for the teaching and to make difficulty for the child who does not know which apparent authority to follow.

It is preferable, on the whole, for the class teacher, rather than an outside lecturer, to give teaching on temperance and alcohol. The teaching is thus a regular part of the health teaching scheme, and, moreover, the class teacher should know his or her own children and how best to appeal to them. Visiting lecturers, too, have been found to be over-lurid and frightening to the children, being sometimes more full of enthusiasm for their cause than skilled in appealing sensibly to a child audience.

CHAPTER XXVII

INFECTIOUS DISEASES—GENERAL
CONSIDERATIONS AND SOME SPECIAL INFECTIONS

THE teacher's concern with infectious diseases is (i) with the incubation period up to the time that characteristic symptoms show themselves, and (ii) with the after-effects, when the child returns to school convalescent. An intelligent teacher can learn to suspect signs and recommend a child for examination, thus minimising discomfort for the child and the likelihood of spread of the disease.

The body may become ill because of some failure of metabolism, as in anæmia or cretinism, or because of lack of vitamin content in the diet, causing deficiency diseases such as rickets or scurvy. A further extensive source of disturbance is from the entry of living parasitic organisms into the body host, where they multiply, live out their life-history, making poison in the body and eventually even killing the host. Disease germs are parasites in this sense.

The largest of such human parasites are the tape and round worms, which get an entry from inadequately washed salad, impure water, uncooked pork, or from children playing with and being licked by infected dogs. They live in the intestine on the host's partially digested food, causing debility and even the formation of abscess in the intestinal wall. Other examples of human parasites are the vegetable fungoid that causes ringworm and the mite that causes itch or scabies.

In the group of diseases loosely termed germ diseases, the invading organisms are microscopic or ultra-microscopic, and commonly termed germs or microbes, but more correctly bacteria or, if ultra-microscopic organisms, viruses (see Chapter I).

Some germ-caused diseases such as rheumatism are of low if of any infective power. In others, spoken of widely as

332

infectious, the germs given out from one person readily cause a similar series of symptoms in other people absorbing doses of the germs in any way. Of infectious diseases, some are local in effects, such as " pink eye " or impetigo, while others produce local symptoms together with a general incapacity, and it is to this latter class that the expression " infectious disease " is usually applied.

Infectious Diseases

Each of such general infectious diseases is caused by a specific micro-organism, without which the disease cannot arise and which always breeds true, that is, the measles virus always gives measles, the diphtheria bacillus, diphtheria, just as on a

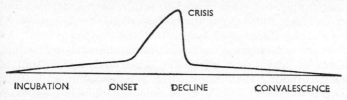

FIG. 140.—Diagram to show the average course of an infectious disease.

larger scale an acorn is always potentially an oak and not an elm.

Thus all general infectious diseases have a fairly constant pattern of development, starting with the incubation period before the symptoms show themselves, followed by the onset when the rash appears, the temperature rises and there is malaise. These symptoms increase in severity to the crisis, after which the patient either dies or, overcoming the germs, passes through the period of decline of symptoms to the longer one of convalescence.

What happens is that once the germs are strongly established, the patient's body becomes a battle-ground. The germs multiply and in doing so give off their particular toxin or poison. During the incubation period the toxin is gradually collecting and the patient seems normal, though towards the end of the incubation period he is likely to be increasingly infectious to people around him. When a sufficient charge of the *toxin* has been manufactured—about a fortnight in measles, three weeks in mumps—definite symptoms show. (Toxin is a general name for bacteria-produced poisons in contrast to chemical poisons such as arsenic and the cyanides.) The patient feels ill, has a higher temperature than normal, a headache, a tendency to shiver or vomit, a sore throat and possibly a characteristic skin rash. The fight inside the body of the germs and toxins against the white corpuscles is fierce, and the body supplies more and more white corpuscles to eat up foreign germs and to manufacture a specific antidote to the symptom-producing toxin, which is called antitoxin.

The patient is isolated because he might give the disease to other people, but often he goes to bed to keep warm and conserve energy, thus helping the body in its fight. The poisoned body cannot digest much heavy food and thus needs less. All effort is concentrated on overcoming the invading germs. Stores of fatty tissue are broken down and used instead of digested food. Thus people while ill become thinner. If the toxin is too strong and the body cannot manufacture antitoxin quickly enough, the patient succumbs. Usually, however, the body, helped by careful nursing, under a doctor's advice, manages to overcome the germs, and the building up stage of convalescence begins.

Defences against Micro-organisms

The body may be said to have three lines of defence against invading micro-organisms :—

    (i) the prevention of successful entry ;
    (ii) the destruction of organisms that have effected entry ;
    (iii) the development of specific immunities.

(i) The *prevention of entry of micro-organisms* can be helped by cleanliness of the skin and by the establishing of a good general resistance. This resistance depends on inborn robustness of health backed up by food, fresh air and sunlight, warmth, exercise and rest, in fact a healthy way of life.

(ii) The *destruction of invading micro-organisms* is effected by the white blood corpuscles and by such defences as the

·2 per cent. hydrochloric acid in the gastric juice of the stomach and the germicidal effect of tears in flowing across the eyeball.

Antiseptic chemicals such as carbolic, have long been known to kill micro-organisms outside the body, but they are harmful to the body tissues. In 1938 Dr. Ewing at Dagenham, at his 693rd experiment, synthesised sulphapyridine, which was found to be highly active against pneumonia. This led on to the

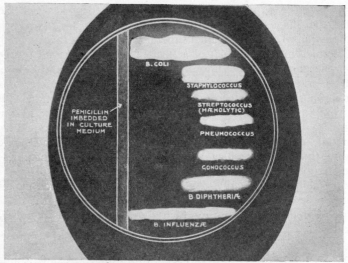

FIG. 141.—This plate shows the differing effects of the trough of *Penicillin* on the different micro-organisms all of which started their growth in a line on the opposite side of the nutrient agar in this petri dish. Which micro-organisms has the Penicillin destroyed? (*From Lacken's " The Story of Penicillin "—Pilot Press.*)

discovery of the Sulphonamide group of drugs. On a separate line of research, Sir Alexander Fleming, at St. Mary's Hospital, London, discovered Penicillin, first used for patients about 1940.

The Sulphonamides and Penicillin

Both the *Sulphonamides* and *Penicillin* kill bacteria, when active and growing (but not when in a resting condition, *e.g.* at a low temperature). They are bacteriocidal not bacteriostatic as was first thought. The Sulphonamides act, on the whole, more slowly than does Penicillin and are more likely themselves to have limited toxic effects on the body than is Penicillin.

The Sulphonamide Group of drugs can be taken by the mouth or by injection. They have been used with success in a number of infective conditions including blood poisoning, middle ear and mastoid disease, septic scarlet fever, pneumonia, meningitis, gonorrhœa, as well as in cases of impetigo, boils, puerperal sepsis. For wounds and burns a powder form is used. So far they have been of little value against most virus-caused diseases. Their use against tuberculosis is being investigated.

Penicillin is a product of a Penicillin mould, related to one of the common green moulds that grow on jam and cheese. It is practically non-toxic to the body cells. One part in a million kills staphylococci which cause wound infections. It promotes healing in burns and ensures the success of skin grafts. It has been successfully used for meningitis, tonsillitis, middle ear disease, scarlet fever, puerperal sepsis and septic sore throat, gonorrhœa and syphilis and against infections such as boils, styes, pimples and abscesses.

Penicillin has usually to be given by injection, which makes its use less easy than if it could be given by the mouth.

Streptomycin is being increasingly used for forms of tuberculosis.

Aureomycin inhibits the growth of a wide range of bacteria, is of low toxicity, and does not seem to produce resistant strains as does Penicillin. It can be taken by the mouth.

Immunity

(iii) *The development of specific immunities.* We are all, for different reasons, probably immune to particular infectious diseases ; that is, however much we come in contact with the causative organisms we do not catch the illness. Such immunity may be acquired in different ways.

(*a*) *Congenital immunity.* Some animals and people are born immune to certain diseases : for example, sheep, which live out of doors, do not get tuberculosis, whereas cattle, which live partly in cow-sheds, do. The Welsh black cattle, which are milked out of doors, do not get tuberculosis.

(b) *Acquired immunity.* An attack of a disease confers a certain measure of immunity to that particular infection, either for a limited period or for life ; for example, having had scarlet fever, a second attack is unlikely because the anti-toxin of scarlet fever remains as a protection in the blood plasma. The strength of immunity varies for different infections ; that for scarlet fever is relatively high, whereas that for the common cold or influenza is low, repeated infections being common. Sucklings get their mother's specific immunities from her milk, a benefit that bottle feeding cannot confer. This immunity lasts for about the first six months of life.

(c) *Artificial Passive Immunity.* Such immunity is acquired by the injection of ready prepared anti-toxin in place of waiting for the patient to make his own. For instance, at the onset of scarlet fever, the patient may be given scarlet fever anti-toxin which shortens the course of the disease. By the same method close contacts may be protected against developing the infection. The immunity, however, where the patient has not made the anti-toxin for himself, passes off in a matter of weeks.

(d) *Artificial Active Immunity.* Immunity can also be induced. An example is the immunisation to diphtheria which is recommended for all children. The child is given, at spaced intervals, some three injections of mixed toxoid-anti-toxin of diphtheria ; the blood serum, thus stimulated, builds up anti-toxin which will prevent the child from catching diphtheria when the infection is encountered. This immunity is lasting. Vaccination is an analogous way of developing an active immunity against smallpox.

How Infections are Conveyed

Infections are conveyed (i) by breathed-out droplets of moisture in, for example, influenza, colds and measles ; (ii) by infected dust, because bacteria can float on dust particles ; (iii) by infected food and drink, such as milk containing tuberculosis bacteria ; (iv) by water fouled by excreta impregnated with germs of enteric fever, for example ; (v) by fleas and other parasites that bite, sucking the blood of one person to inject it with its charge of germs into another (typhus fever and malaria are transmitted in this way) ; (vi) by personal contact, for example, with a person suffering from impetigo ; (vii) and by contact with articles which an infected person has used or been near, such as recently soiled handkerchiefs, dressings and drinking-cups.

The carrying of infections in this last way is probably less likely to occur than was formerly believed, because such contacts are rarely able to give a sufficiently large dose of germs to cause infection. Reasonable care and sanitary precautions are, however, advisable, for a person whose immunity is low might be infected in this way. Many medical authorities now consider the value of spraying with disinfectant to be mainly psychological, in that the smell of disinfectant reminds people of the need for caution and obedience to medical orders. In the *Health of the School Child*, 1929, it is stated that " anything which tends to encourage the belief that infection is spread mainly by inanimate objects is harmful, in that it diverts attention from the more important method of spread, namely, by personal infection, and thereby helps to perpetuate more or less obsolete beliefs " (Appendix C).

Droplet Infection

Everyone exhaling eighteen times a minute or more breathes out continually clouds of minute *droplets of moisture*, usually invisible, though this moisture containing germs can actually be seen to condense into a visible cloud on a frosty day. In a normally healthy person there will not be harmful bacteria in the droplets, but anyone with a cold or other infection continually breathes out droplets, each one impregnated with the germs of the specific infection, for example, cold, influenza, measles or whooping-cough.

Coughing and sneezing without a handkerchief in front of the mouth obviously must make a forcible *spray of droplets*, the spray impetus of which may extend to 9 feet distance. An infectious person may project from one to several millions of germs by each cough. It is not considered that a charge of germs sufficient to do harm can be conveyed beyond a radius of about 12 feet. The atmosphere of a closed room in which someone breathing out infected droplets stays continuously, would obviously become more and more impregnated with germs, whereas if there were a window open and a through draught the concentration of germs present could never become so great, as some would be borne away by the air currents. In addition, bacteria blown about in fresh air soon tend to die.

The body can deal with and nullify small doses of bacteria. White corpuscles are continually destroying foreign germs in the blood and tissues, particularly the lung tissue. If, however, the dose of germs is over large and concentrated, the body cannot destroy them quickly enough, and the germs multiply, make toxin, and an infection has been caught. It takes, in fact, a large dose of germs to start an infection. This is spoken of as a *mass infection*. It is possible to get a mass infection of bacteria in a number of ways, such as from taking heavily infected food or water, or from breathed-in infected " droplets " or even dust. Thus a child sitting by another with incipient measles is more likely to catch it than are those sitting farther away.

Lessening Mass Infections

Besides adequate through ventilation, effective *methods of lessening mass infection* include the use of single and well-spaced desks and the avoidance of over-crowded classrooms. In such sleeping quarters as dormitories, the slinging of hammocks a matter of only a foot farther apart and of putting beds alternately head to feet, instead of having all bed-heads in a row, reduces the spread of infection, by lessening the dosage of germs throughout the nights. Since germs are inhaled in dust, infection can be reduced by keeping living rooms and bedrooms clean and dustless.

" Salting " and Carriers

Given equal dosage of germs, not everyone contracts infections. *Personal susceptibility* varies. Some people are congenitally inclined to catch any infection going while others seem to be practically immune. Besides this, however, a partial immunity is built up by the continual small doses of germs that the body encounters in any crowded civilised community.

Each small dose stimulates the manufacture of the specific antitoxin and a relative resistance to infections is attained. Such a population is said to have become *"salted."*

This " salting " comes partly from the presence of *carriers* of diseases. Such people are healthy themselves and the germs they carry do not affect them. They do, however, breathe them out, and while small doses in a sanitary carefully-run community possibly make for useful " salting," susceptible people may catch an infection such as diphtheria from a carrier and suffer severely. In a diphtheria epidemic probably one child in ten is a carrier, and many people are carriers of cold germs. Further, convalescents may be carriers.

It is recognised that newcomers into a community, being " unsalted " for the particular germs of which everyone of the community must have had at least small immunising doses, are liable to catch readily an infection such as a particular type of cold there prevalent. Newcomers may also bring into a community fresh germs, against which the community is " unsalted," and such a new infection often spreads rapidly. " Unsalted " peoples, such as the Fiji Islanders, were rapidly and severely affected by measles when they first met it, whereas a " salted " population would have taken it lightly if at all.

A *hot enervating atmosphere* in a room lowers the body's resistance and increases susceptibility to infection ; it also probably increases the dosage of germs. Resistance is also lowered by sitting in damp clothes and boots.

Lack of satisfactory *vitamin content* in the diet or of a balanced nutritious diet lowers resistance to infections, as does a run-down, over-worked and worried condition coupled with over-strain and want of sleep. The frequent development of pneumonia on the top of a neglected but seemingly slight cold is an instance. However, some germs, smallpox for example, attack fit equally with less fit people.

Disease *germs vary in virulence* over a series of years. Smallpox and scarlet fever have become milder in type in the last thirty years, whereas measles appears to be getting more severe. As diseases become milder in type, a larger proportion of cases tend to occur, because, relatively, people become neglectful of precautions.

Quarantine

Quarantine is the period of exclusion of contacts with infections until they are considered safe from contracting the disease. A quarantine period is thus always a day or two over the longest limit of the incubation period. Authorities tend to differ slightly in their estimates of lengths of incubation and quarantine periods. The figures given here follow the table drawn up by the Association of School Medical Officers to govern exclusion of school children with infectious disease.

School Closure

School closure is now rarely resorted to because at school children can be intelligently supervised and guarded, and they make fewer contacts with infected children than when they are unsupervised in their homes or in out-of-school play. Closure may be of more value in a school in a scattered rural area, where the children might well not meet out of school. The closing of a school on the head teacher's initiative, because of low attendance, should not be confused with a medical officer's order to close.

Law about Infectious Disease

Certain diseases, mainly infectious, are classed as *notifiable*, that is, there is a legal obligation to inform the public health department of the city or other local authority when a case occurs. With this information in his possession, the medical officer of health is able to order the isolation of the case as seems necessary ; to see that adequate disinfection takes place ; to aim at tracing from what source the infection arose and so guard against the occurrence of further cases by the supervision of contacts. Such procedure is an example of the way the community agrees to guard itself from possible danger. The actual procedure varies for different diseases.

Among the notifiable diseases are diphtheria, scarlet fever, small pox, typhoid, tuberculosis, ophthalmia neonatorum, acute poliomyelitis (infantile paralysis), malaria and, since 1940, measles and whooping cough.

The *law about infectious diseases* provides also, among many points, that no one having an infectious disease may enter a public conveyance or be about a public street, nor may anyone in charge take such a person to such places. No one may let a house without disclosing the fact, if a case of infectious disease has occurred there within six weeks. While laws are necessary, it is far better and more effective to educate a strong health conscience so that people take precautions voluntarily, and not merely because they are compelled by law to do so. This view-point teachers more than anyone else can help to train.

Measles

Of the commoner infectious diseases, *measles*, though so general that many people think it is harmless, is actually of considerable seriousness in its effects, particularly to the pre-school child. The incubation period averages fourteen days, and ends with what appears to be a running cold, on the third day of which a coarse blotchy rash occurs showing first behind the ears and on the face. The child is very infectious during the " cold " stage before the rash appears, but in the time of an epidemic, it is possible for a doctor or school nurse to isolate suspected cases a day earlier by recognising the characteristic round red spots with white centre, called Koplik spots, that occur on the inside of the cheek. There is usually a rise in temperature, headache and loss in weight. In mild cases the rash will have disappeared in four to five days. In normal cases where convalescence is in every way satisfactory, the infected child should be isolated for not less than ten days from the disappearance of the rash ; if, however, discharges are still continuing, this isolation period must be extended.

The child needs careful nursing in a warm, well-ventilated room, for such nursing will do much to prevent incapacitating after-effects. Possible *complications* include, on the one hand, virulent septic infections of the eyes, leading even to blindness, and of the ears and nose, and, on the other hand, the onset of bronchitis and pneumonia and continued chest weakness. At any signs of heavy, rapid breathing and cough, a doctor should be called lest pneumonia is starting.

The old idea used to be that all children were sure to have measles, and the sooner the better. Actually, no child need have it, but if he does have it the older he is when it occurs the better. Deaths from measles are due to ignorance and neglect of nursing, and most occur under five years of age. Half the children entering London infant schools have already had measles, and the poorer the district, the younger the children are when they have had it. More cases occur in November and December than in May and June. Waves of outbreaks, lasting for six months, occur every two years. Some authorities suggest that this interval is due to the fact that children in contact, who do not catch the disease, develop a temporary immunity lasting about two years only. The disease spreads by droplet infection from child to child and disinfection of the school is useless.

Gamma Globulin serum is chiefly used to protect children under two years of age from infection and so postpone attack to a later age when resistance is higher. This has replaced the use of adult convalescent serum. Such passive immunity lasts only for about a month. Active immunisation is still a matter for experiment and is not yet reliable.

Measures of protection, initiated by health authorities, aim at preventing complications due to bad nursing and at delaying the age of incidence. School nurses and health visitors visit homes to give suggestions about nursing and care. In some areas leaflets of instructions are issued to parents, and talks and advice are given at maternity and child welfare centres. The convalescent child may need to go for a holiday or to an open-air school for a month or so. The quarantine period for contacts is at least sixteen days. While school closure during an epidemic is of little use, in the infant school all contacts should be excluded and in the primary and secondary school all who have not had measles. Practice, however, varies. In areas such as Cardigan, where tuberculosis is particularly rife, school closure for measles is still usual.

Whooping Cough

Whooping-cough causes more deaths than does measles or scarlet fever. It occurs mainly during the pre-school and infant school years and about half the deaths from it occur in children under one year of age. The incubation period is from three to ten days. The danger lies in the possibility of

12

heart failure or of wearing out of the lungs so that the weakened child succumbs to pneumonia or tuberculosis.

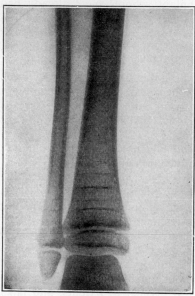

FIG. 142.—*Radiogram of the ankle of a girl of 6 years.* The lines of arrested growth, due to successive illnesses, measles, whooping-cough and several attacks of broncho-pneumonia, from $1\frac{4}{12}$ to 6 years, are seen on the tibia. Similar transverse ridges, due to arrested growth, may occur in the permanent teeth, from severe illness or starvation. Note here the epiphyses of the lower ends of the tibia and fibula. (*From the Report of the Consultative Committee (Board of Education) on " The Primary School," by permission of the Controller, H.M. Stationery Office.*)

The disease starts with what seems to be a common cold, and by the time the characteristic " whoop " has developed, the disease is no longer very infectious. It is spread by droplet infection, by healthy carriers of the germ, by inhaling infected dust, by soiled linen, such as handkerchiefs and by the hands of the patient's attendant.

The reason why it spreads rapidly is that, as in measles, it cannot be differentiated from an ordinary cold in the early infectious stage. Skilled nursing and hygienic conditions reduce deaths. The child needs to be kept warm, though not necessarily in bed, and to have plenty of fresh air and sunlight. Neither school closure nor disinfection is of use, but children under five should not attend school while the disease is prevalent. Its main season of incidence is from November to March.

The child may become worn out with coughing and undernourished because of the tendency to vomit, all continued over a period of weeks or months. A change of air or attendance at an open-air school during convalescence is of value. An attack appears to confer permanent immunity.

Serum from human convalescents can be used to induce passive immunity. Active immunisation can be successfully carried out and should not be delayed beyond the age of one year. It can conveniently be combined with immunisation against diphtheria. The child is considered infectious for four weeks from the onset of the disease. There is no quarantine period, but any child showing cough or catarrh symptoms should be isolated.

Scarlet Fever

In *Scarlet Fever* the greater number of cases occur between five and ten years of age. Spread is by droplet infection. The incubation period is from two to eight days.

The onset shows as a sore throat, a single attack of vomiting without any obvious digestive upset twenty-four hours before the rash appears, headache, a temperature, and redness of the tongue and throat. The bright red rash appears on the second day, first on the chest, rarely on the face; before the rash appears infection is being spread by droplets. In a matter of days only the symptoms decline in severity and peeling of the skin begins. The patient is not considered to be infectious during peeling, but any septic discharges of the throat, nose or middle ear are highly so. The period of communicability is four weeks from onset, if there are no open discharges.

The main risk is of *complications and after-effects*. Rheumatism and heart weakness, if they occur at all, do so early in the course of the disease. Discharge of the middle ear and kidney inflammation may also be serious. Chills during convalescence are specially to be avoided. Infection may be conveyed by contaminated articles, but the main sources of spread are personal contact and apparently healthy carriers of the germs. Milk handled by a carrier has been known to convey infection. School closure is not usually advised. The disease occurs most frequently in October and November.

By the *Dick test*, a small quantity of scarlet fever toxin injected into the skin produces no effect in those immune, but in those susceptible, a pink areola of rash that dies away in about twelve hours.   Repeated small doses of toxin [1] given to such susceptible persons develops active immunity.

Scarlet fever antitoxin, injected early in the course of the disease, lessens the characteristic symptoms, and cases are thought to show less tendency to septic complications.   It also reduces the length of time that must be spent in hospital. Small doses give contacts temporary immunity for from one to two weeks.   Apart from isolation, the child should have at least two weeks' convalescence before return to school, to build up his health.

Diphtheria

Diphtheria is a disease that has become less dreaded owing to the widespread use of (i) passive, and (ii) active immunisation.

Attack is most likely at four to five years of age, so that the longer the infection is postponed the less likely is it to occur severely, or at all.   Incubation varies from two to seven days. The nose, throat, pharynx, tonsils or the larynx may be specially affected, but the sore throat is often not so severe as in tonsillitis.   Stoppage of the windpipe, due to growth of membrane across it, is possible, and the making of an incision in the windpipe (tracheotomy) so that the patient breathes through an inserted tube is still, on occasion, necessary.

Passive Immunisation

Antitoxin of diphtheria injected as early as possible in the course of the disease lessens the further development of symptoms, and is not in itself dangerous.   Early and immediate injection, in a matter of hours, is important, for the disease develops with extreme rapidity.   Paralysis of the limbs felt as pins and needles is a later symptom but passes off, but the child should be kept quiet for at least a month because of the possibility of paralysis of the heart muscle.

Antitoxin is made by cultivating diphtheria bacilli in a nutrient broth, filtering off the germs and injecting the toxin of diphtheria that is left behind into a healthy horse in small

· That is, the toxin, but *not* the live germs are injected.

recurring doses. The horse, without harm to itself, progressively develops antitoxin against the toxin doses. It is then bled, and its blood serum is filtered and standardised and put up in sterilised tubes to be distributed for use.

Diphtheria is transmitted by infected droplets either from a patient or from an apparently healthy carrier. There is some, though not a great, chance of carrying infection by contaminated articles. Sucking infected pencils, or drinking from contaminated cups can cause spread, and should be continually discouraged, not just when an epidemic is prevalent.

It was once thought that diphtheria and other septic throat conditions could be caused by bad smells from drains. Such septic throat conditions actually are due to bacterial invasion. It is now recognised that people working where strong smells are characteristic, as in abattoirs, may have a high general level of health.

The *period of exclusion* is settled by rubbing a sterilised swab on the back of the throat or other infected part; if on cultivation, it is found to have picked up no germs it is said to be negative. Usually three such negative swabs are demanded. The infected person should be isolated for not less than four weeks, or until convalescence is complete *after* negative swabs have been secured.

Active Immunisation

The *Schick test* consists of an injection into the skin of a minute charge of dilute diphtheria toxin. If in a few days a small painless reddened area shows at the puncture, the person is susceptible to diphtheria, and such people can be made immune by a course of inoculations, spread over an average of three successive weeks, of a mixture of toxin and antitoxin.

Immunity begins to develop at once and is at its maximum in about three months. A repetition of the Schick test shows whether immunity is complete or whether, as in some people, four or five inoculations must be made. Inoculations are harmless to children and cause only slight temporary *malaise* in adults.

Local Education Authorities provide this treatment. As £13 provides enough material to protect 100 children, and as in

London it is estimated that each case of diphtheria cost the ratepayers £37, it can be seen that the provision of immunising facilities by authorities justifies itself on economic as well as on humanitarian grounds (Public Health Report, 1927).

In 1943 a publicity campaign about the value of immunisation against diphtheria was sponsored by the Ministry of Health. That this was successful, can be judged by mortality figures. Over the years 1938–41, deaths from diphtheria averaged 2500 a year whereas in 1949 there were less than 100 deaths from diphtheria all told, a new low record.

Chapter XXVIII

FURTHER INFECTIOUS DISEASES

Smallpox

Smallpox is a virus-caused disease, at one time virulent and dreaded, now often milder. Because of sanitary improvements and immunisation by vaccination, the mortality is now small. The disease spreads in the early unrecognised stages from person to person by infected droplets, and is extremely infectious, the incubation period being nine to fourteen days. There is backache, high temperature and rigor, followed in about two days by the appearance of small shotty spots, first on the forehead and wrists, spreading over the body, each of which comes up to a mattery head and leaves the typical pits in the skin's surface. Blindness also may result. The milder non-fatal type of smallpox approximates more closely to chicken-pox,[1] and is little more severe than influenza. There is always the danger, however, that infections may assume a virulent form. Smallpox is not mainly a school-age disease.

Vaccination protects people from catching smallpox. If a vaccinated person does contract the disease, the attack is less severe than it might otherwise have been. Jenner, a Gloucestershire doctor of the eighteenth century, noticed that while people working among cows tended to have a mild disease, cowpox (vaccinia), they rarely caught smallpox, and he experimented by injecting some of the watery fluid from the blebs of people having cowpox into healthy people. He found that this treatment rendered them at least partially immune from smallpox. It is just cause for national pride that this first step of Jenner's in preventive medicine has saved so many lives and made for much increased happiness all over the world, and has led to the discovery of similar preventive measures for other diseases.

Now vaccine lymph for vaccination is got from specially selected and healthy calves, and the quality of the vaccine is standardised and controlled so that no harmful matter is

[1] The two diseases are quite different, however, in spite of the names.

349

included. In England vaccination is not compulsory, but people who so desire can be vaccinated free of charge.

The quarantine period for smallpox is sixteen days, and a patient should be isolated until every scab has fallen and the skin is healed. If anyone has knowingly encountered smallpox infection and is immediately vaccinated, some protection is given against possible attack, as the incubation period of vaccination is some four days, whereas that for smallpox is twelve.

Chicken Pox

Chicken-pox, a mild virus-caused disease of childhood, most prevalent in October and November, is seldom fatal. It is spread, at first, by droplets. It incubates in from eleven to nineteen days. The child does not feel particularly ill, and the rash appears on the body first so that children may well be in school with the rash on them. The red spots turn into watery blebs that dry into scabs in a few days and fall off in about a fortnight. Infection lasts probably for five days. Exclusion until all scabs have fallen off is usual. Particular attention should be paid to the scalp.

Mumps

The incubation period for *Mumps* is from fourteen to twenty-eight days, but is usually eighteen. The virus attacks the parotid glands, so that the swelling shows below the ear and behind the angle of the jaw, one side swelling up first. Other glands, the sublingual and submaxillary, may also be infected and show as a " double chin." Swellings of toothache or of lymphatic glands are more local. The child needs to be kept warm and away from others. Infection, spread mainly by droplets, continues for not less than two weeks after the beginning of the illness, but longer if one clear week has not elapsed since the swelling subsided. Mumps is rarely fatal. Inner ear deafness and sterility in boys may be complications of mumps.

German Measles

German Measles, a virus-caused disease, spread by droplet infection, is most prevalent between March and June, and affects adults more often than does ordinary measles. The incubation period is from nine to nineteen days. A rose-red flushed face is the first symptom. There is a fine pink rash all over the body, and lymphatic glands at the back of the neck are usually enlarged. Infection lasts for seven days from the appearance of the rash, and longer if there are nasal or other symptoms.

Enteric Fever

The *Typhoid and Para-typhoid Fevers* are milder than formerly. Infection is always from the bowel and urinary passages. For infection to take place, excreta must be conveyed to some article of food either by hands which themselves have been fouled during the toilet (i.e. after defæcation) or by sewage as by its access to the water supply. Hence the importance of hand washing after every visit to the water closet.

Healthy carriers and preparers of food spread infection, as for example, in the wide-spread epidemic of typhoid which started at Aberystwyth in 1946 from contaminated ice cream.

The washing of milk vessels with sewage contaminated water can make milk an infecting agent. In country districts the water of shallow wells may be fouled by cesspools after heavy rains, when the ' ground water ' rises. The installation of water carriage systems for sewage disposal produced, in city after city, immediate diminution of water-borne fevers such as enteric and dysentry. Incubation is from seven to twenty-three days and quarantine twenty-five days and the patient is considered to be infectious until convalescence is firmly established.

Routine inoculation was carried out against enteric fever in the 1914–18 and 1939–45 wars. In the South African War, 1898–1901, when such protection was not available, more men died of enteric fever than of wounds.[1]

The Common Cold

The *Common Cold*, cold in the head, is wrongly named. It is not due to cold but to the breathing in of a sufficiently large

[1] The anti-biotic *Chloromycetin* is effective for typhoid fever. Its toxicity is low and it can be taken orally, unlike Penicillin.

12*

dose of infected droplets in a hot, stuffy, crowded atmosphere. The inhaling of infected dust may also be a cause. Out of doors germs of cold are quickly carried away by the wind and rarely if ever are colds actually caught there.

A " cold " is not caught by being cold unless the individual breathes in the " cold " virus. On Sir Ernest Shackleton's Arctic Expedition, in spite of the cold weather and hardship of going to sleep in wet clothes, in spite of having frost-bite, no one in the party caught cold until a fresh bale of blankets was opened. The bale had evidently been packed by some one who had a cold and had coughed or sneezed charges of germs into the blankets, and all the party caught the cold. Similarly, it is the passenger in the moist, heated, germ-laden carriage who catches cold rather than the engine-driver in his open coach. People who walk to and from work are less likely to catch colds and influenza than those who have to travel inside trains and buses.

The incubation period for colds is about two days, and the chilly shivering feeling that precedes the stage of nasal congestion marks actually the end of the short incubation period and is one symptom produced by the cold toxins. A non-constipating aperient such as cascara would help the body to carry away the toxins. Colds can be spread by healthy carriers of the virus.

Soiled *handkerchiefs* may be a source of infection. Handkerchiefs should never be flourished or held in the hand when not in immediate use. Dirty handkerchiefs, retained in use too long or cold-infected pockets, may cause re-infection. Paper handkerchiefs used once and burnt are best.

To avoid catching colds: (i) keep away from people with colds ; (ii) get plenty of fresh air ; (ii) breathe through the nose ; (iv) keep the feet warm and dry ; (v) sleep with the window open ; (vi) do not wear too many clothes ; (vii) have a well-balanced diet of satisfactory vitamin content.

Influenza

Influenza may be of a respiratory, gastric, nervous or febrile type. Its onset is sudden, and uncomplicated cases improve after the third day of illness. It is a virus infection and it is spread by inhaled droplets. Immediate bed on onset is best for the patient and for preventing others being infected. Characteristic after-effects are depression and lassitude ; and the heart may be affected. An attack gives little immunity, though vaccine treatment is sometimes given.

The Ministry of Health's advice in times of epidemic is to avoid crowds and to shield the mouth and nose in coughing and sneezing. The first may not always be possible, and high resistance and lack of fear is perhaps preferable to an over-valetudinarian attitude. Nevertheless, people with colds or influenza should refrain from attending churches, cinemas and public meetings lest they spread their infection.

Infectious diseases of the nervous system include infantile paralysis, cerebro-spinal fever and acute encephalitis (p. 249).

Infantile Paralysis

Infantile Paralysis (Anterior Poliomyelitis) is a virus-caused infectious disease that is most prevalent in hot weather such as in July and August. The incubation period is from two to ten days. The disease is conveyed directly by droplet infection and by the nose and throat excretions, or it may be ingested with food or drink. Not all cases pass to the paralysed stage. The disease may be disseminated by healthy " carriers" as well as by patients who have had mild, even unrecognised, attacks only. The virus, which is excreted with the fæces, is highly resistant and will stand drying, chlorination and very low temperatures.

Adults may be attacked as well as young children. The anterior horn of grey matter in the spinal cord (Fig. 95) is affected in the cervical or lumbar region. From this anterior horn go nerves to muscles to control movement, so that it is the power to make movements that is affected. The patient has a sore throat, is feverish and out of sorts, and there may be temporary pain and stiffness in the neck or waist. At the slightest suspicion a doctor should be called.

In a matter of hours the feverishness passes off, but there is found to be loss of some degree of movement and wasting of particular muscle-groups, which, though it can be lessened by massage, almost certainly leaves permanent defect, leading even to limb deformity. The limb is cold, blue and wasted and lacks power.

Thus the importance of guarding against the infection is because of the disabling after-effects, and this is one of the very few diseases for which school closure, particularly for infants, is still advocated. Contacts should be isolated. Teachers are likely to encounter children in school who are deformed from infantile paralysis.

Venereal Disease

Venereal Diseases are those connected with sex intercourse, and are contagious and germ spread. A good deal of uncertain information is surreptitiously circulated about them, and it is important that teachers should have some accurate knowledge on the matter. Though such infections are mainly transmitted during sex intercourse, innocent people may be infected, and so long as the condition is untreated the infected person is a continuing danger to the community.

The *Gonorrhœa* germ readily attacks the mucous membrane of the genital organs, producing inflammation. It may be passed on during sex intercourse or, rarely, by contact with an infected closet seat. Treated without delay the disease can be cleared up rapidly. Untreated it may produce sterility in either men or women.

Ophthalmia of the new-born caused at birth by gonorrhœal infection has been considered in Chapter XXII. Gonorrhœal rheumatism is a possible disabling complication. The gonococcus is carried by the blood and causes severe inflammation of the joint attacked, often the knee ; it produces pain, swelling and possibly permanent stiffness of the joint. Early treatment minimises the likelihood of this complication.

Syphilis is a chronic disease which, if untreated, runs a typical course in three stages with quiescent intermediate periods. Infection may take place when any discharge containing the germ comes in contact with any mucous membrane, such as the external genital organs or the lips, or with broken skin, and in from ten days to six weeks a comparatively mild sore, which soon dies down, develops at the point of infection.

The secondary stage, which occurs from six to eighteen months later, is important because during it the disease is specially infectious. Infection may be handed on by sex intercourse, by kissing and by common drinking vessels. Children of syphilitic parents may be infected before birth, and syphilitic blindness or deafness or general puny lack of development (marasmic babies) and possibly early death may follow. Mothers infected with syphilis tend to have miscarriages, still- or prematurely-born children. People having syphilis should not marry until definitely cured. The tertiary stage of the disease may appear from three to four years later, or symptoms may be delayed till even thirty years later, and such progressively fatal diseases as general paralysis of the insane and locomotor ataxy are associated with it.

The treatment of both gonorrhœa and syphilis has been considerably shortened by the use of, first, sulphathiazole and more recently still of penicillin.

The treatment of gonorrhœa by penicillin can be completed in eight hours or less, thus greatly reducing social difficulties. At present for treatment by penicillin, syphilis requires residence in hospital for eight days, but it is hoped to perfect a method of treatment by which injections at twelve or twenty-four hour intervals, will obviate this.

It is not yet considered safe to rely entirely on this eight-day treatment, or with penicillin alone, but the total treatment period for syphilis has now been reduced from about a year to approximately ten weeks. This means that patients are less likely than formerly to give up treatment before it is completed. The presence or absence of infection can be determined, even at a quiescent stage, by the Wassermann blood test. Free treatment can be obtained at V.D. clinics, where secrecy of the patient's identity is observed ; for mothers and children treatment is also given at ante-natal clinics.

Opinions differ as to whether venereal diseases should be made notifiable, like some other infectious diseases, and whether treatment should be compulsory, thus further protecting the community. The social slur attached to having venereal disease, however, would probably make people hide infections, leaving them untreated or it would tempt them to have recourse to doubtful quacks who would promise secrecy. Thus the aim of any compulsion would be defeated.

Knowledge of measures to take to prevent infection after sex intercourse exists, but there is a prominent body of opinion that is opposed to the dissemination of such knowledge. They argue that although it would actually decrease the chances of infection for the community, it would make illicit sex intercourse safer and so the more likely to occur, thus weakening individual moral fibre.

It is not expected that *the teacher* will give any direct teaching on venereal disease, nor is it desirable that teachers should be continually expecting evil. Infected children may, however, attend school. The teacher can recommend medical inspection and, meanwhile, take what precautions he can against the spread of infection, always remembering that suspicion may quite well turn out to be groundless and that discretion in such a matter is essential.

Playgrounds should not be used as public passage-ways and short cuts. Outsiders may use and infect school lavatories. Children should be taught never to sit right down on the seat of a public lavatory such as one in a railway train or station or restaurant. Any slight skin abrasion could readily be infected by germs left on the seat. Lavatory seats which are roughly horse-shoe in shape and so not closed in front, and which have a shiny non-absorbent surface are best. To fold a newspaper in four and tear out a quarter circle at the middle corner makes a safe cover for a closet seat that is suspect, particularly if the seat is otherwise too high for the child. Common towels are another possible source of infection.

Finally, teachers need to know about these problems, without dwelling on them. A wise teacher can so train his or her pupils in self-respect, control and respect for others that they develop a balanced attitude in sex matters as in other important aspects of social living. All movements that make for wide interests such as out-of-school activities, sports, games, hobbies, debating and social societies, guide and scout movements, help here. Adolescents, particularly, need opportunities for enjoying each other's company, boys and girls together, in healthy, natural surroundings.

CHAPTER XXIX

TUBERCULOSIS

TUBERCULOSIS is a matter of consequence both for the child and for the teacher personally. It is unlike other diseases many of which tend to affect mainly childhood, before stability is established, or later age when resistance is waning. Tuberculosis, though it may affect any age, kills most people between 15 and 45 years of age, which should be the most productive and healthy period of life. Furthermore, tuberculosis is not over in a matter of weeks as is an uncomplicated case of scarlet fever, or measles. It runs a prolonged course and the average duration of the final illness is three years, during which the patient is continually ailing; earning power is reduced; he needs plenty of relatively expensive and appetising foods, such as butter, milk, eggs and meat; and there is the continual need for care lest other members of the family catch the disease.

The incidence of tuberculosis is decreasing in most civilised countries. In the British Isles in the last fifty years the death-rate from tuberculosis has been halved. This improvement may be partly due to a better standard of living and partly to greater knowledge and care in prevention.

Bovine and Human Strains

There are two distinct strains of the tuberculosis bacillus, the human and the bovine. The human strain is the more virulent, causing twenty times as many deaths as the bovine strain. It affects children and adults.

The bovine strain is conveyed by the milk from tuberculous cows. Children, because their resistance is less, are infected more than adults. Most of the deaths from bovine tuberculosis occur between the ages of one and five years. The majority of bovine infections are non-pulmonary.

357

DEATHS PER 100,000

Year					At all ages	Women 15–24 age
1875	.	.	.	.	. 223	276
1900	.	.	.	.	. 133	115
1913	.	.	.	.	. 99	102
1916	.	.	.	.	. 116	126
1920	.	.	.	.	. 87	115
1925	.	.	.	.	. 79	121
1930	.	.	.	.	. 69	111
1935	.	.	.	.	. 55	93
1938	.	.	.	.	. 48	—
1939	.	.	.	.	. 49	—
1940	.	.	.	.	. 53	—
1942	.	.	.	.	. 48	—

TABLE to show deaths from *tuberculosis of the lungs* in England and Wales. What deductions can you make from the figures? To what factors is the all-over decrease in deaths due? Why are the figures for younger women relatively high?

It is estimated that by twelve years of age, 50 per cent. of children have been infected by one or other form of tuberculosis, but most have been able to overcome the disease by their natural resistive powers and have made for themselves a useful immunity against further attack.

Pulmonary tuberculosis, also termed consumption or phthisis, attacks the lungs. Non-pulmonary forms include tuberculosis of the lymphatic glands, intestines, eyes, ears, bones and joints, lupus, in which the skin is attacked, and meningitis, in which the membranes covering the brain are attacked.

Prevention of Tuberculosis

Tuberculosis should be prevented rather than cured. For children, the following are the chief preventive measures: (i) avoidance of contact with tuberculous adults, (ii) the boiling of milk to protect against bovine tuberculosis, or use of T.T. milk, (iii) the maintenance of a high level of bodily health, and (iv) the attainment of complete recovery after acute catarrhal illness, such as cold, bronchitis or diarrhœa which lower the resistance of the body to the tuberculosis bacillus.[1]

Doses of tuberculosis germs, particularly those of phthisis, may be spread by breathing and coughing out infected droplets ; by the drying up of sputum, the bacilli surviving to be blown about, when they may infect milk or food, or be inhaled again (hence legislation against spitting) ;

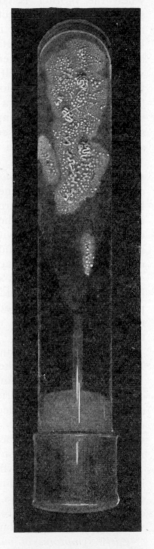

FIG. 143.—Tubercle bacilli growing in large masses on specially nourishing material in a test tube. A smear of sputum or discharge suspected to contain bacteria would be cultivated thus at the optimum temperature, and in the resulting possibility of larger growth, the presence or absence of bacteria can readily be decided.

by the dried discharges of tuberculous lesions and by tuberculous milk, butter and cheese from infected cows (see Chapter IX).

An experiment in which a consumptive coughed on to guinea-pigs proved that this was sufficient to infect them with tuberculosis. Tuberculosis germs may remain quiescent in old upholstery, bedding, curtains, carpets, or cushions for years even, and then when disturbed cause infection. They remain in dark, dirty, damp places, but exposure to direct sunlight kills them (see Fig. 6).

Tuberculosis not Inherited

Tuberculosis is not inherited as, for instance, mental defect is. Babies are not born with it, even

---

[1] Professor Calmette's " B.C.G." strain of attenuated tuberculosis bacilli is now being used in Sanatoria to immunise the nursing staff against tuberculosis.

when the mother is consumptive, but they may catch it soon after birth if subjected to continual large doses of germs, as from a consumptive in the home. What is inherited is a bodily make-up and metabolism that makes one person more susceptible to doses of germs than another, and such make-up will tend to repeat itself in families just as family tendencies to get fat or to live long may reappear. Children whose family histories show a susceptibility to tuberculosis need special care in upbringing, and the type of work they take up should be carefully chosen. But given intelligent nurture they are by no means certain to catch tuberculosis.

Probably 80 per cent. or more of the population have had slight attacks of *tuberculosis*, but the majority get over it without treatment. Routine post-mortem examinations show healed patches of tuberculosis on the lung tissue or in the abdominal glands of the majority of cases examined. The usual seaside holiday with its extra sleep, fresh air and sunshine, plentiful food and lack of worry, must have averted many such incipient attacks of phthisis.

In those who actually consult a doctor, the disease usually has gained a definite hold. The earlier a person infected with phthisis begins treatment the greater the chance of arresting the disease, and of cure, a point to stress in all teaching about tuberculosis.

Mass Radiography aims at early pre-symptom diagnosis. X-ray photographs of the lungs, 1 in. square are taken and 100 people can be examined cheaply in an hour. One per cent. of those examined may show early signs of tuberculosis, and these are re-examined more fully. With early treatment, complete cure is likely. A system of Government maintenance allowances to help patients to undertake early treatment has been in force since 1943.

Predisposing causes which enhance susceptibility to attack, include continual catching of colds and influenza, general debility, alcoholic excess, too little sleep combined with badly chosen and insufficient food, and poor, badly ventilated living, working and sleeping conditions.

Early symptoms of pulmonary tuberculosis may include a slight persistent cough that has gone on for more than three weeks, not a hard stomach cough, but a rather softer throat cough; an unwonted feeling of tiredness without evident cause; loss of weight and appetite and persistent indigestion;

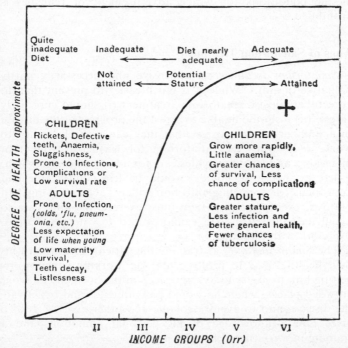

FIG. 144.—It is difficult with the changed values of money to give a satisfactory numerical range for the income groups I–VI, moving as it does from unskilled labour through increasingly skilled artisan and lower professional classes to high earning commercial and professional classes. It is not only amount of income that counts but also sense in spending. Rationing from 1939 onwards has equalised out food supplies so that the lower income groups have been the better nourished. (*From " Biology for Schools, Autumn, 1941 "—B.B.C.*)

and night rise of temperature and night sweats. There is no one specific cure for tuberculosis, like antitoxin for diphtheria or quinine for malaria.

Treatment includes rest, proper food, graduated exercise and fresh air, together with varying specific treatment.

The anti-biotic *streptomycin* gives good results particularly with tubercular-meningitis and miliary tuberculosis. Under the Pharmacy and Medicines Acts, 1941, tuberculosis is one of the conditions for which advertisement of remedies is prohibited.

Aims of Sanatorium Treatment

Sanatorium treatment is expensive and necessarily partly palliative in aim. While it is much easier to prevent than to cure tuberculosis, sanatorium treatment (i) should cure early cases ; (ii) it should be able to arrest the progress of the disease in a number of patients so that they can possibly return to work, re-entering the sanatorium for further treatment at intervals ; and (iii) it provides care for advanced cases, which, if left in their own homes, would be less comfortable and be a focus for spreading infection widely. Once having had phthisis, even a cured patient must exercise life-long care to avoid its recurrence. He cannot afford to catch cold or to overwork with impunity.

The *sanatorium aims* at training the patient to safeguard his own health so as to prolong life and working capacity, by getting him to *prefer* to live and sleep in the open air, to avoid crowded places, where he would pick up colds and re-activate the disease, and to avoid alcoholic and other excess. It also gives him a knowledge of his personal limitations and a training in a routine of healthy living.

It should also teach the patients habits which prevent the spread of infection, thus protecting the community. Spitting is done into a flat-shaped pocket expectoration flask, in which is a little disinfectant ; the flask and the contents are sterilised frequently. On no account is sputum allowed to dry, as germs are thus freed to be blown about.

Paper handkerchiefs that can be burned immediately are also used, and the patient should keep his own utensils, cups, plates, knives, spoons and forks, always using these only ; they should always be sterilised in boiling water after use and not washed up with the utensils of healthy people.

Three to six months' sanatorium treatment should thus repay

both the patient and the community that pays for it, but the value obtained depends much on the intelligence and good-will of the individual patient. Tuberculosis is a notifiable disease, but notification is not always made. Patients are advised to keep in touch with their own medical man or with the local tuberculosis medical officer. Health visitors follow up cases and aim at giving practical tactful advice about precautions for the patient and his family in the more difficult home environment; and after-care schemes give help to ex-patients in grants for living, in getting better housing conditions, and in providing suitable work and workshops and in marketing products.

The Cambridgeshire Tuberculosis Colony at Papworth is one of the best known of these settlements and is self-supporting. Life in such a colony prevents the relapses that are unfortunately so frequent, when patients have to return to unsatisfactory home conditions and strenuous work. Lacking medical supervision, patients at home are apt to become careless and to neglect the treatment and the precautions learnt. At Papworth there is a resident medical staff.

Sanatorium Schools

In *sanatorium schools for children* only, or in connection with an adult sanatorium, education limited to the varying capacities of the children is provided. Methods of teaching have to be largely individual, and the children, apart from the educational work covered, get interest and incentive and feel as far as possible like normal children. Teachers recovering from tuberculosis who may teach in such schools, must not undertake the full responsibility that a fit member of the staff could accept.

In bone or joint infections, the hip, spine or elbow are the most likely places of attack. There may be breakdown of the skin, when open tubercular lesion occurs. Such cases are frequently treated by immobilisation and graduated exposure to sunlight, the ultra-violet rays of which enable the body to overcome the tubercular toxin and germs. Mountain sun is rather more effective than sea-level sun; this partly accounts for the success of treatment centres in Switzerland. This is partly because, at higher levels, ultra-violet rays are less cut

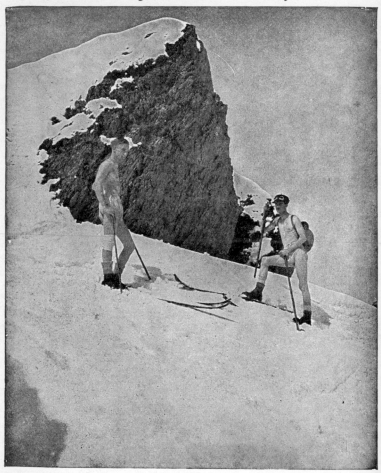

FIG. 145.—Convalescent soldiers ski-ing at a high altitude dressed only in loin-cloth, cap and boots. (*From Hill's " Sunshine and Open Air " —Edward Arnold & Co.*)

off by clouds or smoke. Similar open-air treatment is, however, carried out successfully at the Treloar Homes at Alton, and at Chailey, Sussex, among other places, in Great Britain (see Fig. 156).

The child's skin, beginning with the foot, is exposed partially and later more completely, at first for short and then for increasingly long periods to the early morning sun. This gives ultra-violet rays with less of the infra-red dark heat rays that are felt later in the day, when the sun is higher, too much of such heat being harmful for consumptives. Even frosty air makes no difference to the value of such sunlight. Pigmentation is gradually induced, and the more readily this happens, the better the chance of cure. The children, at first thin and emaciated, increase in tone and vigour through the action of the sun and air. The muscles become firmer, and general body metabolism is stimulated and tubercular ulcers heal up spontaneously. The degree of deformity that remains depends on how far the disease had progressed before the beginning of the treatment.

In later stages of treatment the children play and work in the winter as well as in the summer dressed only in hat, boots and a loin-cloth, for having been gradually acclimatised they do not feel the cold. Artificial sunlight baths which supply ultra-violet rays, can be used as an accessory treatment, where real sunlight is scarce.

Lymphatic glands in the neck and in other regions sometimes become tubercular. Such swollen hard glands should not be rubbed, and early medical advice should be sought, particularly as less unsightly scars result if the abscess of such glands is opened surgically rather than allowed to break down spontaneously.

If full advantage is to be obtained from the very large expenditure of public money that is made in maintaining sanatoria, specialist tuberculosis doctors, health visitors and dispensaries, the public must understand something of the aims of the service and be sympathetic to them. Propaganda, however, may well suffer from its over-enthusiastic adherents, who, by their insistence, alienate those they would convince ; by supplying morbid detail of disease, they either repel their audience or breed undue disease " phobias " in them.

Teaching About Tuberculosis

Teaching about tuberculosis, particularly for children, should be of a robust, positive kind, stressing rather the values and satisfaction of sound health and how to get it than the horrors of the disease.

On the other hand, however, the teacher should have continually in mind the help she can give to the children in her class by educating them to resist tuberculosis. Partly by habit training, partly by teaching, she can influence them to *prefer* fresh air, sunlight and open windows, to know what foods to eat for health, to wear as few light, loose clothes as are compatible with warmth, to keep the teeth and body clean, to avoid spitting and uncovered coughing, and to keep milk clean.

For *older children* who will soon leave school and go to work, more specific teaching should be added. Guidance can well be given about predisposing causes, how germs are spread, how to avoid infection, the value of early treatment and where in the district to get it, and the individual's responsibility in helping to prevent the spread of infection. Many people do not know that anyone can have free advice from the local tuberculosis medical officer. Sound advice wisely given will influence not only the particular boy or girl but very probably the family circle as well.

Tuberculosis has been called a " bedroom disease." It runs " not in the bones but in the blankets." It spreads in dark, dirty workshops and poor housing conditions. The problem of preventing it is partly medical and partly social, and with an enlightened public opinion there is not a doubt that it could be entirely stamped out. Teachers can, if they will, play a large part in creating such an opinion.

Chapter XXX

RHEUMATISM

It is considered that rheumatism is caused by a streptococcus of low infective power. Three forms in which rheumatism occurs in children are (i) rheumatic heart disease (carditis) ; (ii) acute rheumatism, popularly called rheumatic fever ; and (iii) chorea or St. Vitus' Dance. In children the danger of rheumatism is that there may result heart disease, permanent invalidism and even early death, unless prolonged care is taken.

First attacks of rheumatism are most prevalent from 8 to 10 years of age. They are less likely to occur after puberty, although relapses may occur. Unlike infectious diseases, rheumatism is more and not less likely to recur after a first attack. Girls are more susceptible to rheumatism than boys.

Rheumatism occurs in temperate regions, rather than in the tropics and it is a disease, on the whole, of the less well-to-do. Cold and damp combined with any conditions that lower general resistance make the onset of rheumatism more likely. Children living in jerry-built houses, which are likely to be damp, and who are coddled by wearing too many clothes of the chest-protector type are likely to become rheumatic. On the other hand, children of the lowest wage-earning class, such as gipsies who are hardy and sleep out of doors, and children of well-to-do homes, show less rheumatic tendency. Hereditary make-up is probably a predisposing cause.

Rheumatism shows itself as joint inflammation, muscular pain, rheumatic nodules, rashes, chorea, dry pleurisy, sore throat and tonsillitis, and inflammation of the lining, muscle or surrounding membrane of the heart. This carditis is important because it may permanently affect the valves of the heart.

The toxin of rheumatism tends to destroy the red blood corpuscles and so to produce anæmia.

Normal growth is painless, but Shelton considers " growing pains " are not necessarily rheumatic. Such pains occur

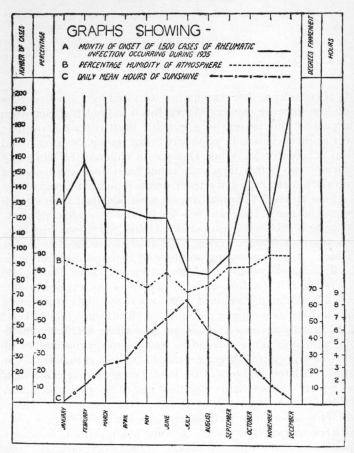

FIG. 146.—From the graph, decide in what months the air is damp and cold from lack of sunshine. What can you find out about the onset of cases of rheumatism at these times ? What are the conditions when the onset of rheumatism cases was least ? (*Courtesy of L.C.C.*)

chiefly in the legs, between the ages of 6 and 10. Asthmatic and tubercular children and those who have recently had measles and influenza get such pains. Rest, warmth, and tonics for the general health, are indicated.

Acute Rheumatism

Acute Rheumatism (*Rheumatic fever*) is a condition of non-suppurative inflammation of the joints. It hardly ever occurs before the age of five years and is less frequent after the age of fifteen. Its onset tends to be most frequent in the cold wet months of the year—November to February. Its danger lies in the possible complication of carditis (inflammation of the heart. The history of such cases shows continual relapses and return for treatment with the heart more damaged. At first the heart seems to recover completely, but after the next relapse a slight permanent defect is observable, although the child will be able to support himself. Later there is permanent disability, and with further relapses premature death, which may have been delayed for from ten to twenty years from the first infection. (See note on page 373.)

Chorea

Chorea is a nervous disorder related to rheumatism. It is characterised by (i) involuntary movements and fidgetiness, (ii) incoördination of voluntary movement and apparent clumsiness, and (iii) emotional disturbances. It is most prevalent round about the age of ten and it is approximately twice as common in girls as in boys.

Alert, intelligent children who are making headway at school are more likely to be affected than are dull, placid children. Anxiety about a scholarship examination, a fright or a shock, may be exciting causes. Again the condition is less common in the children of well-to-do parents.

The child affected drops things, fidgets, makes faces, cries readily, and cannot concentrate. The writing tends to be characteristically angular. The teacher must aim at recognising and bearing with such children, and should arrange for medical treatment as soon as possible.

Chorea must not be confused with habit spasm (tic), in which one or two movements, such as blinking or screwing up the face, are continually repeated. Choreic movements are more generalised.

The illness lasts for from five to six weeks and unless convalescence is prolonged, relapse is likely. The danger, as in acute rheumatism, is that the heart may be affected. Choreitic children are irritable and difficult to manage both at home and in school.

Rheumatic Heart

Immediately a case is diagnosed as *rheumatic carditis* the child should be removed from school and, if the attack is acute, he should receive special treatment in a hospital or in a special *Home of Recovery for Cardiac and Rheumatic Children*. It is essential for the heart to have complete rest, which entails staying recumbent in bed for weeks and possibly for months on end. Such rest treatment is difficult to carry out, particularly in the straitened homes from which such cases too often come. There may be no bed available for the patient's sole use, the mother may well be single-handed, and she may have other children to attend to ; the patient may be disturbed by the other children and she may even have to look after them ; and rheumatic children are apt to be alert, sensitive, quarrelsome and temperamentally difficult to keep in bed at all.

The *aim of treatment* is to prevent recurrence of the acute attack, to avoid heart defect, or, if this has occurred, to prevent it becoming worse. Treatment would, therefore, include complete rest in bed till three weeks *after* symptoms of acute illness had ceased, together with the removal of foci for septic infections, such as tonsils or teeth.

There would be a graduated return to normal activity with country air and sunlight and constant medical care, with satisfactory food, sleep and special educational arrangements. Children who have to stay in bed for so long get backward and possibly valetudinarian in attitude. Some four hours' school a day helps them to make up what they have lost and gives interest and occupation. Classes may be taken while the children are reclining in chairs in order to give the heart as much rest as possible.

The teaching is done out-of-doors in summer and a feature

is made of handwork; there are indoor and outdoor games and physical training and dancing for the fitter children. There must be *no competitive element*, nor must the children be pushed to cover assignments of work. To stimulate an

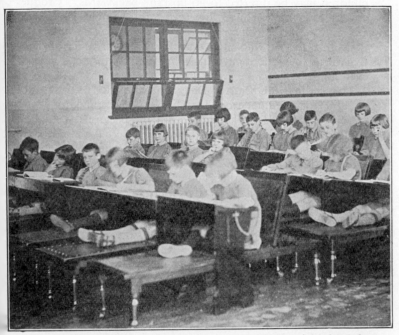

FIG. 147.—Semi-open-air classroom in a residential special school for *Cardiac and Rheumatic Children*, showing the special reclining couches, the use of which rests the heart. Note in the background the window with lower panes in the form of a hopper-shaped opening, which directs the incoming air upwards into the room, thus preventing direct draughts. (*From " Acute Rheumatism " (Public Health Report, No.* 44), *by permission of the Controller of H.M. Stationery Office and the Birmingham Education Committee.*)

interest in reading is of value. Knitting and card games and dominoes are useful to help choreitic children to re-establish muscle co-ordinations. Suitable vocational training is supplied for elder children who are handicapped in their choice of work in later life and need help. There is a teaching and a nursing staff, and classes are not larger than twenty to twenty-five in number.

Gain in weight is a sound indication of progress in health in these children. To avoid heart-strain from hurrying, children may be directed to go upstairs backwards. Croquet and clock golf are played, but few if any ball-chasing games. Choreitic children will not usually start school work until after their first month and then only for an hour a day. They remain at the school anything from six months to a year or even longer.

The ordinary Open-Air Day School of Recovery is not suitable for rheumatic children because the standard would be too competitive and happily active, and because the children would have to sleep in their own homes where the atmosphere would probably be hot and stuffy, and so equal to a harmful change of temperature. Convalescent Residential Homes also give too stimulating and boisterous an environment. Schools for Physically Defectives may take children crippled by permanent heart defect as an after-effect of rheumatism, but for children actually rheumatic, the environment is again over-stimulating and competitive.

After Care

The value of the Home of Recovery is almost entirely lost unless there is efficient *after care*. Voluntary workers follow up the patient, give advice and induce parents to let children attend an out-patient department of a hospital or a rheumatism clinic, and find openings in suitable types of work.

Preventive measures include the education of parents by the distribution of leaflets and by talks at welfare centres ; early enucleation of tonsils, the keeping of a rheumatism register in school of children likely to become rheumatic and the examination of them at Rheumatism Supervising Centres. The *pre-rheumatic child*, debilitated, sub-normal and malnourished (*not* the child actually with rheumatism) benefits by attendance at an ordinary open-air day school.

In adults, rheumatism reduces industrial efficiency. It costs the National Insurance Health Scheme £5,000,000 a year, and the workers in lost wages some £17,000,000 a year. Relapses due to return to old conditions are frequent. Patients may, for example, return to intemperate habits such as over-eating, to predisposing work, such as stoking or gardening, or to bad conditions such as damp houses, mental anxiety and overwork. There are 2400 deaths a year from rheumatic heart disease, and practically every death from heart disease under forty-five is reckoned as being due to rheumatism. Prevention here, as in tuberculosis, is better than cure, and prevention depends on better housing and food and more knowledge, in the spread of which enlightened teachers can take their part.

Note to p. 369.

The giving to rheumatic convalescent children of massive doses of *penicillin* by the mouth is found to prevent the recurrence of acute rheumatism and tonsilitis. The penicillin is taken in glucose three-quarters of an hour before breakfast over periods of years.

Chapter XXXI

MATERNITY WELFARE
AND THE PRE-SCHOOL CHILD

The first compulsory medical inspection of school children occurs when they enter school. This inspection, when first instituted, quickly made clear that already by this age a large number of preventable defects had developed. These arrest and upset the child's rhythms of growth, make him less happy and more fractious to deal with, lessen his ability to profit by school, are expensive to treat and may well, to some extent, affect his development as a child, an adolescent, and even as an adult.

The principal remediable defects found in school entrants include skin diseases such as impetigo, sores, ringworm, scabies and eczematous conditions ; external eye diseases such as blepharitis and conjunctivitis ; defective vision and squint ; enlarged tonsils and adenoids ; ear discharges ; anæmia and malnutrition ; deformities from tuberculosis, infantile paralysis and rickets ; tubercular glands of the neck and decayed and defective teeth.

It is obvious that these defects are often produced through carelessness and ignorance, carelessness as to the spread of infection, ignorance as to the need for adequate food, sleep and cleanliness. In addition, more than half the school entrants have already had measles and nearly as many whooping-cough, both diseases calling for long and careful convalescence to avoid severe after-effects.

The children examined are those who have weathered the impeding difficulties to growth and health. Numbers of the babies born never do reach school age, succumbing to conditions that maim so many school entrants. The most dangerous year of life is the first, and every year a child can survive after that makes it more likely that he will reach maturity.

374

Infant Mortality Rate

The *Infant Mortality Rate* is the death-rate, per 1,000 live births, of children under one year of age. In 1944 the rate was 45. This is among the best measures of the health of any

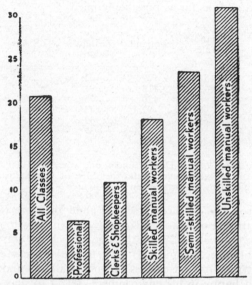

FIG. 148.—Column graph of Infant Mortality in differing social groups. *Infant Mortality* records do not usually state the actual number of deaths but indicate the number of infants, out of every 1,000 born, who die between the ages of 3 and 12 months. The last five columns therefore show the relative infant death rate in the various social classes in 1930–32, not the actual number of deaths in any one class. (*Based on a graph in " A Charter for Health "—George Allen & Unwin, Ltd.*)

community, because a low Infant Mortality Rate correlates highly with good general education in the parents with which goes the intelligence to realise the value of and to make use of maternity and infant welfare facilities. Ignorant people will not take the necessary trouble. The Neo-mortality Rate is the death rate per 1,000 live births of infants during the first month

13

of life. Premature births account for about half of these deaths.

Community health can be thus compared over a series of years or city by city, and wherever the rate is lowest the methods there used to produce the good result can be investigated and, as far as possible, copied.

	England & Wales	Scotland	New Zealand (Whites)	U.S.A.	Holland
1871–75	151	127	102	..	..
1881–85	139	118	91	..	181
1901–05	138	120	75	..	136
1921–25	76	92	43	74	64
1936–40	55	76	32	51	37
1941	59	82	36	45	..
1942	49	69	29	40	..

Infant Mortality Rates.—Deaths under one year per 1000 live births. This kind of table demonstrates the value of vital statistics. What deductions can you make from these figures?

The problems of the pre-school child then are (i) how to preserve the life of infants up to one year, (ii) how to safeguard the pre-school child up to the age of school entry against preventable defects, and (iii) how to make every child, not just free from obvious illness but physically fit and mentally alert, and happy in his environment, ready to play and with that natural vigour that everyone recognises readily enough in puppies and kittens.

Causes of Infant Mortality

The *chief causes of infant mortality* are abortions, still and premature births, wrong feeding and respiratory disease, measles and whooping-cough.

Wrong feeding tends to take its toll more in summer when flies are plentiful and milk goes sour readily, when kept in a hot ill-ventilated place. Epidemic infant diarrhœa, and enteritis (inflammation of the intestine) are also prevalent at this season. The installation of a water carriage instead of a pail and closet system of sewage disposal has a marked effect in reducing the incidence of infant diarrhœa.

Respiratory conditions such as catarrh, bronchitis and pneumonia are more prevalent in the winter, and they may be related to the after-effects of neglected measles and whooping-cough. Proprietary soothing syrups for babies often contain opium or laudanum and, if given ignorantly in too frequent doses, may even cause the child's death. The fractiousness for which the syrup is given is probably due to improper feeding, and the cause, whatever it may be, should be found and treated. Infant welfare centres combat such dangerous and expensive ignorance.

It has been said that the child's early environment is the mother. Thus, if the mother's health and welfare is supervised so that she has the vigour to do the best for her child, and if she can be taught how to treat herself and her child, and can be encouraged to emulate the standard of nurture of other careful mothers she meets, then infant mortality will decrease, and there will be more healthy happy babies growing up.

The Pre-natal Clinic

The care of the mother should begin before the child's birth. The *ante-natal or pre-natal clinic* gives advice to pregnant women about the management of their health, and acts as a centre for social health service and education about maternity welfare. Possibilities of difficulty at birth can be foreseen and guarded against to the advantage of both mother and child. Permits for extra food are given. The mother is also further advised after the birth about re-establishing her health.

The *Midwives Act* (1900) established a register of midwives, similar to the medical and legal registers, of women authorised to attend a woman at a normal birth, without calling in a doctor, save in certain eventualities. Midwives attend about half the births in England and Wales. Until this Act, any woman could undertake the responsibility however ignorant or lacking in skill. No midwife can now be put on the register without passing a recognised examination and thus showing evidence of having attained a certain degree of skill. The county councils and local authorities supervise the work of midwives, and any midwife having a case of ophthalmia neonatorum or of puerperal fever, or guilty of other negligence, may be reported to the Central Midwives Board and her name, for repeated carelessness, struck off the register, thus causing her to lose her right to practise and her livelihood.

The *Notification of Births Act* (1907 and 1915) made it obligatory for births to be notified to the district medical officer of health (in addition to registering the birth) within the first thirty-six hours. This enables the *health visitor* to follow up the case by a friendly personal visit within two or three days of birth. The health visitor aims at consulting with the midwife before the latter ceases to attend the case, and the health visitor makes some eight visits during the first year after birth, continuing the visits at intervals up to school age. Advice needs to be practical and personal, to be given in an authoritative yet unassuming way and to be reiterated tactfully. The health visitor may combine the work of a school nurse and tuberculosis visitor. She is usually a trained nurse and possibly a certificated midwife or maternity nurse (a nurse who attends only births supervised by a doctor), and she may have had training as a sanitary inspector.

Child Welfare

Post-natal work includes that of maternity and child welfare centres, baby clinics, schools for mothers and mothers' clubs in connection with nursery schools, at all of which, in varying degrees, talks and advice are given on the baby's and mother's health. A good deal depends on the personal contacts and interest of the staff, doctors, nurses, voluntary workers with the mother and child, and on the social interest of meeting other mothers with similar problems. Facilities for buying dried milk, fish liver oil and orange juice, free or at cost price, classes for simple sewing of children's garments, and homely addresses, followed by questions and discussion, on the value of ante-natal care, food and cooking, fresh air and sunlight, thrift devices, breast and artificial feeding, teething, sleep, sex teaching, are only some of the possibilities. Infant Welfare Centres are grant-earning if established by a local authority.

These welfare activities, under whatever name, are primarily educational and aim at keeping healthy babies healthy. The Baby Clinic, however, is for the treatment of children who are ill. The one service works closely in touch with the other. Mothers are asked to bring all children under five to the welfare centres. The Pre-natal Clinic is usually conducted as a department of the Infant Welfare Centre.

Aims of Mothercraft Teaching

An indirect but important way of spreading mother-craft knowledge is by *the teaching of mothercraft in the schools to older girls.* This is of value because the older girls often help with the younger children at home, and they may put into practice the teaching given to them at school and tell their mothers about it. Also, though they will not probably set up a home of their own for some years after leaving school, and by this time may well have forgotten much of the mothercraft taught them, yet the impression of its value and interest may be sufficiently lasting to induce them to take advantage of the maternity and child welfare facilities that exist.

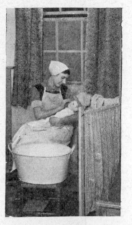

FIG. 149. — Secondary school girl learning mothercraft by bathing and dressing a life-size baby doll. (*Courtesy of L.C.C.*)

The teaching should be as practical as possible. Every girl should have a chance to make up a bottle for a baby, and undress and dress and bath the life-sized model baby doll. With this should go teaching on such topics as the value of scrupulous cleanliness and care of the baby, the dangers of dust and of using a comforter, and the signs of indigestion in a baby. Some ordinary household routine such as how to make a bed, how to light a fire, and how to lay the weekly money out and administer to the best advantage might also be included.

The work can be taken in connection with the domestic science course or by a member of the school staff who has a special interest and training in the subject. Occasional visiting teachers are less valuable because they cannot know the home circumstances of the girls, nor get into such personal touch with them, nor give sufficient time for each girl to have her turn at the various forms of practical work—at washing the baby, for instance.

It is sometimes possible for the girls following the school course to give time to helping in a crèche or day nursery, thus getting experience with real babies. To transfer the teaching

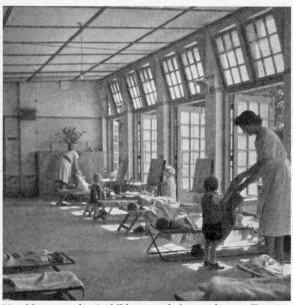

FIG. 150.—Nursery school children at their rest hour. Two kinds of beds are shown. The wooden kind is the more satisfactory, because it allows more clearance from the floor. (*Crown copyright reserved.*)

to the crèche is a mistake, as a busy day-nursery staff has not the time to teach the girls as well as to do their own work.

The infant welfare centre supervises the health of the infant in arms. The Nursery School, or Nursery Class, bridges the gap from 2–5 years, when the child enters the Infant School proper.

The *Day Nursery or Crèche* is a centre where mothers, who go out to work during the day, can leave their young children to be cared for, in some cases on payment. The nursing staff feeds and tends the children, but does not pretend to offer teaching. Such provision is grant-earning.

The Nursery School

The *Nursery School*, for children from two to five years of age, of which the Rachel Macmillan School at Deptford was the pioneer, aims at giving that nurture and training in health habits, with the chance to grow up happily, mentally and physically, that a good home gives. Its work is thus partly medical, partly educational in the broad sense and partly social, and it is much more than a place where children are " minded," as in a crèche, though actually it does relieve harassed mothers.

Some nursery schools are held in adapted private houses with large gardens, others in buildings designed for the purpose but again with plenty of surrounding space. To be useful the school must be in the centre of the district from which it draws its children, and this sometimes makes it difficult to provide essential garden space. At first it was thought desirable to limit the size of the nursery school to from forty to fifty children for fear of the rapid spread of epidemics, but by doing most of the work out-of-doors this danger can be obviated, and schools up to 160 children are now used. The larger numbers make for considerably cheaper running costs per head than in a smaller school.

There must be easy access from the buildings to the gardens, and all possible sun be caught. Verandas may here be useful so long as they do not obscure light. The playground should be partly paved for use in damp weather, and there should be bright flower beds, a sand pit, and provision for keeping pets. Each classroom, which may be used for play, sleep or meals, needs floor space of at least 15 square feet per child. Floor heating is an expensive but satisfactory form of heating. An even temperature of from 56° to 60° F. is desirable.

The hours vary in different schools, but are usually from nine till four. A midday rest of up to two hours compensates for the children's often disturbed or late nights at home. All rest and work are taken out of doors in the sun and air whenever possible. The child usually gets a light meal (milk and biscuits) on arrival, a two-course midday meal and a light tea before going home. There are plenty of chances for games and physical activities that foster unhampered growth. A jungle gym for climbing, a slide or chute, bouncing board and see-saw meet the children's natural age interest. To prevent rickets children need exercise as well as sunshine and food containing Calcium. It is difficult for tenement and flat dwellers to give sufficient exercise in the open air to their toddlers.

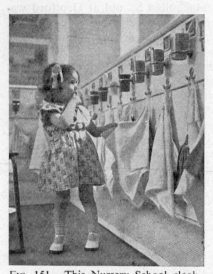

FIG. 151.—This Nursery School cloakroom is light and airy. It shows the children's individual pegs with towel, mug, tooth brush. The child's height shows that the pegs are so placed that the children can use them themselves without adult help. (*Courtesy of Dr. Hamilton Hogben.*)

The children are examined medically on admission, and, before they pass on to the elementary school, such defects as squint, external eye infections, enlarged tonsils and adenoids, faulty teeth, middle ear defects, rickets, ringworm and general states of debility receive treatment so that the effects are lessened or eliminated.

" Skilled Neglect "

The expression " skilled neglect " sums up the nursery school teacher's objective. The average adult attitude to a child's early and inept efforts to do simple things for himself is to do them for him, either from a feeling of impatience or from the rather patronising pleasure in being omnipotent. The nursery school teacher's aim is to let the child do everything that he can for himself, to give him confidence, thus making him an easier and pleasanter small person to have in the home. He is used to trying to do things for himself, and since he is at least beginning to feel self-reliant and able, he does not cry for help at any slight difficulty. The example of other children helps here.

The child is encouraged to enjoy and take an interest in bathing, washing and teeth cleaning ; he helps to lay the tables (some 17 inches high only) for meals, to clear them afterwards, and to keep the room tidy. Though some suggestions about activities are given, as far as possible each child chooses his own, and no child is forced to use particular apparatus or to join in specific playing or singing. Every child, however, is guided to put away for himself apparatus he gets out.

The fact that all the furniture is small size gives confidence ; the child feels that he lives in an environment of his own and not in a giant adult-size environment. In cloakrooms pegs rather less than a yard up from the ground allow each child to hang up his own clothes without help. Pedestal water closets, 6 to 9 inches from the ground, are provided with chains long enough for the children to reach and pull them. Shower baths are advised, both because they are bracing and because they help to avoid the spread of infection.

The regularity of the small routine of a nursery school, as of being seen by the nurse on arrival, of carefully set meals, of washing and teeth cleaning, of tending pets and of group singing, all help the child to fit himself readily into such regularity in later life, to prefer it and to be self-controlled about it, without feeling coerced or misunderstood. Speech training is given, and the children are encouraged to talk, to use words, and to get over shyness and be friendly. Any teaching of reading and counting is quite subsidiary to the school's main aim, and may well be omitted.

The teachers need to be satisfactorily qualified so that the child is not just minded but is guided to develop socially, physically and mentally by his own experiments and interested activity. The nursery school may have a mother's club connected with it. It certainly should be linked with one, and do its part in educating the parents in the care of their children.

13*

The Nursery Class

The *Nursery Class* is one for children under the Education Act, 1944, from two to five. It is run in conjunction with an infant school. The children are trained in health habits and have something of the same routine as in the nursery school, but they go home at midday, coming back to a camp-bed rest. A good deal of difference of opinion existed as to whether development should be by way of nursery schools or of nursery classes. The classes are cheaper to run, and have been widely and quickly developed.

The *Nursery School* provision is more comprehensive but dearer. It has to be run as a separate institution, and at present children enter such few nursery schools as exist by recommendation of the school medical officer, and are mostly delicate or from specially difficult homes. In 1939 there were nursery school places for approximately 10,000 children only in England and Wales.

The matter lies rather between practical immediate but lesser benefits of the nursery class against more expensive, ultimately better, but more likely to be deferred benefits of the nursery school.

Under the Education Act, 1944, it has become the duty of the Local Education Authority, in the words of the Act, " to have regard to the needs for securing that provision is made for pupils who have not attained the age of 5 years " by the provision of Nursery Schools or Nursery Classes. Medical Inspection and free treatment must also be provided under the Acts. This should benefit the children directly and also by increasing the spread of knowledge among mothers of how to care for the infant and toddler.

Chapter XXXII

PUBLIC HEALTH—THE SCHOOL MEDICAL SERVICE—SPECIAL SCHOOLS

It can readily be recognised that the health of the school child is bound up with the health of the community and that many aspects of health have been touched on in this book that are outside the strict boundaries of any school medical service. Hence a short summary of the responsibilities that the State accepts for community health follows as an introduction to the consideration of the School Medical Service.

The Minister of Health, who changes according to the government in power, is responsible to Parliament for the work of the Ministry of Health. The Ministry's function, through its permanent officials, is to advise and exhort Local Authorities as to what the law requires of them and to try to get a uniformly high standard of health practice throughout the country. Money grants from taxes are payable to Local Authorities, if the services they maintain are of a satisfactory standard. These grants have to be supplemented by money from the local rates.

It is therefore the Local Authorities (City, Borough, County, Urban and Rural District Councils) who, through their Public Health Departments, implement the rulings of the Ministry of Health.

Public Health Departments

The Local Authority *Public Health Department* is presided over by the Medical Officer of Health, who, with his staff of Assistant Medical Officers, Sanitary Inspectors, Health Visitors, Midwives, Food Inspectors and other officials, carry the Ministry's rulings into effect. The main activities of any Public Health Department can be summarised under six heads.

(i) *The Collection of Vital Statistics.* These include the

385

			I	II	III	IV
1.		Date of Inspection				
2.		Age				
3.		Standard				
4.		Attendance				
5.		Height (inches)				
6.		Weight (pounds)				
7.		Clothing				
8.		Footgear				
9.		Cleanliness—Head				
		,, Body				
10.		Nutrition				
11.	Skin	Ringworm, Head				
12.	Skin	,, Body				
13.	Skin	Scabies				
14.	Skin	Impetigo				
15.	Skin	Other Diseases				
16.	Eye	Blepharitis				
17.	Eye	Conjunctivitis				
18.	Eye	Other Conditions				
19.	Eye	Vision R.				
20.	Eye	,, L.				
21.	Eye	Squint				
22.	Ear	Hearing				
23.	Ear	Otitis media				
24.	Ear	Other Diseases				
25.	Nose & Throat	Tonsils				
26.	Nose & Throat	Adenoids				
27.	Nose & Throat	Other Conditions				
28.		Cervical Glands				
29.		Speech				
30.		Teeth—Number decayed				
31.		,, Condition				
32.		Heart and Circulation				
33.		Anæmia				
34.		Lungs				
35.	Tuberculosis	Pulmonary				
36.	Tuberculosis	Non-Pulmonary				
37.	Nervous System	Epilepsy				
38.	Nervous System	Chorea				
39.	Nervous System	Other Conditions				
40.	Deformities	Rickets				
41.	Deformities	Spinal Curvature				
42.	Deformities	Other Forms				
43.		Other Defects and Diseases				
44.		Mental Conditions				
45.		Initials of Medical Officer				

FIG. 152.—A sample School Medical Record card. Can you decide why piece of information is wanted? (*By courtesy of E. J. Arnold & Son,*

Birth, Death, Infant Mortality, Maternal Mortality and Marriage Rates. These rates are stated per 1000 of the population and are a measure whereby the health of any community can be assessed and compared (i) with its own figures for former years or (ii) with communities with like problems. Vital statistics prevent feelings of complacency and show where a higher standard of effort is needed.

(ii) *Control of Infectious Diseases.* This comprises the organisation of Isolation Hospital services, vaccination, immunisation, the care of Tuberculosis patients in the home and in sanatoria, and the treatment of venereal disease.

(iii) *Maternity and Child Welfare Services.* This embraces the provision of Ante-natal Clinics, maternity beds in hospital, a " home " midwifery service, day nurseries and infant welfare centres.

(iv) *Supervision of Food Supplies* to ensure clean, healthy, good quality food. This comprises the taking of food samples to check that they are (i) up to the required standard as food and (ii) not carrying infection (*e.g.* milk, meat), and the regulation of the handling, storing and marketing of foods.

(v) *Supervision of Environment.* This includes the control of sanitation factors in and around dwellings, that might be detrimental to health—technically " nuisances." The provision of satisfactory water supplies and the disposal of sewage are included here.

(vi) *Housing.* The condemning of slum property, the removal of slums and re-housing is a responsibility of the Public Health Department. The Medical Officer reports to the Local Authority, which must then decide on what action shall be taken.

(vii) The *School Medical Service* is at present administered by the Local Education Authority but often the area Medical Officer is also the School Medical Officer. Under the new Health Service proposals these services merge.

None of these Health Services will be effective unless the general public are sufficiently enlightened and informed to know their value and to support them in practice. Legal sanctions are essential for strength but people who only carry out what they are legally compelled to do, do only a grudging minimum. In combating ignorance and in forming public opinion, teachers have had and can have an important place.

L.A. " Powers " and " Duties "

It should be noted that there is considerable difference in law between what is a " power " and what is a " duty " for a Local Education Authority. A " power " need not be exercised and whereas progressive and wealthy authorities are likely to use their " powers," poorer smaller authorities may not choose to do so. Under the Education Act, 1944, a number of " powers " have now become " duties " as, for example, the provision of free medical treatment for school children. The *School Medical Service* was inaugurated legally by the Act of 1907 which introduced the medical inspection of school children. The widespread disabilities that it revealed made arrangement for treatment necessary. The aim of the service is to fit the child to benefit by education and to build up a robust population.

The Education Act, 1944, has made Medical Inspection of all school children compulsory and has made it a duty of every local education authority to secure the provision of free medical treatment for pupils. Treatment, however, is not compulsory.

The School Medical Service

The school medical service employs school doctors, dentists and nurses, who give treatment and advice in school clinics, and at special schools. They also deal with and minimise school outbreaks of infectious disease, and give general supervision and advice on school sanitation and building as far as these affect the health of the school population. Each child is inspected at least three times during his school life : on entrance, after attaining the age of eight, and after twelve or on leaving. Kerr considers a yearly inspection desirable, the teacher possibly making the first selection, the school nurse reviewing these, and the doctor seeing those she finally puts forward.

The *medical inspection* must be held during school hours. A card record of each child is kept. The school nurse may test

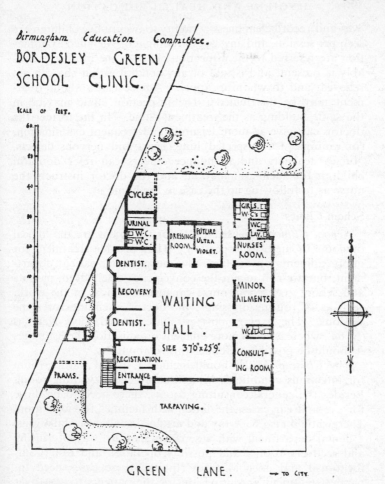

Birmingham Education Committee.
BORDESLEY GREEN
SCHOOL CLINIC.

FIG. 153.—A typical small school clinic. The children recovering from dental treatment do not return immediately to the waiting hall to produce fears in those still to be treated. (*By courtesy of City of Birmingham Education Department.*)

eyes and record cleanliness ; twenty to twenty-five children are seen per session, and any cases needing more detailed examination are referred to the inspection clinic. The mother preferably is present, and is told of any condition that she can get relieved, and to whom to apply. Advice cards about treatment may be distributed. The inspection clinic may be in the same building as the treatment clinic. In the former the doctor can give a more leisurely and frequent examination, for example, for suspected lung, heart and nervous defects. Nurses, teachers and attendance officers can refer doubtful children for such examination, and the doctor instructs the nurse as to following up the case in the home.

School Clinics

School Clinics (legalised 1921) for treatment are the logical outcome of medical inspection. They provide treatment for minor ailments on the lines of a hospital out-patient department, but are run to suit the convenience of children, parents and school. A school nurse can manage most of the work, such as of routine dressings, the doctor attending for some sessions. The average cost per case treated, says Kerr, is 7s. 6d., whereas, with more efficient organisation, he estimates it should be possible to reduce this to about 2s.

The *Clinic premises* should include a special waiting-room for infectious conditions, as well as a general waiting room. Besides the general consulting rooms, there need to be those for eye and ear cases, the latter with facilities for ionisation. There should also be X-ray and artificial sunlight installations, a dental department with a separate exit by way of rinsing and recovery rooms, and possibly operation and rest rooms for tonsil and adenoid cases (though these cases need in-patient treatment and provision for the patients to stay over night).

The *conditions treated* include (i) minor ailments, such as vermin in children, scabies, impetigo, ringworm (for which one sitting plus attendance for a month is usually sufficient) ; (ii) eye diseases, such as blepharitis, pink eye, squint, short- and long-sight and astigmatism (the authority is empowered to supply glasses free or at cost price, and nearly all now do so) ;

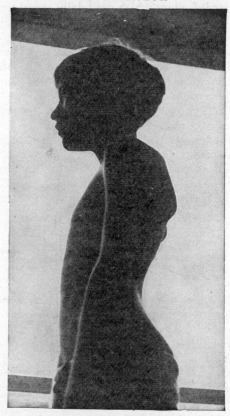

FIG. 154.—*Round upper back* and some degree of hollow back in the waist region. Notice the forward thrust of the head, the slack abdominal muscles and the general loss in height (contrast Frontispiece). Such a posture might be caused by muscular weakness, rapid growth, and accentuated by bad furniture and ventilation. It might also be aggravated by bad eyesight and mental weakness. Hollow back causes decreased inspiration and fatigue in standing and walking. Such postural deformity cannot be spontaneously outgrown. (*From " School Orthopædics "—George Simpson & Co., Devizes, Ltd.*)

(iii) middle ear infections which need daily expert treatment to clear them up; (iv) crippling from tuberculosis, rickets, infantile paralysis; slack posture or flat-foot for which massage, remedial exercises and electric treatment needs to be provided; (v) tonsils and adenoids; (vi) dental decay; and (vii) first stages of such diseases as rheumatism, chorea, heart defect and tuberculosis.

Certain children will be recommended for appropriate special school education. Not all authorities, however, maintain so fully equipped a clinic as this. Massage and X-ray treatments may, for instance, be given in conjunction with local hospitals, as may also treatment for adenoids and tonsils. Some county areas provide caravan clinics, mostly dental; some employ peripatetic doctors, dentists, and nurses who spend three or four days at different small centres. Under the Education Act, 1944, it is the duty of every local education authority to secure that comprehensive facilities for free medical treatment are available.

Results of School Medical Service

The *results of the school medical service*, after nearly forty years' working, show that the average school-leaver is taller and heavier and better nourished than he was. The handicaps of defects of vision and hearing are lessened, there are fewer children with crippling deformities and more children of cleanly habits. Less school time and education was lost now from neglected inflammatory conditions of eyes, ears and skin; the teeth are in better condition.

Thus the leaver has a better chance of turning out a healthy, self-respecting, happy citizen, who will keep himself and be unlikely to become a charge on the community. Such inferences are not the results of the unreliable, but common, method of arguing from the particular to the general on insufficient data, but are conclusions based on statistics collected over the whole country over a series of years. One function of the school medical service is to collect statistics, which show where weakness lies and where public money needs to be spent.

There are still backward authorities who ought to bring the facilities they offer up to standard, so that children in all areas may benefit equally ; and there is need for better teaching of hygiene and health education in schools, and for still more complete understanding and co-operation with the school medical service by the parent and the general public. It is the local authority that finally co-ordinates the health services of any area.

Everyone possibly shares the natural tendency to be excited to sympathy by cases of acute distress or disease ; preventive health work is less spectacular and excites less interest because it aims at eliminating such crises, which upset family life, cause undue expense and may result in permanent individual disability. The family as well as the country that lacks history is, in fact, relatively fortunate.

Special Education.—Part of the duty of the school medical officer is, as has been noted, to recommend defective children for special education and, under the Education Act, 1944, it is the duty of the Local Education Authority to provide such special education facilities. The sanatorium school, home for recovery for rheumatic children, mentally defectives' school, and schools and classes for the blind and deaf have been dealt with already. Other special education for which the authority provides facilities includes the day open-air recovery school and the school for physically defectives.

Open Air Recovery School

The open-air school ideal arose from early methods of treating tuberculosis, and it benefits normal equally with delicate children. The trend of school building design is towards the open-air type. Open-air arrangements include classes taken in the playgrounds, in parks or in a bandstand, classrooms that can be converted by opening up the sides, school camps and school journeys as well as the open-air recovery school for delicate children, which may be residential or day, more often the latter.

The aim of the *day open-air recovery school* is to provide nurture and education for children who are temporarily delicate. The school gives nourishing food, fresh air and sunlight, with the opportunity for keeping up educationally with the age standard so that the delicate child can regain strength and vitality to return to the ordinary primary or secondary school. The school population is thus continually changing, the children staying for from six months to a year, but longer or shorter periods are possible.

The children found to benefit from open-air school attendance include (i) those suffering from malnutrition, anæmia and rickets ; (ii) pre-tubercular children and those with tubercular glands of the neck, and delicate children living in the same house as a consumptive patient ; (iii) children convalescent after long and debilitating disease, such as whooping-cough, measles and pneumonia, or after an operation for adenoids or tubercular glands of the neck ; (iv) children with chronic and stubborn external eye disease, such as blepharitis when associated with malnutrition ; (v) certain types only of crippled and myopic children ; (vi) nervous and pre-rheumatic children.

The *school site* should allow of spacious gardens and playing space, and should preferably be on the city outskirts where air is purer and sunlight the less obscured by smoke. The children often come to school by special bus or tram, in which latter case the site must not be too far from the tram terminus. Light dry soil and a south aspect protected by trees from winds are desirable.

The buildings may be an adapted private house, an existing school building or a new building, possibly prefabricated. There must be provision for teaching, dining and resting ; and the building should be so far compact as to facilitate service while keeping the advantage that spread-out plan gives ; for example, classrooms that can be thrown open on three, or even on all sides. The use of light trestle tables and folding desks allows rooms to be readily adapted for different purposes, such as dining, resting or teaching. Each child needs a locker in lieu of a fixed desk.

The continuous classroom arrangement, as in the Staffordshire type of school (see p. 79), allows opening on only two sides, usually north and south. The twin classroom plan, each room opening on three sides, or the individual classroom opening on all sides, is preferable. Glazed french windows all round, or a low surrounding wall with canvas protection above as necessary, are provided, the latter being cheaper.

The essential point is to have quick, easy methods of closing and opening the sides of the classroom to meet changing weather conditions and to avoid draught round the feet. Verandas, because they make classrooms dark and add to initial costs, are not advised.

Heating is of value rather to dry unpleasantly damp air than to provide warmth and, in bad weather, for its comforting

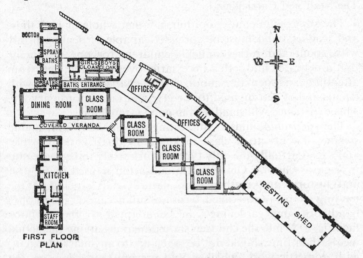

FIG. 155.—Plan of *an Open-Air School*, showing classrooms able to be opened on three sides. Note (i) that only the ground floor is used by the children, (ii) that there are verandas and paved ways to the offices and resting shed, (iii) that the planning of the buildings ensures quietness during rest periods, and (iv) which part of the school gets the sun during school hours. (*Buildings adapted from Clay's " Modern School "—B. T. Batsford Ltd.*)

psychological effect. Any heating method is possible, but a modern type of slow combustion stove, which in an ill-ventilated classroom would be condemned, is a cheap and possible heat source under open-air conditions. Some authorities prefer under-floor heating by low-pressure pipes.

Ample *lavatory and cloakroom* accommodation is necessary, as children are in school all day and will all need to use it before meals. Training in health habits is part of the school's work, and each child should have his own towel, hair and tooth-brush and be supervised in using them. Each should have his own blanket, cane or stretcher rest-bed and mackintosh cape. Spray or shower baths with dressing-rooms are necessary, and there must be examination and treatment rooms for minor ailments. If there is a rest shed, it can be used also for physical exercises and games in wet weather.

The Staff and Curriculum

The *staff* include, a school nurse, either whole or part time, and teachers who must be specially capable of dealing firmly with spoilt and rather difficult children, for one advantage that a delicate child, often necessarily over-cosseted, gets from attending an open-air school, is the chance of mixing with equals and of getting used to the give and take of ordinary life. This experience will stand him in good stead later.

The *curriculum* aims at interesting the child, without undue strain. Twenty to a class makes individual work possible, and this is actually the only type of work likely to be successful in such a school. Outdoor dramatisation is used in English and history, and mathematics, nature study, including the tending of pets (not caged birds in small cages), geography, handwork and gardening can be adapted to the outdoor facilities. While the children should help in serving the actual meals, their time should not be taken up, to any marked extent, with domestic work, which would prevent them from getting full benefit from the open-air conditions they need. Physical exercises, dancing and games are included as the child's health allows him to benefit.

The school doctor and dentist attend, the former weekly. Children are usually weighed fortnightly, and careful medical records are kept. Three meals a day, breakfast, dinner and tea, are generally given, and the diet should include first-class protein, fat and vitamins. Additional milk may be ordered for particular children, but soups and liquid foods, as a substitute for solids, are on the whole to be avoided. Meals should be appetising and well served, and behaviour at them supervised.

A feature of the open-air school is *the midday rest* after

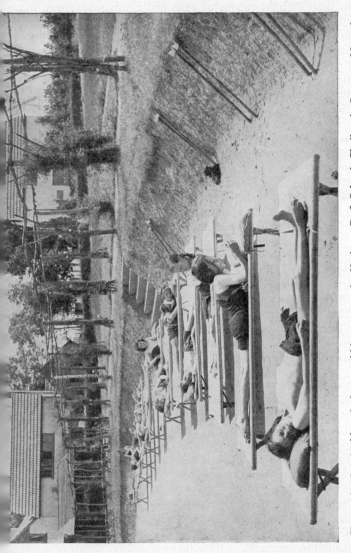

Fig. 156.—Sun-bathing during a midday rest at the Heritage Craft School, Chailey, in Sussex. Note the light type of bed with a washable and removable cover. (*Reproduced by kind permission of the Heritage Craft School, Chailey.*)

dinner for from one to two hours, in the open air whenever possible. A light canvas or cane bed is advisable ; rest in a deck chair is less valuable. Extra clothing, a jersey or overcoat, is generally provided for sitting work. Clogs, felt lined, may be supplied, and there should certainly be arrangements for drying damp shoes. However, the less clothing worn the better, ultimately.

Results show that improved metabolism gives a sense of well-being and happiness, combined with a ready interest in school activities rather than in a self-centred interest in their own ailments. In the open-air school colds and infections rarely spread, and bad school attenders attend regularly. Open-air classes, in connection with the ordinary school, are less valuable than Open-Air Schools because of the lack of provision for (i) rest, (ii) meals, (iii) baths and showers, and (iv) routine medical supervision.

Many local education authorities support a modified form of open-air education in *a school camp*, often with semi-permanent buildings in country or seaside surroundings, and here normal children come in batches, staying for longer or shorter periods. Teachers volunteer to accompany children from their school, and a modified educational programme is carried out. The parents may be asked to contribute towards the cost. The benefits of nutritious food, a health habit-forming regime, an outdoor country holiday and an enjoyable community life are given.

School for Physically Defective Children

The School for Physically Defective Children may be day or residential, more usually the former. It makes provision for children to the age of sixteen, as in a school for retarded children. The school gives treatment and education with suitable vocational training in the last years of the course. After-care committees help leavers to find work and supervise its conditions.

Children attending the physically defective or cripple school include those disabled through tuberculosis of the bones or joints, or through infantile paralysis, rickets, congenital deformity or accident, or those permanently disabled by heart defect, often of rheumatic origin. Advanced tuberculosis cases with open wounds are not suitable for day schools.

Arrangements are often made to collect the children, who stay all day in school, by motor. There may be full-time nursing and massage members of the staff to give remedial and sunlight treatment. Apart from actual mental defect, physically defective children tend to be mentally retarded and possibly to indulge in self-pity. In a cripple school they need not feel inferior and at a disadvantage, and the aim should be to treat them as normal children, making reasonable demands as to conduct and behaviour. They should be made to feel self-reliant and reasonably ambitious, and as far as possible they should be trained to be self-supporting. Spare-time hobbies are of special value to them. A wide range of interests and opportunities for self-expression must be given. The regime of meals, midday rests and outdoor work whenever possible resembles that of an open-air school. All rooms must be on the ground floor.

Some children may improve so that they can return to the ordinary school, but the majority stay at the physically defectives' school throughout their school life. They are more likely to do well in after-life, given reasonable health, than are the dull children.

Asthma Clinics

In Asthma there is extreme difficulty in breathing out. Treatments that have been successful in individual cases vary widely. It is important to find out what protein causes the attacks in each individual. De-sensitisation against the protein causing the allergy is possible.

In Asthma Clinics the work includes:

(i) Teaching of specific breathing exercises to encourage lower costal breathing and correct and relaxed expiration.

(ii) Remedial exercises to encourage mobility of the shoulder girdle and chest.

(iii) General exercises and games.

(iv) Teaching of correct posture.

An effort is made to build up the general health of the children without coddling and too solicitous care.

CHAPTER XXXIII

THE SCHOOL BUILDING

A GOOD many points in connection with the design of school buildings have already been touched on in considering the child's make-up, how his eyesight can be guarded, how habits of cleanliness can be formed and how fatigue may be combated. The ordinary class teacher cannot alter and must necessarily accept the school building conditions of the department to which he or she is appointed. Many buildings are old-fashioned, but while the teachers should know what constitutes adequate buildings and what they would like to have, they must also know how and on what lines to make the best of conditions already there, with goodwill and intelligence.

It is now generally recognised that school buildings have, in the past, been built too solidly and permanently; so great an amount of capital has been laid out on them that they are not replaced even when they have become out of date. The tendency now is rather in favour of building schools that may be expected to last only about twenty years so that the next generation will not be tempted to retain buildings that by then may very well have become obsolete in design. Development will thus be less hindered than it now is by heavy, dark, badly ventilated buildings, often pseudo-gothic in style, that are left over from the well-meant but misguided enthusiasms of 1870 onwards.

It is, for instance, generally recognised that an extension of the open-air school type of building, cheap, light, and with classroom walls able to be closed or opened rapidly, would benefit the health of children and teachers, but authorities are reluctant to demolish expensive old buildings, many of which are still sound. Many old-type schools were built to accommodate more than one class in a room. The " big room " meant that several teachers had to teach against each other, thus increasing the strain for the teachers and making attention more difficult for the children.

Many schools have been damaged during 1939–45 and, under the Education Act, 1944, many additional school buildings will be needed. Schools serving the same age groups tend to need the same standard accommodation all over the country ; for instance, separate classrooms for each class, a hall, a gymnasium, a library, kitchen, art, craft, laboratory and domestic science rooms, as well as cloak rooms, changing rooms, drying rooms, store rooms, medical inspection room and domestic offices.

Prefabricated School Buildings

In order to hasten the provision of school buildings, it is proposed to construct *prefabricated school buildings* in quantity and on a standard plan. In the same way that on a small scale a greenhouse or garage or fowl pen can be bought in sections, brought to the site and there erected, so on a larger scale it is proposed to erect prefabricated schools.

This will allow of (i) standardisation of construction and fittings, (ii) quick erection and (iii) lessened cost per head of the school population. It will do away with the long-drawn-out procedure necessary to get a school planned on individual lines including, as it does, the making of plans, the passing of these by a committee, the getting of estimates from builders and the agreeing on the cost before the actual building can even start.

Prefabricated school units can be fitted together in varying ground patterns to suit the site available and can be in one or two storeys. Also as a district grows and more school accommodation is needed, additional classrooms can be added as they are wanted. Steel, concrete and timber are materials suggested for use in these prefabricated schools. The outside walls are faced with brick or other customary building material so that the buildings do not look unsightly. The net effect is to get the schools into use at a much earlier date than would be possible under the older system of individual planning.

Chosing Sites for Schools

While *the school site* should be central because of convenience to the children attending, it should preferably not be too near slums or a heavy traffic area or a railway station because of noise, dust, squalor and risk of street accidents. It should have unobscured lighting. A dry site prevents the building being damp, and so reduces the risk of rheumatism. Gravel, sand and chalk soils are best because rain-water drains rapidly through them and the foundations remain dry. Sandstone is moderately porous, whereas clay soils are impervious and they remain damp for a comparatively long period. A damp site is always colder than a dry site because of the evaporation of water which is going on continuously.

Ground Water

Rain-water percolates through the top layer of the soil until it reaches an impervious layer, such as clay, on the surface of which it forms a continually moving body of water, always tending to drain downwards towards the nearest stream. This is called *ground water* and obviously, should there be much rain, the level of ground water would rise until the foundations of any buildings above it were reached.

To combat the dampness of walls from " ground water," in every building there is put *a damp-proof course* of specially prepared brick or slate with a layer of tar above the ground level of the foundations, but below the building's floor level. Other ways of preventing dampness of walls are by digging out the soil, where a building might otherwise impinge on the soil of a hill-side, to make a passage round the building, and also by leaving an air-space inside the wall between the outer and the inner bricks of the wall, so that they do not touch. In jerry-built houses such precautions against damp are often scamped, to the detriment of the people who live in them.

Of the types of school plan, the *central hall school* had considerable vogue at the beginning of this century. Here the classrooms are grouped round the hall either in one or more storeys. The head teacher was supposed to be able to supervise easily from the central hall, but there was the defect that any hall activity, such as dancing or singing, disturbed all the surrounding classrooms, and such halls and the rooms round them, are difficult to ventilate. It was to combat this latter difficulty that the plenum system of ventilation came prominently into use (see Chapter VI).

The better type is the *Pavilion or Staffordshire school*, in

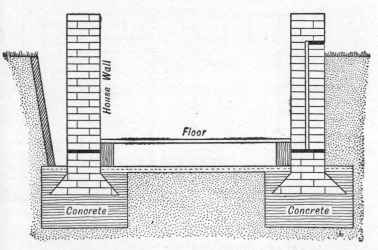

FIG. 157.—Diagram to show two damp-proof courses. The black layers in the brick, of lead or asphalt, prevent damp from travelling to the bricks above. On the left, the earth has been cut away, so that water draining from it reaches the house *below* the damp-proof course. This method is often used for houses built on a hill-side. On the right, two damp-proof courses and an air-space between the outer and inner bricks, keep the inner bricks dry. Note that the floor level is *above* that of the damp-proof courses.

which the classrooms are offset from a fresh-air corridor. The hall adjoins, jutting out from the main block, so that activities in the hall do not disturb work in the classrooms. This building can be spread out to catch the sunlight, and it allows adequate cross ventilation and even favours the conversion to open-sided fresh-air classrooms. No school is now built without a dining-room and kitchen to provide for school meals.

The Playground

The *playground* should be spacious and with all the space in one individual area to allow of seniors playing larger team games. The division of a small but adequate space by a barrier, as is sometimes done in a small mixed school, makes the

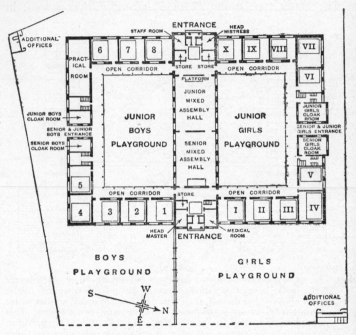

FIG. 158.—Plan of *a Court type of school*. The classrooms of the two schools are numbered in Roman and in Arabic numerals respectively. Note that the two halls are both centrally situated and yet work in them does not disturb that in the classrooms. (*Adapted from Clay's " Modern School Buildings "—B. T. Batsford, Ltd.*)

teaching of games unnecessarily difficult. Gravel or asphalt surfaces have their advantages, for they dry quickly and are hard wearing ; if possible, however, there should be both a covered play space and an area for grass. Jet, cupless drinking fountains, operated by the foot, are desirable. There should certainly be drinking water available either outside or in school, preferably both.

Single storey schools are preferable, but if departments must be one on the top of the other, the infants should have the ground floor, and *stairs* should be at least 4 feet wide, well lighted, walled both sides to prevent accidents, and with frequent landings, at least every fifteen steps, again to break falls and prevent accidents and rest the adolescent heart. There should be hand-rails both sides of the stairs, and two of them, one above the other, for the bigger and smaller children.

Wide exits should allow of emptying the school quietly within three minutes or less. The angle between the wall and floor should be rounded to facilitate cleaning and prevent dust accumulation, and cornices and any fancy decorations that would collect dust are to be avoided. Inset blocks are preferable to plank-length wood floorings. Cork tiles are relatively expensive, but they wear well and are quiet. Rubber flooring is also used.

Cloakrooms should be well lighted and airy. White tiles and paint conserve light and can be readily washed. The pegs must be 18 inches apart, numbered and not arranged one above another so that one child's clothes are on the top of another's. There ought to be facilities for drying clothes as well as hot water for washing, and adequate towels, preferably small individual ones. Paper towels are possible. Continuous flow basins give the children less training than do spring taps that only flow when pressed. The children should be trained to keep and leave the basins clean, a matter that needs supervision (see Chapter XIV).

Heating

Heating must be considered apart from ventilation. It may be by low or high-pressure systems of hot-water pipes, heated panels, electric, coal or gas fires, or by stoves.

Of these, *fires* heat by radiant heat, that does not heat the intervening air (see Chapter VI), but the heat is distributed unequally so that a fire when used must usually be considered as an accessory to some other heating system. Heating by gas and electric fires is expensive but clean. Coal fires make dust and need replenishing, but they give a stimulating variable heat that is healthier, apart from other considerations, than the regular level of heat from gas or electricity.

Stoves are relatively cheap in first and in annual cost, and probably distribute heat better in a room than do open fires. With the exception of anthracite stoves they have to be made up often and need more regulating than open fires and, even if regulated, they may tend to get out of order and smoke more readily than fires, adversely affecting ventilation. The wide use and success of stoves on the Continent suggest that more could be done with them here.

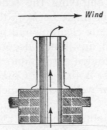

FIG. 159.—As the wind passes over, the pressure of air in a chimney is lessened and air is drawn out of the room below. This shows the value of open chimneys for ventilation even without a fire in the grate.

For heating by hot-water circulation, low-pressure pipes have displaced high-pressure pipes.

Low Pressure Heating

In the *low-pressure system* the water is heated in a boiler to boiling-point (212° F.) ; as it is heated, it rises and circulates through 3 to 4-inch diameter pipes round the building, returning to the bottom of the boiler again. Low-pressure pipes are arranged to enter a room, led round it and double back on themselves so that it is possible to tell by feeling (by relative warmth) which pipe carries the water into, and which out of the room. The rate of flow can be accelerated by a mechanical pump. At intervals in either system are placed radiators (which should be called " convectors ") through which water circulates and which increase the warming surfaces for the room.

The pipes are often arranged in panels in the walls or even

the ceiling, thus making the system less obtrusive. The difficulty about any hot-water system is that it is the air that is heated, not the person directly, as with a fire, and this has an adverse effect on the action of the skin in giving off heat and moisture, and conduces to catarrh. Another point is that as hot air rises, the head tends to become hot and the feet cold, whereas the reverse is desirable for maximum comfort and mental effort. Hot pipes running under the floor partly overcome this.

Windows

The problems of lighting are dealt with in the chapter on eyesight. Considered as ventilating mediums, windows need to be made so that they can be opened at the top, wide middle and the bottom, so that all kinds of weather and wind can be allowed for. Air in the narrower top and bottom sections is best diverted upwards by hopper-shaped glass-winged openings. Thus direct down-draughts are obviated. The wide middle section may well swing on a central vertical pin, as in the Chaddock windows.

All windows should be easy and quick to open and shut, and the fitting should be of a type unlikely to get out of order ; the amount of opening should be easy to adjust. High hoppers controlled by noisy slow cords that are inclined to stick, break and to get into knots, result in neglect of ventilation control (see Fig. 52).

The aim should be to have a larger number of windows to open a little way rather than a few fully open, for by this means fresh air will be diffused widely and no one will be in a direct draught. If a few windows are wide open the people near them are cold and inclined to urge that all the windows should be closed. Too large an area of window space to the room space cools the room unduly in winter, making heating over-expensive and people by the windows cold. The allowance of classroom capacity in primary schools is 120 cubic feet per head, with a window area at least one-fifth of the floor area in rooms about 13 feet high.

Light flat-topped tables with a separate, comfortable chair are better than desks. Children's legs should never dangle,

14

and the chair legs should be short enough for the children to have their feet on the ground. Foot rests are unnecessary and collect dust. Single " desks " prevent over-crowding and the possibility of mass infection from germs breathed out.

Drainage

Drains in a school or a house are all planned to have a slight slope sufficient to help in carrying away sediment ; they have

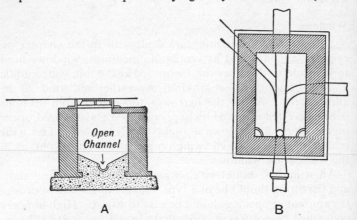

FIG. 160.—A manhole or drain-inspection chamber viewed (A) in vertical section, and (B) from above. Such manholes are arranged at all junctions of drains and where corners are turned, and as many drains as possible are planned to empty into each one. This means that drains run between manholes without bends, and this and the oblique entrance of the drains into the chamber allow of obstructions being dealt with by the insertion of long rods.

no sharp bends, so that should they get stopped up they are easy to free. In addition, they are arranged to meet at intervals (as when corners are turned) so that a number empty themselves into a space called a manhole ; here the flow of each drain (rain-water from the roofs, surface water from round the building, water from slop-closets, water-closets, baths and showers) can be checked when necessary, to see that it is flowing correctly.

Soil pipes which drain water-closets are usually at the back of any building, and are distinguished because they alone of all house spouts pass direct into the ground and have a ventilating shaft opening above the roof or highest window.

All other drains open into some form of open outdoor *gulley trap*, into which there must be a free fall for the water, which thus gets aerated. The trap is an arrangement by which the level of the water, though the actual content of water changes, always remains at a set height, thus blocking the rise of drain smells. The water is actually the trap. The siphon trap found

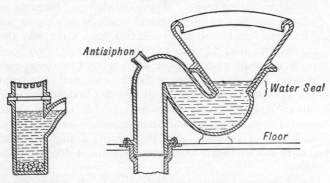

FIG. 161.—A gulley trap. All drains except soil pipes open into such a trap. The grating at the top can be lifted and the sediment cleared out. The water-seal prevents drain smells from rising.

FIG. 162.—A wash-down closet. The water-seal or trap prevents drain smells from entering the building. Were it not for the anti-siphon, the rush of water and variations in air pressure on flushing would empty the water-seal.

often under washing basins works on a similar plan, an opening at the lowest point of the ∽ bend facilitating removal of any sediment that may collect.

The type of *water-closet* almost universally used now is the " wash-down " which, on the water-trap plan, prevents drain smells from entering the building. The water-carriage system for sewage is always more satisfactory than earth-closets, though these may be necessary in the country. The closet seats should be of the pedestal type with as little woodwork about them as possible, and that washable and non-absorbent.

Low seats, 10 inches high in infant schools and 12 inches in the primary and secondary schools, are essential, and each closet should have its own long flushing chain, which the child should be taught to pull. This is better training and more sanitary and pleasant than the trough-closets, which the caretaker flushes only at intervals. Flushing cisterns should fill rapidly enough to allow of the quick reflushing necessary during such times as recess. Closets should be well lighted.

A teacher should supervise the *conduct of the children round the offices* during recess. There should be no loitering near the offices, and two children should never be in a closet together. The head teacher should constantly check the way the caretaker looks after the offices. Children should never be allowed to write their names on the walls (glazed or rough-cast walls prevent this, but it is better for the children not to want to). The children's co-operation should be obtained in keeping the offices well. The way in which people use or abuse such sanitary facilities is a revealing index of their ingrained standard of decency, and by keeping a high standard, the school can do much to promote a sense of decency and cleanliness.

Earth-closets must be emptied daily or they soon form a breeding-place for flies. The " Elsan " chemical sanitary closet, that can be fitted indoors and needs no drainage system, is a useful substitute for the old-fashioned earth-closet in the home. The cost is about £5, and the closet needs emptying and the chemicals renewing about every six months, or more often according to use. Cess-pools are to be avoided. The necessary scale of provision is as follows : two closets for every seventy boys and three for every seventy girls, together with, for boys, urinals in the proportion of 10 feet per hundred boys.

School Cleaning

Apart from health considerations, proper *school cleaning* is essential to the development of a good school tone. In a school luncheon room with 500 or more pupils in it a count of *dust particles* showed that there were 258,000 per cubic foot ; with windows opened and the room nearly empty it fell to

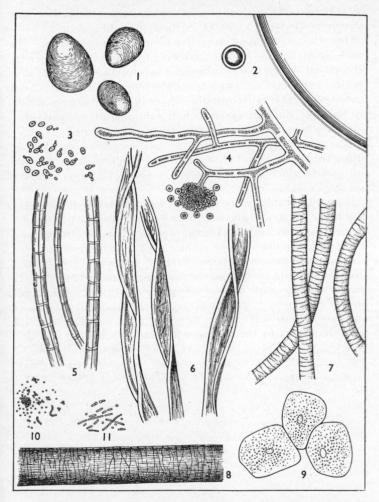

FIG. 163.—Structures observed in room dust when placed in a drop of water magnified 250 diameters under the microscope. 1, starch granules ; 2, a small air bubble and portion of a larger air bubble ; 3, yeast cells, some " budding " ; 4, a mould (aspergillus glaucus) ; 5, linen fibres ; 6, cotton fibres ; 7, wool ; 8, human hair ; 9, epithelial cells from the skin ; 10, bacteria, cocci ; 11, bacteria, bacilli. (After Schafer.)

97,000 particles per cubic foot ; while when the janitor was sweeping it rose to 1,090,000 particles per cubic foot.

Indoor air contains more *bacteria* than outdoor air. In mid-ocean, four or five bacteria were found in 10 cubic metres, compared with 910,000 in a clean school and 1,080,000 in a poorly kept school. Fan ventilation reduced the clean school count to 30,000 fairly rapidly. Not all these bacteria would be harmful, but they would include a number of cold and other infective bacteria in the resistive dry " spore " state.

Vacuum cleaners have helped to establish a new standard of dust freedom. Dust-binding oils on floors last well. Spindle oil gives a mat surface and needs to be applied once in every six weeks.

Finally, cleanliness is not all. Every school should have attractive and well-chosen pictures that appeal to children rather than to adults. Decoration by curtains, friezes and flowers is valuable so long as they are used with restraint. In such beautiful surroundings children unconsciously develop good standards of taste. On the other hand, shabby, dirty paint, a stuffy smell, papers about the classroom, apple cores in the playground, dirty washing basins and dirty windows indicate a poor school tone largely due to the acceptance of poor standards by the head and assistant teachers.

Chapter XXXIV

SCHOOL EMERGENCIES AND ACCIDENTS

TEACHERS have to be prepared to deal effectively with major and minor injury emergencies that occur in the classroom, kitchen and science laboratory, playground or field, or on a school journey or at a school camp. In any emergency, the teacher needs to control signs of personal worry and uncertainty, and to send away children crowding round, briefly giving them, if possible, something definite to do. Simple cases, as of nose bleeding or a slight abrasion, can be dealt with at once, but if there is any doubt it is best to send a child for the head teacher and to get a doctor as early as possible. Parents are naturally quick to say that their child was not treated rightly, and apart from the more skilled treatment they apply, the doctors rightly take the responsibility of the situation from the teacher.

After any injury it will usually be necessary to treat for shock by keeping the patient warm and quiet for a time, and giving a stimulant such as sal volatile or black coffee. The teacher, however, knowing the pupils, will appreciate which are likely to make a good deal of a small injury and which not, and will act with this in mind. It is better, however, to be too careful than not careful enough.

Causes of Unconsciousness

Unconsciousness may be due to fainting (see page 60), an epileptic fit (see page 253), hysteria (see page 225), carbon monoxide poisoning (see page 54), concussion, sunstroke, collapse from electric shock or stroke or apoplexy. No stimulant should be given during unconsciousness, because of the danger of choking the patient.

Concussion or stunning is due to a blow or fall on the head. The child is temporarily unconscious, chilly and pale and the

413

breathing shallow. There is often vomiting on regaining consciousness. Send for a doctor. The patient should be kept lying down and as quiet as possible, and even though on recovering consciousness he is able to walk he should not be encouraged to do so. A wet cold towel round the head may be useful, and no stimulant should be given. Even in mild cases of bumped heads without any unconsciousness, such as occurs in play occasionally, it is wise to keep the child out of the game, even though he protests his ability to go back, for any knock on the head jars the brain, which needs time to recover.

Sunstroke results from prolonged exposure to excessive heat from the sun, heat stroke from exposure to extreme heat whether from the sun or not. The effect is that the body cannot lose heat quickly enough and the " first-aid " aim is to induce heat loss by sweating. The patient may feel sick and giddy and even become unconscious. Removal to a cool place is desirable, clothing should be loosened and removed, and the head and neck bathed in cold water. The patient should be given tepid water to drink but no stimulant. If recovery is delayed unduly, a doctor should be called.

Collapse from *Electric Shock* is treated by getting the patient into the fresh air or by opening the windows near by, giving sal volatile, and as soon as possible a hot bath. Artificial respiration may have to be applied. A doctor should be summoned.

Apoplexy or *Stroke* is due to a breaking of a small blood-vessel in the brain. The face is flushed and the breathing stertorous. The patient should be kept quiet, with no stimulants and a doctor should be called. A hot bottle to the feet and cold applications to the head may be useful.

The Arresting of Bleeding

In minor wounds, bleeding is from capillaries and the problem is (1) to stop bleeding and (2) to keep the wound clean. This also applies to venous bleeding.

Bleeding can be stopped by pressure by the thumbs on a clean pad over the wound or by a pad and firm bandage.

Direct pressure on the wound cannot be used if there is any

foreign body, such as glass, in the wound. Pressure points must then be used to control bleeding (Fig. 165).

In addition (i) the patient should sit or, better, lie down to slow the heart's action and to minimise shock, and (ii) the limb should be raised to reduce the flow of blood to the wound.

If a cut finger is held up, not down, and pressed firmly on either side below the wound, the finger arteries are compressed and bleeding is lessened.

Bleeding from an Artery is less likely to occur than venous or capillary bleeding because the arteries are well protected. It is the most severe type of bleeding, however, and needs prompt and effective action to stop it. The blood is bright scarlet and comes from the wound, if the artery cut is large, in jets or spurts as the heart beats. Immediate vigorous pressure with the thumbs over the side of the wound nearer to the heart is essential, if life is to be saved. As pressure cannot be maintained thus indefinitely, someone else should make and

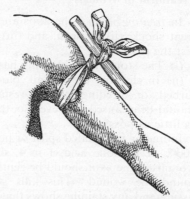

FIG. 164.—The tourniquet has been applied to the brachial artery that passes down the inner side of the upper arm. No tourniquet should be kept on longer than can be avoided, a doctor being called immediately. Compare Fig. 165.

apply a *tourniquet* above the thumb pressure point, before that pressure can safely be released. A doctor must be called.

A temporary tourniquet can be made by knotting a handkerchief tightly, possibly with a stone in the knot, and with the knot over the point where the pressure is needed on the limb, twisting a pencil, pocket-knife or poker put through the other side of the handkerchief, so that the handkerchief becomes tighter and tighter, until the pressure of the knot is sufficient to stop the bleeding without the thumb pressure. The patient should lie down to ease the beating of the heart and the

14*

bleeding part be raised. Any tourniquet must be cautiously released (but not removed) every 15 minutes, so that circulation in the limb is not entirely stopped. If bleeding continues, the tourniquet is re-applied. The points at which pressure should be applied may be learned from the accompanying diagram. Attendance at a First Aid course is better still.

Treatment of Wounds

In *treating wounds* the aims are (i) to stop bleeding and to treat shock, (ii) to clean, and (iii) to dress the wound and to rest the part.

(i) The stopping of bleeding has already been considered.

(ii) In cleaning the wound, blood clots should not be disturbed, or bleeding may be restarted. The helper's hands should be cleansed and, even so, the wound should be touched as little as possible.

Iodine or methylated spirit or potassium permanganate, 1 in 1000, or carbolic acid, 1 in 4, should be poured *round* the wound or the skin should be gently swabbed to about 3 in. all round the wound. This kills germs without injuring the tissues and any staining shows that all the wound area has been covered.

The cleansing of large wounds or that of a compound fracture should be left to the doctor, who should have been summoned.

(iii) The dressing is to prevent germs from increasing in the wound or from entering from outside.

Gauze, pink boracic lint or white lint—the plain side to the wound—can be used. If linen or cotton material is used it should, if possible, be scorched first to kill germs.

Dressing should be handled by the corners only and dropped gently on to the wound, which should then be covered with cotton wool and bandaged.

No ointments, vaseline, creams or plasters should be applied to a recent wound, as they make the tissues sodden and delay healing. Another objection to their use is the fact that they are not sterile.

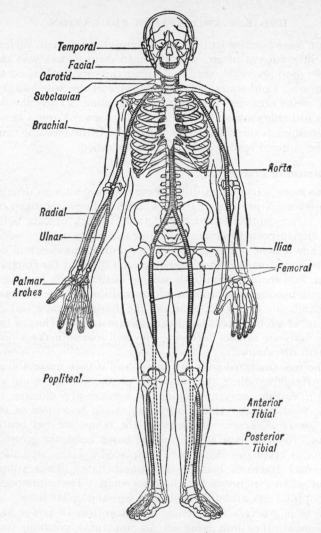

Temporal
Facial
Carotid
Subclavian
Brachial
Aorta
Radial
Ulnar
Iliac
Femoral
Palmar Arches
Popliteal
Anterior Tibial
Posterior Tibial

The small rings (o) show pressure points

FIG. 165.—Diagram of the main arteries of the body. The small rings (o) show the most advantageous points at which to apply pressure to control arterial bleeding. At any of these, it should be possible to locate a pulse. The dotted lines show where arteries pass behind bones, as the figure stands.

For *Nose bleeding* let the child sit upright in a chair, preferably in a current of air, with the head thrown back and the arms raised above the head to decrease the supply of blood to the head. Cold-water pads to the bridge of the nose and the back of the neck may help to stop the bleeding. There should be as little blowing of the nose or leaning forward over a basin as possible, as these accelerate bleeding. If the bleeding cannot be stopped readily a doctor must be called.

Treatment of Fractures

Fractures.—It is often difficult even for a doctor to decide, without an X-ray examination, whether a bone is broken or not. Over-caution is much preferable to lack of care here, and any suspected fracture should be treated as one.

When a bone is fractured, the antagonistic muscles pull on the two ends so that they over-ride each other at the fracture point, and there is definite shortening of the limb. In setting it, these two ends are brought into apposition ; the periosteum or membrane round the bone and the marrow form a sort of jelly in which bone cells lay down calcium again. Thus, if the bone ends are not set correctly, they will join to make a permanent deformity.

The free fractured ends are sharp, and if they move about, as in rough handling, they may well pierce the skin or cut an artery, causing severe bleeding or unnecessary damage to muscles or nerves. Hence *a fracture should be treated on the spot where it occurs.* In children, the bones are not brittle enough to snap, as in adults, but the bones bend, the growing points or epiphyses being partly displaced. These are called *greenstick* fractures because the bone behaves like a young green shoot ; it bends but does not snap. The commonest school fractures are of the arms and legs and collar-bone.

Signs of fracture are swelling and pain, loss of power and movement, the limb lying in an unnatural position, and shortening in long bones. Any suspected fracture must be handled very gently lest the extent of the injury be increased. If possible get a doctor, but if he is likely to be delayed for some time the teacher must carefully apply interim treatment. This becomes specially important if a child with a leg injury is lying on a wet playground surface, but he should not be moved until the limb has been immobilised.

The limb is very gently pulled to straighten it and prevent shortening, and in the case of fracture of the thigh bandaged to the other by a figure of eight round the ankles, the sound leg acting as a partial splint. A suitable splint for the thigh, one reaching from the arm-pit to the foot, such as a broom handle, must be improvised, and having been well padded, it should be used to fix the limb in the corrected position, by a series of firm bandages above and below but not over the site of the fracture.

The weight of a fractured arm should be taken by a sling,

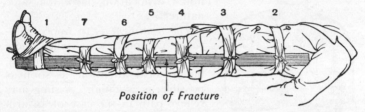

Position of Fracture

FIG. 166.—Diagram of the method of splinting and bandaging a fractured thigh bone. The splint reaches from the feet to the arm-pit ; and the actual site of the fracture is unbandaged. The splint is unpadded, so that it shows the more clearly. The numbers show the order in which bandages should be applied.

and a patient with a broken leg or thigh should be carried on a stretcher, door or blackboard. If there is any wound, it must be dressed previously. Gentleness of movement is essential. Here, as in all bandaging, tie reef knots, which hold better than granny knots. *A reef knot* is made by tying the right end over the left and the same, now left, end over the right ; the two ends then lie parallel to the line of the bandage, not at right angles to it, as in a granny.

In a broken collar-bone or clavicle, the patient tends characteristically to support the elbow of the injured side and bend the head to that side. Put a firm pad under the arm-pit and bandage the elbow-joint and flexed arm to the body. In all cases of fracture, keep the patient quiet and warm, treating for shock.

Sprains and Dislocations

A Dislocation occurs when the ends of the two bones that usually move on one another become displaced, the commonest joints affected being the shallow shoulder-joint, the elbow, the thumb in boxing, finger-joints and the lower jaw. There is pain, swelling, loss of power and deformity. Once a dislocation has occurred it is likely to happen again, for the tendons and

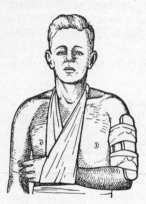

ligaments around the joint are stretched and torn and tend to lose their elasticity, like worn elastic. The slipping of the inner semilunar cartilage of the knee-joint, though not a dislocation, is of the same nature.

The treatment is to apply cold-water compresses or, when these fail to give any relief, fomentations, but medical attention, as soon as possible, is essential. A sling may relieve pain in the case of an arm by taking the weight.

FIG. 167.—The method of splinting for a fractured upper arm. The small arm sling allows the splinting to be seen. Actually a large arm sling, which would give greater support, would probably be used.

Sprains are really half dislocations. A sudden wrenching or twisting of a joint forces the joint surfaces apart on one side, and though they immediately come into place again, there is tearing of the joint ligaments and the muscle tendons round the joint. "Turning of the ankle" is common, and occurs rather more readily in people who lead an inactive, sedentary life and are out of training and relatively flabby, their muscles and ligaments softer and less tense and resilient than they could be with more use. Sometimes it is difficult to tell a sprain from a fracture except by an X-ray examination. Pain is intense, the joint cannot be used, and there is swelling and discoloration from bruising.

If a sprained ankle occurs some distance from home, bandage the foot firmly, with the shoe on, with strips of handkerchief or anything available, first padding with wet moss round the injured part. Then wet the bandage, which will tighten it. Even so, the patient should use the foot as little as possible, because further strain on it will increase the tearing of the tissues round the joint. Application of cold-water compresses or of lead and opium relieve pain. Severe sprains need splinting and a doctor's examination. In any event, a sprain should be rested with the foot up for some days at least; massage usually hastens recovery. Children who sprain a joint during games should be forbidden to continue to play, lest they make a slight injury worse, for which the teacher would rightly be held responsible.

The discoloration of *bruises* is due to the breaking of capillaries under the skin. Cold or hot applications may be made, but a routine application of witch hazel or arnica for slighter school bruises relieves pain and is psychologically comforting.

Cramp is a painful spasm of a muscle or muscle-group, due to over-contraction and fixing. It can be rapidly relieved by stretching the contracted muscles, for example, by pressing the toe upwards firmly to stretch cramped calf muscles. " Stitch " is a form of cramp which is relieved by touching the head to the knee.

Burns

A Burn is caused by dry heat, corrosive acid, or alkali, or by electric current, a *scald* by a hot liquid or steam.

Burns or scalds produce reddening of the skin, pain, blisters or actual destruction of tissue, which is less painful immediately because of the destruction of nerve endings. There is always danger that shock may cause collapse, which shows as paleness, coldness, shallow breathing and feeble pulse. If not properly treated death might ensue.

If a person's *clothes catch fire* he should lie down on the ground and roll, thus preventing the flames from getting to the face, and if possible wrap himself in a rug, curtain, or blanket to stifle the flames. Anyone present should do this for him. To run about increases the fire by supplying more oxygen still.

It is better to crawl on all-fours. This also protects the face and head from being burnt.

Treatment of burns and scalds. Burns differ in degree:

(i) If the skin is reddened but not broken, a dressing of boracic ointment or a solution of bicarbonate of soda—a dessert-spoonful to a pint of warm water—is soothing.

(ii) If the skin is broken, the aim in any treatment is to exclude air, relieve pain and minimise shock.

If treatment in a hospital is possible within five to six hours, a dry dressing and light bandaging, with immobilisation of the limb, is used or the burn may be covered with a dressing which has been wrung out in bicarbonate solution, a teaspoonful to a pint. The patient should be hurried to hospital. In this way treatment in hospital is not hindered by earlier First Aid work.

In dressing a burn, the wound does not need cleansing because bacteria will have been destroyed by the heat. Clothing should be cut away, but any material that has stuck to the wound should not be removed. The wound is covered with sulphonamide impregnated gauze. Tannic acid jelly [1] is also used. It has an astringent effect, coagulating the superficial tissues and helping healing. No oil should be applied. It is not sterile and delays healing.

Blisters should not be pricked except by a doctor who should have been summoned.

Dressings, if the burn is large, should be put on in overlapping strips, so that on renewing, a small surface only is exposed to the air at one time. Cotton wool and light bandaging completes the dressing.

It a child gets *corrosive acid* on his skin, as in a laboratory, the first thing is to put the part under the tap, and then to bathe it with a weak alkali solution of washing or baking soda, of magnesia, slaked lime, corrosive alkali with diluted lemon juice, or vinegar (acetic acid), finishing with a dressing.

Insect Stings should be bathed with weak alkali, such as ammonia or washing soda, and if the sting has been left in, it should be squeezed out.

---

[1] Tannic acid jelly needs regular renewing because of deterioration.

The Eye and Ear—Choking

Foreign bodies in the Eye generally lodge under the upper lid. The patient should blow his nose sharply and try opening his eye several times under water or in an eyebath of water or boracic lotion. The upper lid may be lifted gently away from the eye and the lids closed so that the under lid brushes against the inside of the upper eyelid, possibly removing the irritating particle. If the irritation is still there, put a spot of oil in the eye, bandage lightly to prevent continual rubbing and get the child to the doctor. Delay, causing unchecked inflammation, can lead even to loss of sight.

If children poke beads or hard *objects in the ear*, these can possibly be floated out by filling the ear with oil. Beware, however, of trying to wash out such an object as a pea, which will absorb liquid and swell up. On no account should the child's ear be poked or the drum may be injured permanently. Take the child to a doctor. Beads or peas up the nostrils can sometimes be got rid of by inducing the child to sniff pepper and sneeze. Blowing the nose hard, with the free nostril closed, may also be successful.

Choking may be caused by swallowing food, bones or sweets whole, or such objects as pennies or pins. If the child cannot breathe prompt action is essential. Open the mouth and hook the finger as far down the throat as possible, trying to hook out the object. If the child vomits, so much the better. Failing this, a smart slap between the shoulder blades may help; with a small child, this may be done while holding him up by the feet. If suffocation seems imminent, start artificial respiration. In any case send for a doctor.

If a child swallows an open pin, drawing pin, or paper clip and is not choking, do not give an emetic or aperient but, rather, stodgy food in which the object can be embedded. An X-ray examination makes the exact location of such objects possible. Consult a doctor without delay.

Poisons

Poisons may be roughly classed as those corroding the lips and mouth, for which no emetic is given, and those not burning the mouth, for which an emetic to induce vomiting is the right treatment. If poisoning is suspected, prompt action is essential. Find out the poison taken and keep the remains. Send for a doctor, giving such particulars of the case as are possible.

Acids and alkalis, which burn the lips, need an antidote to neutralise the poison. For acids give whiting, common chalk, powdered washing or baking soda, or soap suds, and follow with oil, butter or milk to protect the membrane of the stomach. The drinking of large quantities of water will dilute this type of poison, if specific antidotes are not available at once.

For alkalis, such as caustic soda, potash or ammonia, give abundance of weak vinegar and water, or lime juice, and later milk, white of egg in water, or a wineglassful of olive oil in a pint of warm water.

If the mouth is unburnt, give *an emetic*, or tickle the back of the throat. Effective emetics are a tablespoonful of mustard to a tumbler of warm water, or two tablespoonfuls of salt to a tumbler of warm water repeated until sickness occurs. Signs of collapse should be looked for and treated.

If a child is sleepy, he may have taken a *narcotic poison*, such as opium, chlorodyne, or laudanum, and must be kept awake at all costs by being given strong black coffee, walked up and down briskly and flicked with a wet towel ; anything to keep him awake. The pupils become of pin-point size. Meanwhile, as in all poison cases, send for a doctor, who may apply a stomach pump to empty the stomach of its contents.

If match heads have been sucked giving phosphorus poisoning, there is violent vomiting and thirst. " Safety matches " have the phosphorus on the striking surface of the match box. Give no oil but an emetic of magnesia. For coal-gas poisoning let in fresh air and start artificial respiration. Smelling-salts to the nostrils are also useful. Call a doctor.

Artificial Respiration

Artificial Respiration is used for unconsciousness from drowning and suffocation, and even if a person has been immersed up to fifteen minutes, artificial respiration should be started at once and should continue for at least an hour ; some authorities advise continuance for five to six hours. Clear the mouth and nostrils of any obstruction, and turning the patient on his face, lift him up, standing astride him, at the hips, to try to drain any water out of the lungs. To roll the body prone over a barrel is effective. Artificial respiration will be of little use unless this is done first. Draw the tongue forward if necessary, an assistant holding it, and start artificial respiration without delay. Send for a doctor and for hot bottles and blankets.

In the *Schafer method*, the operator kneels astride, or on one side of the prone patient, and puts his hands in the small of the patient's back, thumbs parallel and nearly meeting. By bending forward, elbows straight, the weight of the operator's body falls on the wrists and makes a steady pressure downwards, emptying the lungs. By leaning back, pressure is relaxed, though the hands are still in contact, and air can rush in. Repeat this rhythm twelve to eighteen times a minute until natural breathing re-starts.

There must be no delay in starting artificial respiration, because if the neurones of the brain are deprived too long of oxygen they cannot be revived. Assistants should apply warmth to the patient by vigorous rubbing of the limbs, by covering the patient and, if possible, by using hot bottles. Once breathing is restored, wet clothing can be gently removed and the patient encouraged to sleep. Rubbing the limbs briskly upwards towards the heart, helps to restore circulation.

In the *Sylvester method*, the patient lies on his back with a pillow under his shoulders, and the operator, kneeling behind his head, grasps the forearms and alternately raises the arms above the head, expanding the lungs, and brings them down to make strong steady pressure on the chest, expelling air. Move the arms on a plane parallel with the floor rather than up into the air, repeating twelve to eighteen times a minute. Too fast a rhythm is less valuable. Apply methods making for warmth.

The inhaling of CO_2 is used to stimulate breathing in suffocation. Firemen have frozen CO_2 " snow " in their axe handles, which, when allowed to volatilise, can be inhaled.

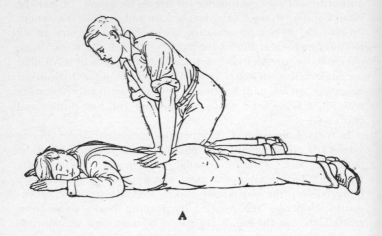

A

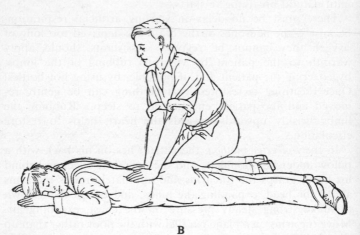

B

FIG. 168.—Artificial respiration by Schafer's method. A, operator leans forward, pressing air out of the lungs; B, he leans back, letting air enter the lungs. This should be repeated at the rate of eighteen times per minute. The operator can also kneel astride the patient. Elbows should be kept straight throughout the movement.

Every school should have a first-aid box which should be kept replenished and in order. In addition to attending to the child's comfort and dealing satisfactorily with any crisis, the teacher needs to recognise his own responsibility to take such precautions continually, and by forethought prevent the occurrence of accidents at all.

BIBLIOGRAPHY

" Health of the School Child." The yearly reports of the Chief Medical Officer of the Board of Education. H.M.S.O.

" Public Health." The yearly reports of the Chief Medical Officer of the Ministry of Health. H.M.S.O.

" Health Education." Board of Education. H.M.S.O.

" Infant and Nursery Schools." H.M.S.O.

" The Primary School." H.M.S.O.

" Elementary School Buildings." H.M.S.O.

" Standard Construction for Schools." Post-War Building Studies, No. 2. H.M.S.O.

" Manual of Nutrition." Ministry of Food. H.M.S.O.

" Sex Education in School and Youth Organisations." H.M.S.O.

" Sex Education." Cyril Bibby. Macmillan.

" Outline of the Practice of Preventive Medicine." Sir George Newman. H.M.S.O.

" Fundamentals of School Health." J. Kerr. Allen & Unwin.

" The Body and Its Health." W. Cullis and M. Bond. Allen & Unwin.

" Science of Life." Wells and Huxley. Cassell.

" Biology and Mankind." S. A. McDowall. Cambridge University Press.

" Health Facts for College Students." Maude I. Etheredge. Saunders.

" School Education in Hygiene and Sex." G. O. Barber. Heffer.

" Fundamentals of Bio-Chemistry in relation to Human Physiology." T. R. Parsons. Heffer.

" Ground-work of Bio-Physics." Wishart. Bell.

" Conditioned Reflexes." I. P. Pavlov. Oxford University Press

" Functions of the Body." V. H. Mottram. Nesbit.

" Design of Nursery and Elementary Schools." H. Myles Wright and R. Gardner Medwin. Architect Press.

" The Battle of Health." Stephen Taylor. Nicholson & Watson.

" A Charter of Health." Committee of the British Medical Association. Allen & Unwin.

" The Nation's Health." James Mackintosh. Pilot Press.

" Molecules Against Microbes." E. S. Duthie. Sigma.

" Human Problems in Industry." N. M. Davies. Nicholson and Watson.

" Health Services and the Public." Stella Churchill. Douglas.

" Recent Advances in Preventive Medicine." J. F. C. Haslam. Churchill.

" Health and Social Evolution." Sir George Newman. Allen & Unwin.

" The Virus." Kenneth Smith. Cambridge University Press.

" Special Education Services in London." University of London Press.

" Acute Rheumatism." Ministry of Health. H.M.S.O.

" Modern School Buildings." Sir Felix Clay. Batsford.

" Health of the Mind." J. R. Rees. Faber. (2nd Ed.)

" Endocrin Disorders in Childhood and Adolescence." H. S. le Marquand. Hodder & Stoughton.

" The Nervous Temperament." May Smith. H.M.S.O.

" The Nervous Patient." M. Culpin. Lewis.

" Guide to Intelligence and other Psychological Testing. Haut and Smith. Evans Bros.

" Mental and Scholastic Tests." C. Burt. King.

" The Will to Work." G. H. Miles. Routledge.

" The Sub-normal Child." Cyril Burt. University of London Press.

" The Backward Child." Cyril Burt. University of London Press.

" Diseases of Children." R. Hutchinson. Arnold.

" Diseases of Infancy and Childhood." W. Sheldon. Churchill.

" The Young Delinquent." C. Burt. University of London Press.

" Child Welfare Outside the School." Michael Kaye. Oliver & Boyd.

" Your Mind and Mine." R. B. Cattell. Harrap.

" Intelligence of Scottish School Children." University of London Press.

" School Life and Nervous Instability." National Council of Mental Hygiene.

" Mental Deficiency (Amentia)." A. F. Tredgold. Baillière, Tindall & Cox.

" Report of Committee of Enquiry into Problems relating to Children with Defective Hearing." 1938. H.M.S.O.

" Handbood for Assistant Medical Officers of Health on School Welfare and School Medical Work." F. J. G. Lishman. Lewis.

" Report of the Commission on Mental Deficiency," 1939. H.M.S.O.

" Diagnosis of Mental Deficiency." H. Herd. Hodder & Stoughton.

" The Mental Defective." Berry and Gordon. Routledge.

" Survey of Child Psychiatry." R. G. Gordon. Milford 1939.

" Alcohol.—Its Action on the Human Organism." Central Control Board. H.M.S.O.

" Nutrition and the War." Dr. Geoffrey Bourne. Cambridge University Press. 1940.

" Food, Health, Vitamins." R. H. A. and V. G. Plimmer. Longmans.

" Food Values at a Glance." V. Plimmer. Longmans.

" The Vitamins in Medicine." F. Bicknell and F. Prescott. (2nd Ed.). Heinmann.

" Nutrition and National Health." Sir Robert McConison. Faber.

" Diets of Boys During School Age." H. Corey Mann. H.M.S.O.

" Hygiene of the Mouth and Teeth." Dental Board. Constable.

" A Handbook of Health Teaching." Rose Bland. Faber.

" Nursery School Buildings and Equipment." Pamphlet 17. Nursery Schools Association.

" Spread of Droplet Infection." Dudley. H.M.S.O.

" Schick Test, Diphtheria and Scarlet Fever." Dudley. H.M.S.O.

" Recent Advances in Laryngology and Otology." Scott Stevenson. Churchill.

" A Code of Rules for the Prevention of Communicable Diseases in Schools." Medical Officers of Schools Association. Churchill.

" Sunshine and the Open Air." L. Hill. Arnold.

" Six Talks on Heredity." Mary Adams. Heffer.

" Heredity." A. F. Shull McGraw Hill.

" Being Well Born." M. F. Guyer. Constable.

" How You Began." A. Williams Ellis. Howe.

" How a Baby is Born." K. Schweinitz. Routledge.

" Personal Hygiene for Women." C. D. Mosher. Mills & Boon.

" Womanhood and Health." Christine Murrell. Mills & Boon.

" Health Compendium." T. Crew. Reader Printing Co.
    (A reference book on health propaganda, including addresses of societies, lists of films, journals and posters.) (2nd Ed.).

The British Film Institute, 4, Great Russell St., London, W.C.1, supplies information about Health and Scientific film sources.

INDEX

A

Abdomen, 62–3
Abscess, 12, 336
Accessory food factors, 106
Accommodation, 261–3
Accredited milk, 124–5
Achilles, tendon of, 38
Acid poisons, 424
Acne, 157
Acute rheumatism, 369
Adenoids, 40, 71–2, 285, 374
Adrenal glands, 185–6
Adulteration, 115
Aerated water, 118
Agglutinins, 56
Albumen, 124
Alcohol, 352–31
Alkali poisons, 424
Allergy, 228–9
Alopecia, 157
Amino-acids, 93, 101
Anæmia, 60–1
Aneurine, 108–9, 117
Ankle, sprained, 420–1
——, weak, 30
Antagonistic muscles, 38–9
Ante-natal clinic, 377
Anterior poliomyelitis, 353–4
Anti-toxin, 334–7
Anvil bone, 284
Aorta, 48
Aperients, 99
Apoplexy, 413–4
Appendix, 7
Appetite juice, 89
Aqueous humour, 258–60
Arachnoid membrane, 194
Arch of foot, 28–30
Artery, 50–1
Artesian well, 119
Artificial respiration, 424–6
—— selection, 323–4
—— sunlight, 85
Ascorbic acid, 110–1, 117
Association fibres, 204

Asthma, 229, 399
Astigmatism, 228, 267–8
Audiometer, 290–1
Auditory nerve, 285–6
Auricles of heart, 48–50
Axon, 192

B

Bacilli, 12–13, 357
—— coli, 125
Bacon, 88
Bacteria, 11–13, 83, 335
Ball and socket joint, 22–5
Ballast, 88
Banana, 88
Bath, 155, 177
——, swimming, 178–9
B.C.G. strain of T.B., 359
Beans, 101
Bedroom, 217, 366
Bemax, 109, 117
Benzyl benzoate, 159, 161
Beri-Beri, 108, 117
Bicuspid teeth, 137
Bifocal vision, 264, 274–6
Bile, 96
Binet and Simon, 234
Binocular vision, 273
Biscuit, 88, 109
Bismuth, 95
Black currant juice, 111, 117
Bleeding, 414–6
Blepharitis, 277–8
Blindness, 282–3
Blind spot, 264
Blood, 53–6
——, functions of, 58
Blushing, 59
Body temperature, 74
Boots, 167
Boredom, 214
Bovine tuberculosis, 123, 357
Braille type, 282–3
Brain, 190–6; damage, 207
Bread, 88, 104

Breathing, 62-5
Bronchi, 66-7
Bronchitis, 377
Bruises, 421
Buildings, school, 400-10
Bunions, 168-9
Burns, 421-2
Butter, 104, 112

C

Caffeine, 118
Calciferol, 112, 117
Calcium, 104-6, 141-2
Calmette, Professor, 359
Calorie, 127
Cancellous tissue, 15
Canine tooth, 137-8
Capillary vessels, 51-2
Carbohydrate, 88, 102-4
Carbon dioxide, 58, 425
—— monoxide, 54-5
Care Committee, 252
Carious teeth, 138-46
Carpel bones, 17, 22
Carrier of infection, 339-40
Carrotene, 107-8, 117
Carrots, 107, 117
Cartilage, 15
Casein, 120
Cataract, 277
Celery, 142
Cell division, 303-5
Cellular cotton, 164-5
Cellulose, 88, 104
Cement, tooth, 136-7
Central hall school, 80
—— nervous system, 192
Cerebellum, 191
Cerebral palsy, 206
Cerebro-spinal fluid, 194
Cerebrum, 194
Chaddock windows, 78
Chair and posture, 42-3
Cheese, 88
Chicken pox, 350
Chilblains, 169-70
Child guidance, 231-2
Chimney, 406
Chocolate, 104
Choking, 423
Cholesterol, 112, 117
Chorea, 369-70
Choroid coat, 260

Chromosomes, 303-7, 315
Chyme, 93
Ciliary muscles, 260
Classification tests, 238
Classrooms, open air, 394-5
Clavicle, 18, 21
Clinic, school, 389-92
Cloakroom, 382
Closets, 409-10
Clothing, tight, 165-6
Clotting, 56
Coal gas, 54
Cochlea, 285-6
Cocoa, 118
Coffee, 118
Colds, 69-70, 351-2
Compact bone tissue, 15
Concussion, 413-4
Condensed milk, 126
Condiments, 129
Conditioned reflex, 202-3
Conduction of heat, 74
Conjunctiva, 257
Conjunctivitis, 278
Constipation, 99
Convalescence, 333
Convection currents, 74
Convergence, eye, 261, 264
Cornea, 257-62
Corns, 168
Corpuscles, blood, 53-6, 60
Corsets, 166
Cortex, cerebral, 195
Cory Mann, 120-1
Cotton, 162-4
Cough, 229, 288, 338
Court school, 404
Cows, 123-5
Cramp, 421
Cretin, 181-3
Curvature, spinal, 46

D

Damp-proof course, 402-3
Dancing and flat foot, 29
Day nursery, 380-1
D.D.T. powder, 161
Deafness, 288-9
Decay of teeth, 138-46
Decline of infection, 333
Deficiency diseases, 106, 332
Dehydrated foods, 116

Delinquent children, 231–2
Dendrites, 192–3
Dermis of skin, 149–50
Desk, positions, 41–3, 269
Diabetes, 97, 186
Diaphragm, 62–3
Diarrhœa, infant, 376
Dick test, 345
Diets, 127–31
Diffusion, 33
Digestion, 89–99
Dinners, school, 131–2
Diphtheria, 346–8
Dirt diseases, 157–60
Dirt, habitual, 154
Dislocation of joints, 420
Dominant factor, 309–13
Dorsal region of spine, 20–21
Drains, 408–9
Dried milk, 126
Droplet infection, 338–9
Drosophila, 305, 307
Drum of ear, 284–8
Ductless gland pattern, 189
Ductless glands, 189
Dull children, 247
Dumbness, 293
Duodenum, 96
Dura mater, 194
Dust, 410–12
" Dutch courage," 326
Dysmenorrhœa, 301

E

Ear, 284–8
Earache, 288
Eggs, 101, 117
Elbow, 16
Electric shock, 414
Emetic, 424
Enamel of teeth, 136–8
Encephalitis lethargica, 249
Endocrine glands, 181–9
Enteric fever, 351
Enzyme, 91
Epidermis, 149–50
Epiglottis, 92
Epilepsy, 253–5
Epiphyses, 16–17
Ergosterol, 112
Eruption of teeth, 137, 144
Eugenics, 322

Eunuch, 188
Euphoria, 327
Eustachian tube, 284–8
Expectation of life, 329
Extensor muscles, 38
Extractives, 102
Eye defects, 266–79
Eyelid, third, 8
Eye strain, causes of, 268–9
——, structure, 257–65

F

Face, bones of, 19
Factory Acts, 209
Fæces, 98
Fainting, 60
Fallopian tubes, 295
Fatigue, muscular, 47
Fats, 104
Femur, 22
Ferment, 91
Fibrinogen, 56
Fibula, 18, 22
Fires, 405
First aid, 413–27
Fish, food, 88, 101, 106
Fish liver oils, 108, 112, 117
Flannelette, 165
Flat bones, 14
—— foot, 28–30
Fleas, 161
Flies, 116
Flexor muscles, 38
Fluorescent lighting, 270
Fœtus, 5
Follicle of hair, 149–50
Fontanelles, 19
Food fads, 130
Footgear, 167–9
Foreign bodies in eye, 423
Fossil-forms, 2–5
Fowls, inheritance in, 308–9
Fulcrum, 35–8

G

Gall bladder, 96
Games, value of, 40–1
Gamete, 305
Garters, 165
Gastric juice, 93–5
Gelatin, 101
General Intelligence, 233–4

Genes, 305, 313–6
German Measles, 350
Germs, 11–13
Gland, endocrine, 181–9
———, liver, 96
———, lymphatic, 57–8
———, Meibomian, 257
———, pancreas, 96–7, 186
———, parathyroid, 183–5
———, parotid, 89
———, pineal, 186
———, pituitary, 188
———, supra-renal, 185–6
———, sweat, 140–50
———, thymus, 186
———, thyroid, 181–3
Glucose, 32, 102
Gluten, 101
Glycogen, 96
Goitre, 181–3
Gonads, 187
Gonorrhœa, 354
Grape sugar, 102
Greenstick fracture, 418
Ground water, 402
Growing points of bones, 16
Growth, stages of, 27–8
Gulley traps, 408–9

H

Habit formation, 201–4
———, length muscles, 39
——— spasm, 227
Hæmoglobin, 54
Hammer bone, 284
Hamstring muscles, 34, 38
Hay fever, 229
Head ringworm, 155
Headaches, 134, 229
Health education, 221–2
——— visitor, 378
Hearing, 284–8
Heart, 48–53
——— disease, 61, 370–1
Heat loss by body, 74–8
Heating, school, 80, 405–7
High heels, 30, 168–9
Hinge joint, 22
Hip joint, 24–5
Hollow back, 46
Honey, 102
Hopper opening, 78

Hormone, 181
Hot-water systems, 405–7
Housing, 330, 387
Humerus, 18, 22
Hump-back, 45
Hybrid, 318
Hydrochloric acid, 93
Hysteria, 225–6

I

Immunisation in diphtheria, 346–8
Immunity, 336–7
Impetigo, 157–8
Incubation period, 333
Indigestion, 128–31
Infant mortality, 375–7
Infantile paralysis, 353–4
Influenza, 352–3
Infra red rays, 82
In-growing toe nail, 170
Inhibited action, 200–1
Inner ear, 285
Inset tests, 240
Insulin, 97, 186
Intelligence quotient, 234
——— tests, 233–44
Involuntary muscles, 31
Iodine, 106
Ionisation, 289, 390
Iris of eye, 258
Iron, 106
Itch, 158

J

Jam, 109
Joint stiffness, 40
Joints, 22–5
Jukes family, 320
Jungle gym, 382

K

Kallikak, Martin, 320–1
Kata-thermometer, 77
Keratitis, 278
Kidneys, 148–9
Knee jerk, 198
Knickers, 165
Koplik spots, 342

L

Lachrymal glands, 257–8
Lacteal, 97–8
Lactic acid, 34–5
Larynx, 65–7
Lean meat, 101–2
Legumin, 101
Lemonade, 118
Lemons, 111
Lens of eye, 258–61
" Lethane 384," 161
Leucocytes, 55
Levers, principles of, 35–8
Ligaments, 22
Lighting, school, 268–270
Linen, 165
Lip-reading, 291, 293
Liver, 96
Long bone, 14
—— sight, 266
Low pressure heating, 406–7
Lungs, 62–5
Lupus, 358
Lymph system, 57–8
Lymphatic glands, 57

M

Macrocephatic, 248
Maize, 101, 110
Malnutrition, 132–4
Malphigian layer, 149–50
Manhole, 408–9
Margarine, 104, 115
Marmite, 109, 117
Marrow of bone, 14–15
Mass infection, 339
—— radiography, 360
Maze tests, 238
Measles, 342–3
Medical inspection, 388–90
Medicines, patent, 134
Medulla oblongata, 196
Meibomian glands, 257, 277
Mendel, 306
Mendelism, 306–18
Menstrual period, 299–302
Mental fatigue, 211–14
—— ratio, 234
Mercury vapour lamp, 114
Metabolism, 88
Microcephalic, 248

Middle ear, 284
Midwives Act, 279, 377
Milk, 112, 118–126
—— teeth, 137, 144
Minerals in food, 104–6
Mitral stenosis, 61
Mongol defective, 248
Mothercraft teaching, 379
Motor nerves, 196–8
Mumps, 350
Muscular fatigue, 47
—— tone, 38–9
Mutations, 317–8
Myopia, 267, 271–2

N

Nails, care of, 170
Narcotic poisons, 424
Neo-mortality rate, 375
Neurasthenia, 108
Neuritis, general, 108
Neurones, 192–3
Neurosis, 226–7
Nicotinic acid, 110, 117
Night blindness, 277
Nitrogen, 62
Nits in hair, 160–1
Nose bleeding, 418
Notifiable diseases, 341, 363
Notification of Birth Act, 378
Nurse, school, 390
Nursery school, 378, 381–4

O

Ointments, 416
Olive oil, 104, 117
Onset of disease, 333
Open air recovery school, 372, 393–8
Open windows,
Ophthalmia neonatorum, 279, 354
Opsonins, 55
Optician, 280–1
Oranges, 111, 117
Orthoptic clinics, 275
Osteoblast, 16
Osteomalacia, 113
Otitis media, 288
Otorrhœa, 288–9
Outer ear, 284
Ovary, 187, 295–6
Overwork, 214
Oxygen, 62

436 INDEX

P

Pancreas, 96-7
Papworth, T.B. Colony, 363
Paralysis, 206-7
Parasites, 160-1, 332
Parathyroids, 183-5
Paratyphoid, 351
Parotid glands, 89
Partially sighted children, 272-3
Pasteurised milk, 125
Patella, 22
Patent foods, 131
—— medicines, 134
Pavlov,
Peas, 101
Pediculosis, 160-1
Pellagra, 110, 117
Pelvis, 16
Penicillin, 335-6, 355
Pepsin, 93
Peptones, 97
Performance tests, 237-8
Periostium, 418
Peristalsis, 98
Permanent teeth, 138
Perspiration, 149-51
Phagocytes, 55
Pharynx, 286
Phlyctenular conjunctivitis, 278-9
Phosphorus poisoning, 424
Phthisis, 358
Physical training, 40-41
Physically defective children, 398-9
Pineal gland, 186
Pink eye, 278
Pituitary gland, 188
Plasma, blood, 53-8
Play therapy, 231-2
Playground, 404-5
Plenum system, 80
Pleura, 65
Pneumonia, 336
Poisons, 423-4
Poked head, 44
Polyneuritis, 109
Porteus maze, 238
Potato, 88, 104
Posture, good, 38-41
Pregnancy, 144
Prefabricated schools, 401
Pre-molar teeth, 138
Pre-natal clinic, 377

Pre-rheumatic child, 372
Pre-school child, 374-84
Pressure points, 417
Print, size of, 270-2
Prism, 82
Protein, 101-2
Protozoa, 13
Ptyalin, 89, 103
Public Health Departments, 385-88
Pulp cavity, 136-7
Pulse, 49
Pus, 55
Pylorus, 93
Pyorrhœa, 146

Q

Quarantine, 341

R

Radiation of heat, 74
Radiography, mass, 360
Rashes, 333
Reading, 41-3, 269-71
Reasoning tests, 241
Recapitulation theory, 5-7
Recessive characteristics, 309-10
Red corpuscles, 54, 60
Reduction division, 305
Reef knot, 419
Reflections, 269
Reflex action, 198-9
——, conditioned, 202-3
Relief drill, 43
Rennin, 93
Reproduction, 295-302
Rest, 214-5
—— Pauses, 210-1
Retarded children, 245
Retina of eye, 261
Rheumatism, 367-73
Riboflavin, 109, 117
Rice (unpolished), 109, 117
Rickets, 113-5
Ringworm, 155-7
Rods and cones of eye, 262
Rose hip syrup, 111, 117
Roughage, 106
Round shoulders, 44-5

S

St. Vitus' Dance, 367
Sal volatile, 413

Salads, 88
Saliva, 89, 91
" Salting," 338–40
Sanatorium aims, 362–6
Scabies, 158–60
Scald head, 157–8
Scalds, 422
Scarlet fever, 345–6
Schafer method, 425
Schick test, 347
School closure, 341
—— for the blind, 283
—— for deaf, 293
—— for mothers, 378
—— heating, 405–7
—— meals, 131–2
—— medical service, 387–8
—— nurse, 390
—— nursery, 381–3
—— open air, 393–8
—— prefabricated, 401
—— sanatorium, 363–5
Sclerotic coat, 257
Scurvy, 112, 117
Sebaceous gland, 149–50
Secretin, 97, 181
Semicircular canals, 285–6
Sense of touch, 151–3
Sensory nerves, 196–7
Sex determination, 314–6
—— linked characteristics, 316
—— teaching, 297–9
Shivering, 151
Shoes, 167–8
Short sight, 266–9, 271
Shoulder straps, 44
Shower baths, 177–8
Sight-saving classes, 271–3
Sight testing, 280
Sinus in bone, 70
Site of school, 402
Sitting posture, 41–3
Skeleton, 18
Skim milk, 122
Skin, 149–54
Sleep, conditions for, 215–7
Sleeplessness, 218
Sling, 420
Smallpox, 349–50
Smoke, effects of, 85–7
Sneeze, 338
Snellen's sight test, 280–1
Soap, 154–5

Soil pipe, 408
Soothing syrups, 377
Sore throat, 345
Soup, 131
Spastic paralysis, 207
Special education, 393
Spectacles, 280–1
Spectrum, 82–3
Speech therapy class, 228
Spinach, 106
Spinal curvature, 46
Splints, 418–19
Sprains, 420–1
Sputum, 359
Squint, 273–6
Staffordshire type of school, 79
Stairs in school, 405
Stammering, 228
Starch, 88, 102–4
Steapsin, 96
Stings, insect, 422
Stirrup bone of ear, 284
" Stitch," 421
Stomach, 92–5
Stoves, 406
Streptomycin, 362
Structures, vestigial, 7–8
Stuffy room, ill effects of, 76–8
Stye, 277
Sugar, 88, 102
Suggestion, use of, 220–1
Sulphonamides, 335–6
Sunlight, values of, 82–5
Sunstroke, 414
Suspensory ligament, 260
Sweat glands, 140–50
Sweets, 128
Swimming baths, 178–80
Sylvester method, 425
Sympathetic nerve system, 192
Synapse, 193
Syphilis, 354

T

Tannin, 118
Tape worm, 332
Taste, 256
Tea, 118
Tear duct, 257–8
Teeth, 136–47
Temperament, tests of, 234
Temperature, body, 74
Tendons, 34, 38

Testes, 187, 296
Tests, intelligence, 233–43
—— of hearing, 290–1
Thiamin, 108, 117
Thoracic duct, 97
Thorax, 62–3
Thymus gland, 186
Thyroid gland, 181–3
Tic, 227
Tinned food values, 111
Tocopherol, 117
Tone, muscular, 38–9
Tonsils, 72–3
Tooth brush, 143
Torolopsis ulitis major, 101
Touch corpuscles, 151–2
Tourniquet, 415
Toxin, 334
Trachea, 66
Trichinosis, 115
Tuberculosis, 357–66
Typhoid, 351

U

Ultra violet rays, 82, 112–13
Unconsciousness, causes of, 413–4
Underclothing, 167
Under-nutrition, 133
Uranium, 9
Urea, 148
Uterus, 295
Uvula, 72–3

V

Vaccination, 349
Vaccines, 349
Valves of heart, 49–50
Variation, 316–7
Varicose veins, 52–3
Vegetables, 88, 107–8
Veins, 52–3
Venereal disease, 354–6
Ventilation, 78–82
Ventricles of heart, 48
Venus di Milo, 45
Verruca, 170
Vestibule of ear, 287
Vestigial structures, 7–8
Villi, 98
Viruses, 11–13

Vision, bifocal, 264
——, tests of, 280–1
Vitamin A, 107–8
—— B complex, 108–10
—— C, 110–1
—— D, 112–3
—— E, 114
—— K, 115
—— P, 112
Vitreous humour, 260
Vocal folds, 65–6
Vocational guidance, 243–4
Voluntary muscle, 31

W

Walking, economical way of, 29–30
Wash-down closet, 409
Water in body, 106
—— closet, 409
—— supplies, 119
Wax in ear, 288
Weak ankles, 30
Wells, 119
Wheat germ, 109, 117
White corpuscles, 55–6
—— of egg, 127
Whooping cough, 343–5
Windows, school, 79, 407–8
Windpipe, 66
Womb, 295
Wool, 162–4
Word blindness, 206
—— deafness, 206
Writing, position for, 42, 270–11

X

X-Chromosome, 314–6
Xerophthalmia, 107
X-ray, 81, 156, 392

Y

Y-Chromosome, 314–6
Yeast, 109–10, 117
Yellow spot of eye, 262
Yolk of egg, 127

Z

Zinc ionisation, 289